GERIATRIC NURSE PRACTITIONER

Certification Review

JoAnn Zerwekh, EdD, RN, FNP, CS

University of Phoenix
Carondelet Health Network Community Services
Tucson, Arizona
Nursing Education Consultants
Dallas, Texas

Jo Carol Claborn, MS, RN, CNS

El Centro College
Nursing Education Consultants
Dallas, Texas

W.B. SAUNDERS COMPANY

A Division of Harcourt Brace & Company

Philadelphia   London   Toronto   Montreal   Sydney   Tokyo

W.B. SAUNDERS COMPANY
A Division of Harcourt Brace & Company

The Curtis Center
Independence Square West
Philadelphia, Pennsylvania 19106

Library of Congress Cataloging-in-Publication Data

Zerwekh, JoAnn Graham.
   Geriatric nurse practitioner certification review / JoAnn Zerwekh,
Jo Carol Claborn.
      p.   cm.
   ISBN 0−7216−7742−8
   1. Geriatric nursing—Examinations, questions, etc.   2. Nurse
practitioners—Examinations, questions, etc.   I. Claborn, Jo Carol.
II. Title.
   [DNLM: 1. Geriatric Nursing examination questions.   2. Geriatric
Assessment examination questions.   3. Drug Therapy—in old age
examination questions.   4. Nurse Practitioners examination
questions.   WY 18.2Z58g   1999]
RC954.Z47   1999
610.73′65′076—dc21
DNLM/DLC   98-34771

GERIATRIC NURSE PRACTITIONER CERTIFICATION REVIEW

ISBN 0−7216−7742−8

Printed in the United States of America

Last digit is the print number: 9   8   7   6   5   4   3   2   1

To Tom, my soul mate,
who brings a smile to my face and
a warm glow in my heart.
JoAnn

To Robert, my friend and partner,
whose love and patience keeps me going.
Jo

Series Contributors

Susan E. Chaney, EdD, MS, BSN
Professor, Family Nurse Practitioner
   Coordinator
Texas Woman's University
Family Nurse Practitioner
Homeless Outreach Medical Services
Parkland Health and Hospital System
Dallas, Texas

Cynthia Churgin, RN, FNP, CNM
Casa Blanca Medical Group
Mesa, Arizona

Sharon I. Decker, RN, CS, MSN,
   CCRN
Professor of Clinical Nursing
Director, Clinical Simulation Center
Texas Tech University Health Sciences
   Center
Lubbock, Texas

Nicolette Estrada, RN, MS, FNP-C
Chief Research Coordinator
Carl T. Hayden VA Medical Center
Phoenix, Arizona

Mary Jo Gagan, RNCS, FNP, PhD
Assistant Professor
University of Arizona College of Nursing
Nurse Practitioner
Campus Health
University of Arizona College of Nursing
Tucson, Arizona

Ela-Joy Lehrman, MS, MAEd, PhD
Program Manager for Nursing, Counseling,
   and General Studies
University of Phoenix
Tucson, Arizona

Beverly McCoy, BSN, MS, FNP
Clinical Director/Family Nurse Practitioner
Breaking the Circle Children's Health Care
Arizona State University
College of Nursing
Tempe, Arizona

Jacquelyn McGlamery, BSN, FNP
Family Nurse Practitioner
Sierra Tucson
Tucson, Arizona

Loretta Manning, RNC, MSN, GNP
Educational Consultant, Sylvia Rayfield &
   Associates
Executive Director, I CAN, Inc. Publishing
Atlanta, Georgia

Kathleen T. Ogle, RN, MS, CFNP
Instructor
Bowie State University
Department of Nursing
Bowie, Maryland;
Family Nurse Practitioner
Maryland Primary Care Physicians
Arnold, Maryland

Alice B. Pappas, BSN, MSN, PhD
Associate Dean for Academic Affairs
Baylor University School of Nursing
Dallas Texas

Jodi Pelusi, RN, MS, FNP
University of Phoenix
Phoenix, Arizona

Patricia J. Pinckard, MS, ANP
Adult Nurse Practitioner
Occupational Health
Desert Samaritan Medical Center
Mesa, Arizona

Sylvia M. Root, EdD, RNC, FNP
Associate Professor
Arizona State University
Tempe, Arizona

Patricia Scully, RN, MS, JD
Nurse Attorney Consultant
Tucson, Arizona

Patricia A. Shannon, RN, MS, CS, PNP
Faculty, University of Phoenix;
Director of Nurses and Nurse Practitioners
North Valley Pediatrics PC
Phoenix, Arizona;
Adjunct Faculty
Arizona State University
Tempe, Arizona;
President/Consultant
Pediatric Nursing . . . PLUS
Phoenix, Arizona

Linda Stevenson, RN, PhD
Baylor University School of Nursing
Dallas, Texas

Gail Tucker, RN, MS, FNP
BMT Nurse Practitioner
Good Samaritan Regional Medical Center;
City of Hope/Samaritan Bone Marrow
   Transplant
Phoenix, Arizona

Gayle P. Varnell, RN, CPNP, PhD
Assistant Professor
Nurse Practitioner Program Coordinator
The University of Texas at Tyler
Tyler, Texas

John Walter, RN, BS, CPNP
Guest Lecturer
Family Nurse Practitioner Program
University of Arizona College of Nursing;
Pediatric Nurse Practitioner
University Physicians
Tucson, Arizona

Pamela Becker Weilitz, AD, BSN,
   MSN(R)
Assistant Clinical Professor, Graduate
   Program
St. Louis University School of Nursing;
Adult Nurse Practitioner
Washington University School of Medicine
University Care
St. Louis, Missouri

Margaret "Pegi" Yancy, RN, MS,
   OGNP
Faculty Associate
Arizona State University
Tempe, Arizona;
Women's Health Nurse Practitioner
Department of Reproductive Medicine
St. Joseph's Hospital and Medical Center
Phoenix, Arizona

Preface

With the dawn of the role of the nurse practitioner, there is an increasing need for additional reference information and study materials for the certification examinations. Nurse practitioners are playing a vital role in the changing health care delivery system in the United States. The numbers of candidates for the certification examinations is rapidly increasing as more nursing programs implement the nurse practitioner curriculum in their graduate programs. *Geriatric Nurse Practitioner Certification Review* has been developed to assist the advanced practice nurse to prepare for the GNP certification examination. Extensive efforts have been made to include current information that is representative of the content based on the blueprints for the certification exams. This book of questions is not intended to be an exhaustive review of the content, but an adjunct to the review process. Over 850 review questions are included in all.

Test-taking strategies are included in Chapter 1. As a candidate prepares for the examination, it is vitally important to be familiar with and to practice good testing strategies. Testing strategies can prevent the candidate from making mistakes and selecting the wrong answer. As the review process begins, a review of the testing strategies chapter and the practice of good testing strategies is critical. With many years experience in the field of testing, we have consistently identified the importance practice testing plays in the review process. Practice questions give the candidate an opportunity to review questions written from different perspectives. To enhance the review process, answers with complete rationales are provided at the end of each chapter. Not only does the candidate increase their knowledge of the subject area, but with more practice, testing skills become fine tuned. Good testing skills make the candidate more comfortable and help to decrease the stress associated with certification exams.

This book also includes chapters reviewing important concepts related to Growth and Development and Health Promotion and Maintenance. These chapters provide questions that test information related to growth and development, general health supervision, and health maintenance. The clinical chapters are developed using a systems approach, i.e., cardiovascular, respiratory, endocrine, etc. In each of these chapters, the test questions are divided into three areas: Physical Examination and Diagnostic Tests, Disorders, and Pharmacology. This format assists the candidate to easily locate specific questions. The last three chapters in the text are on Theory and Research; Issues and Trends; and Legal and Ethical aspects of nurse practitioner practice. The test questions in these chapters focus on professional competencies inherent in the role and function of the GNP.

Our thanks to the many nurse practitioners across the country who provided questions and insight into the role of the nurse practitioner. We wish to thank Robin Carter, our editor at W.B. Saunders, for her support and suggestions in our preparation of the manuscript. Thank you also goes to all the nurse practitioners who took time from their busy schedules to review the questions for content and clarity.

Acknowledgments

We are continually grateful for the contributions and efforts of our test item contributors who provided their expertise and knowledge for this nurse practitioner certification review series.

We thank the manuscript reviewers for their suggestions and insights as we tackled this large project:

Harvey Baker, RNCS, ARNP
Oswego Family Medical Clinic
Oswego, Kansas

Susan Appel, RN, MN, CCRN, CS
Carolinas College of Health
    Sciences
Charlotte, North Carolina

Genell Lee, BSN, MSN, JD
Hauth & Lee, LLC
Birmingham, Alabama

Stephanie A. Batalo, RN, BSN,
    MSN, FNP
Trinity Health System
Steubenville, Ohio

Dorothy J. Stuppy, RN, PhD
University of Texas at Arlington
Arlington, Texas

Lynette M. Wachholz, MN, RN,
    ARNP, IBCLC
The Everett Clinic
Everett, Washington

We thank the staff at W.B. Saunders Company: Robin Carter, Senior Editor, and Marie Pelcin and Ross Landy, editorial assistants for their calmness and patience. Joan Sinclair, who managed the book's production. It was such a pleasure to work with you again on another publication. Berta Steiner for copyediting and typesetting the manuscript. What a job to keep track of thousands of questions!

Last, but certainly not least, we want to thank: Our children, Tyler and Ashley Zerwekh, Jaelyn Claborn, Michael Brown, and Kim Aultman, for teasing their mothers about writing 5 books!! Our parents, Charles Graham and Hazel Cooper, for their continued support and encouragement. Tom Gaglione and Robert Claborn for their encouragement, support, and love. We love you all.

Contents

Test-Taking Strategies

Testing Strategies

Knowing how to take an examination is a skill that is developed through practice and experience. Being able to take an examination effectively is almost as important as the basic knowledge required to answer the question. Everyone has taken an examination only to find in the review of the exam that questions were missed due to inadequate testing skills. Nurse practitioner programs provide the graduate student with a comprehensive base of knowledge; how you utilize this knowledge will determine your success on a certification examination. The certification examination is an objective test that covers knowledge, understanding, and application of professional nursing theory and practice. When you register for the examination, you will receive a "Candidate Handbook" or information materials from the Certification Board administering the examination.

Read the information in this chapter carefully and make sure you understand the strategies discussed. This chapter is designed to help you identify problem areas in testing skills and learn how to use strategy and judgment in selecting correct answers. It is important for you to practice testing skills, if you are going to be able to utilize these skills on the certification examination.

Question Characteristics

A. Multiple-choice questions.
  1. Scene or scenario—establishes the setting of the question. Not all questions will have a scenario; if a scenario is included, consider the appropriateness of the answer to the information provided.
  2. Stem—states the question that is being asked.
  3. Options—there are four options from which to choose an answer.
    a. Distractors—designed to distract you from the correct answer.
    b. Correct answer—correctly answers the question asked in the stem.
    c. There are only four options in any item; there are no combinations of options to consider.
    d. There is only one correct response; no partial credit is given for another answer.
B. Questions are derived from clinical situations common in the practice setting.

Strategies for Multiple-Choice Questions

1. Cover the options with your hand or a piece of scratch paper.* This strategy makes you focus on the content of the question and prevents your eyes from "darting" to look at the distractors. If you peruse the distractors before you completely understand the question, key words in the distractors will influence your interpretation of the question.

2. Do not read extra meaning into the question. The question is asking for specific information; if it appears to be simple "common sense," then assume it is simple. Do not look for a hidden meaning in what appears to be an easy question.

EXAMPLE:

The nurse practitioner understands that the most common form of facial paralysis in the adult client is:

1. Facial nerve fasciitis.
2. Trigeminal neuralgia.
3. Bell's palsy.
4. Herpes zoster.

Correct answer is Option #3. Be careful not to "read into" the question and add pain to the facial paralysis symptom. The most common form of facial paralysis is Bell's palsy, which is a disorder affecting the facial nerve and characterized by muscle flaccidity of the affected side of the face. Trigeminal neuralgia is a disorder of cranial nerve V characterized by an abrupt onset of pain in the lower and upper jaw, cheek, and lips. Herpes zoster affects the dermatomes and does not cause a paralysis, but pain is possible with postherpetic neuralgia.

EXAMPLE:

When administering skin tests to an immunocompromised older client, the nurse practitioner must consider:

1. The importance of not applying more than one skin test at a time.
2. The skin test may react more aggressively than expected.

3. The use of a known allergen for the client and utilize it as a control.
4. The immunocompromised client should not be skin tested.

The correct answer is Option #3. Do not read into the question and make it more difficult by trying to make the client sicker (i.e., full-blown acquired immunodeficiency syndrome [AIDS]). It is important to remember to apply controls when skin testing the immunocompromised client. Ask clients what diseases they believe they have immunity to, such as measles. Apply the "known" allergen and the skin test to be tested. If the client is unable to mount an immune response at all, the known allergen will not react. By not applying the controls, the nurse practitioner may assume a skin test is negative, when in fact the client's immune system is unable to respond.

3. Read the stem correctly. Make sure you understand exactly what information the question is asking.

EXAMPLE:

An older client with a history of Parkinson's disease has a positive TB skin test and isoniazid (INH) is ordered as a prophylactic medication. Prior to beginning INH, it is important for the nurse practitioner to determine:

1. Is the client's Parkinson's condition being treated with levodopa (Larodopa)?
2. How long has the client been diagnosed with Parkinson's disease?
3. How much respiratory compromise is the client currently experiencing?
4. How adequate is the client's urinary output and renal function?

The question asks you to determine if giving the INH to an older client with Parkinson's disease is a problem. The correct answer is Option #1. This question requires the nurse practitioner to think critically about possible medications the client may be on and whether they would interfere with the ordering of INH. In this case, INH requires concurrent administration of vitamin B_6 to prevent problems of optic neuritis. Vitamin B_6 will decrease the effectiveness of levodopa. If the client is to receive the INH, his antiparkinson medication needs to be re-evaluated.

---

*This testing strategy of covering the distractors is from Phoebe K. Helm, EdD.

4. Before considering the options, formulate in your mind possible answers to the question. If none of the options fit in the pool of answers you anticipated, go back and re-evaluate the question. Assess each of the options with regard to your pool of possible answers.

E X A M P L E :

The usual clinical presentation of an adult client with cystitis is:

1. No chills, fever, headache, malaise or discomfort noted.
2. Acute onset of chills, fever, flank pain, headache, malaise, and costovertebral angle tenderness.
3. Complaints of dysuria, urgency, frequency, nocturia, and suprapubic heaviness.
4. Signs and symptoms of fever, irritability, decreased appetite, vomiting, diarrhea, constipation, dehydration, and jaundice.

Formulate in your mind possible answers to the question. Think to yourself, "Which of these symptoms are normally seen with cystitis? What is different about pyelonephritis? Is the usual presentation without symptoms? Is there involvement of the GI tract" (as eluded to in Option #4)? If you are unsure, go back and reassess the question. In this instance, Option #3 is correct. An adult with cystitis usually presents with dysuria, urgency, frequency, nocturia, and suprapubic heaviness. Acute onset of chills, fever, flank pain, headache, malaise and costovertebral angle tenderness are common adult symptoms of pyelonephritis.

5. Identify what type of response the question is asking. A positive stem requires identification of three false items and one positive as the correct answer.

E X A M P L E :

Clients who believe they have been exposed to human immunodeficiency virus (HIV) should have an HIV antibody test how soon after the exposure?

1. The next day and 2 months later.
2. 6 months after exposure and again at 12 months.
3. 6–12 weeks after exposure and again at 6 months.
4. 4 weeks and 12 weeks.

The correct answer is Option #3. This question requires you to identify three incorrect responses and one correct response. The HIV antibody develops between 6 and 12 weeks after exposure. Because of the variability of antibody development, it is recommended that the test be repeated in 6 months to confirm the findings.

6. Identify questions that require identification of something the practitioner should not or would not do (i.e., unsafe action, contraindication, inappropriate action).

E X A M P L E :

The nurse practitioner is prescribing astemizole (Hismanal) for a geriatric client's allergy problems. When considering the client's current medications, which medication would be a contraindication to the administration of astemizole (Hismanal)?

1. Erythromycin ethylsuccinate (E.E.S.).
2. Verapamil (Calan).
3. Propanolol (Inderal).
4. Captopril (Captoten).

The correct answer is Option #1. Macrolides and Hismanal should not be administered concurrently. Thus, the nurse practitioner is required to identify a medication that should not be ordered.

7. Questions may also be analytical. These questions may ask the nurse practitioner to identify findings, statements, and the like that are consistent/inconsistent with the client's presenting problem and/or differentiate between them.

E X A M P L E :

Dementia can be distinguished from delirium by:

1. Dementia lasts days to weeks compared to delirium, which lasts months to years.
2. Dementia is often associated with medications or systemic illness.
3. Dementia exhibits a disturbance in attention that is not present in delirium.
4. Dementia does not include altered perception, such as illusions.

Before you examine the options in this question, it is important to think about the differences between dementia and delirium. The correct answer is Option #4. Adults with dementia do not usually have altered perceptions that include illusions. They may experience hallucinations and delusions. Dementia does last months to years. Delirium is often associated with medications or systemic illness and a disturbance in the ability to pay attention.

8. Identify key words that affect your understanding of the question. Make sure you understand exactly what information the question is asking. Be aware of questions in which the stem includes words such as *except, contraindicated, avoid, least, not applicable,* and *does not occur.* These words change the direction of the question. It may help to rephrase the question in your own words in order to better understand what information is being requested.

E X A M P L E :

Clients with arteriosclerotic heart disease (ASHD) go through several stages before becoming severely compromised. Which **does not occur** in the early stages of ASHD?

1. Decreased urine output.
2. Dyspnea on exercise.
3. Anginal pain relieved by rest.
4. Increased serum triglyceride levels.

Rephrase the question: In early stages of ASHD, which of the following does not occur? It is important that you identify the key point "early stages of ASHD" and the key words "does not occur." If you miss these essential points, you do not understand the question, and chances are you will not choose the correct answer. The correct answer is Option #1: a decrease in urine output occurs when cardiac disease is advanced enough to cause a severe decrease in cardiac output and renal perfusion.

9. As you read the options, eliminate those you know are not correct. This will help narrow the field of choice. When you select an answer or eliminate a distractor, you should have a specific reason for doing so.

E X A M P L E :

A 45-year-old female complains of knee pain when kneeling and a "clicking" noise when walking up steps. On exam, there is a slight knee effusion and tenderness when palpating the patella against the condyles. The diagnosis for this client is:

1. Anterior cruciate tear. (*No, the client generally cannot bear weight on the extremity without it buckling or giving way.*)
2. Dislocated patella. (*No, there would be considerable effusion and locking of the knee in flexion.*)
3. Chondromalacia patella. (*Yes, there is clicking and anterior knee pain around or under the kneecap aggravated by knee extensor stress.*)
4. Tendinitis. (*No, there would be no clicking sound with movement.*)

After systematically evaluating the choices, Option #3 is the correct answer.

10. Identify similarities in the distractors. Frequently, the distractors will contain similar information, but one will be different. The different one may be the correct answer.

E X A M P L E :

An elderly client is to be encouraged to increase her intake of protein. The addition of which of these foods to 100 ml of milk will provide the greatest amount of protein?

1. 50 ml light cream and 2 tbsp corn syrup.
2. 30 gm powdered skim milk and one egg.
3. One small scoop (90 gm) ice cream and 1 tbsp chocolate syrup.
4. Two egg yolks and 1 tbsp sugar.

Options #1, #3, and #4 all contain a simple sugar. The correct answer, Option #2, has more protein. Notice that three of the options are similar; the one that is different may be the correct answer. This strategy is not a substitute for basic knowledge but may help you figure out the answer.

11. Select the most comprehensive answer. All of the options may be correct, but **one** will include the other three options or need to be considered first.

E X A M P L E :

Diagnostic studies used in the differential diagnosis of systemic lupus erythematosus (SLE) include:

1. Complete blood count (CBC), SMA-12, and erythrocyte sedimentation rate (ESR).
2. Chest radiograph and coagulation profile.

3. Antinuclear antibody (ANA), ESR, and C-reactive protein.
4. CBC, urinalysis, and chest radiograph.

The correct answer is Option #3. Although all of the tests included in the answer may be included in a complete physical examination, laboratory tests specific or inclusive for the diagnosis of SLE include the ANA, ESR, and C-reactive protein. During flares, the ESR and C-reactive protein are elevated. The ANA titer in a client with SLE is positive at a 1:80 ratio.

12. Select the best answer that is most specific to what the question asks. All of the options may be correct, but **one** is more specific or essential.

E X A M P L E :

When taking the history of a client with known allergies, what is the most important information to determine?

1. Reaction associated with each allergen.
2. Drug allergies.
3. Food allergies.
4. Environmental exposure.

It is absolutely essential that the reaction to each allergen is known. The other options are important but are not most important during the taking of the history. Recognize key words that identify the question that is asking for a priority of care—first, initial, best, most. The correct answer is Option #1. The other alternatives may be correct but should be prioritized. Often clients will indicate they have an allergy to a particular food or medication, such as nausea, stomach pain, or diarrhea, and consider it an allergy. The signs and symptoms of the reaction, speed of onset, how long it lasts, and what successful treatment has been used in the past are important information. Both drug and food allergies should be explored.

13. Watch questions in which the options contain several items to consider. After you are sure you understand what information the question is requesting, evaluate each part of the option. Is it appropriate to what the question is asking? If an option contains one incorrect item, the entire option is incorrect. All of the items listed in the selection must be correct, if it is to be the answer to the question.

E X A M P L E :

When evaluating an electrocardiogram (ECG), which characteristics most clearly indicate atrial tachycardia?

1. Heart rate of 96, P waves present on each QRS complex, T wave every other beat.
2. P waves present on every other beat, heart rate of 100, and irregular.
3. Heart rate of 110, P waves present prior to each QRS complex, and regular.
4. P waves for every third QRS complex, adequate P-R interval, rate of 90.

The correct answer is Option #3. In a methodical evaluation of the items in the options, you can eliminate items in options #1, #2, and #4. Sinus or atrial tachycardia is characterized by a rate at or above 100, P waves are present for each QRS complex, the P-R interval is below 0.20, the T wave occurs after each QRS complex, and the beat is regular.

14. Be alert to relevant information contained in previous questions. Sometimes, as you are answering questions, you will find information similar to the information being tested in previous test questions. Previous questions may assist you in identifying relevant information in the current question.

E X A M P L E :

The American College of Physicians (ACP) recommends that healthy adults receive a tetanus-diphtheria (Td) booster vaccination:

1. Every 5 years.
2. At age 75.
3. At age 65.
4. Every 10 years.

The ACP recommends that adults receive a Td booster every 10 years or a single booster at age 50 for clients who have completed full pediatric series, including teenage and young adult boosters. The correct answer to this question is Option #4. In another question involving immunizations, you read the following question.

EXAMPLE:

In taking the history of an alert, older adult, the nurse practitioner determines the client is an avid gardener and spends a great deal of time outside. He had a pneumococcal vaccination last year and states he cannot remember when he had a tetanus vaccination. A health maintenance recommendation for this client would be to obtain:

1. Pneumococcal vaccine.
2. Tetanus vaccine.
3. Hepatitis B vaccine.
4. No recommendation.

The correct answer is Option #2. A clue to the answer to this question may be found in the previous question. Older adults who enjoy gardening and outdoor activities should have a Td booster once every 10 years, as the ACP recommends this practice.

15. Multiple-choice mathematical computations may be included in the exam. Mathematical computations may include calculations of

IM, PO, and IV dosages; calculations of pediatric dosage; determining creatinine clearance; and conversion of units of measurement.

EXAMPLE:

The nurse practitioner is ordering digoxin (Lanoxin) 0.25 mg for a client who has difficulty swallowing pills. How would the order be written?

1. Digoxin 0.25 mg Sig: 5 ml elixir PO qd.
2. Digoxin 0.25 mg Sig: 1 tab PO qd.
3. Digoxin 0.25 mg Sig: 2.5 ml PO elixir qd.
4. Digoxin 0.025 mg/5 ml Sig: 5 ml PO qd.

First, you must know the typical dispensing of oral digoxin, which is 0.05 mg/ml for the elixir. To receive a dose of 0.25 mg, the correct answer would be Option #1.

16. Evaluate priority questions carefully. Frequently all of the answers are appropriate to the situation. You need to decide which of the actions you should do first.

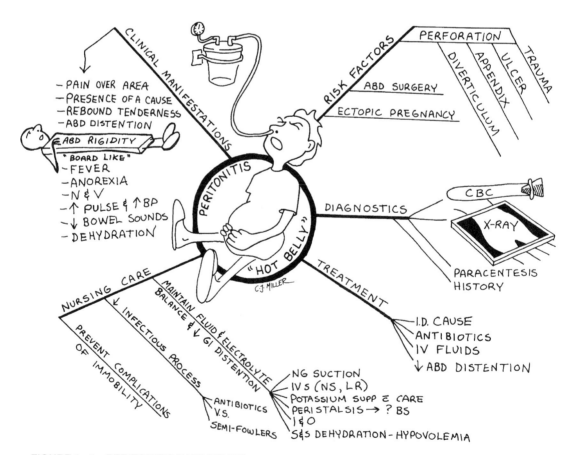

FIGURE 1–1 PERITONITIS "HOT BELLY"
From Zerwekh J, Claborn J, Miller CJ: Memory Notebook of Nursing, Vol I. Dallas, TX: Nursing Education Consultants Publishing, Inc, 1994, p 85, with permission.

EXAMPLE:

While working in her garden, an older adult was bitten on the hand by a raccoon. Her last Td was 4 years ago. At the rural clinic, the nurse practitioner cleansed the wound. The next action is:

1. Administer tetanus antitoxin.
2. Contact local animal control authorities.
3. Administer rabies immune globulin (RIG) and human diploid cell vaccine (HDCV).
4. Teach the client how to do hourly soaks to the hand using normal saline and peroxide.

Correct answer is Option #3. Any type of animal bite that might be associated with an animal that may potentially harbor rabies (skunks, bats, raccoons, foxes, coyotes, rats) should be treated with both active and passive rabies immunization. The priority action is to prevent rabies. Tetanus antitoxin would be indicated, if the adult was not current on the Td immunization. Animal authorities would be called after the initial treatment to locate the animal and sacrifice it, so that the brain can be examined for rabies.

Techniques to Increase Critical Thinking Skills

Memory aids and mindmapping are tools that assist in drawing associations from other ideas with the use of visual images. Mnemonics are words, phrases, or other techniques that help you remember information. Imagery is a tool that helps you identify a problem and visualize a mental picture. Learning content utilizing these techniques will assist you in recalling information more effectively.

Mindmapping™ is a method of organizing important information that is in sharp contrast to the traditional outline format. A thought or concept is written in the center of the page, and images and color are added to information as ideas begin to flow from the center focus (see Fig. 1–1).

Acronyms help you to recall information via word association or arrangements of letters to recall specific information. Examples of these are the 6-Ps of dyspnea (see Fig. 1–2), the 5-Ps of circulatory assessment (see Fig. 1–3), or the ABCs of malignant melanoma (see Fig. 1–4).

Acrostics are catchy phrases in which the first letter of each word stands for something to recall. For example, in remembering the use of canes

FIGURE 1–2 6 Ps OF DYSPNEA
From Zerwekh J, Claborn J, Miller CJ: Memory Notebook of Nursing, Vol II. Dallas, TX: Nursing Education Consultants Publishing, Inc, 1997, p 22, with permission.

FIGURE 1–3 CIRCULATION ASSESSMENT: THE 5 Ps
From Zerwekh J, Claborn J, Miller CJ: Memory Notebook of Nursing, Vol II. Dallas, TX: Nursing Education Consultants Publishing, Inc, 1997, p 27, with permission.

and walkers (see Fig. 1–5) think of "Wandering Wilma's Always Late" (**W**alker **W**ith **A**ffected **L**eg). Everyone remembers the cranial nerve mnemonic (see Fig. 1–6).

Memory aids or images are pictures or caricatures that help you to recall information more effectively (see Fig. 1–7).

Rhymes are phrases or words spoken in a rhythmic or musical manner that increase recall. A helpful musical rhyme for hypoglycemia versus hyperglycemia is "hot and dry, sugar high; cold and clammy, need some candy" (see Fig. 1–8). Another rhyme, "fingers, nose, penis, toes," identifies the areas where lidocaine with epinephrine is contraindicated as a local anesthetic. Or, "two is too much," may help you to remember toxic levels of the following three drugs, which have a narrow margin of safety—lithium, digoxin, theophylline (see Fig. 1–9).

Note: These are just examples. There are entire books on these helpful aids (see the list of references).

Testing Skills for Paper-and-Pencil Tests

1. Go through the exam and mark all the answers that you know are correct. This ensures you have adequate time to answer the questions you know. Go back and evaluate those questions for which you did not readily recognize the answer.

2. Do not indiscriminately change answers. If you go back and change an answer, you should have a specific reason for doing so.

HINTS TO MALIGNANT MELANOMA

FIGURE 1–4 HINTS TO MALIGNANT MELANOMA (ABCD)
From Zerwekh J, Claborn J, Miller CJ: Memory Notebook of Nursing, Vol I. Dallas, TX: Nursing Education Consultants Publishing, Inc, 1997, p 137, with permission.

Sometimes you remember information and realize you answered the question incorrectly. Frequently, test-takers "talk themselves out of" the correct answer and change it to an incorrect one.

3. After you have completed the exam, go back and check your booklet and make sure all of the questions are answered. Answer all of the questions, even if you must guess.

Testing Skills that Apply to Both Paper-and-Pencil Tests and Computer Testing

1. Listen carefully to the instructions given at the beginning of the examination. Make sure you understand all of the information given and exactly how to mark your answers, and/or how to use the keyboard.

2. Watch your timing. Do not spend too much time on one question. It is very important that you practice your timing on the sample exams. When you begin to take a paper-and-pencil test, plan on finishing within the first three fourths of the allocated time. It is not necessary to review all of the questions after you have completed the test. Do it right the first time and there is no need to review the entire test again. Go back and answer the questions that you left blank. Watch your timing on computer tests—make use of a computer clock, if it is available.

3. Be aware of your "first hunch." It is frequently the correct answer. Sometimes information is processed by the brain without

FIGURE 1–5   CANES AND WALKERS
From Zerwekh J, Claborn J, Miller CJ: Memory Notebook of Nursing, Vol II. Dallas, TX: Nursing Education Consultants Publishing, Inc, 1997, p 8, with permission.

you being aware of it. If something about an answer "feels right" or you have a "gut-level feeling," pay attention to it.

4. Eliminate distractors that assume the client "would not understand," or "is ignorant" of the situation, or those that "protect them from worry." For example, "The client should not be told she has cancer because it would upset her too much."

5. Be aware of distractors that contain the words *always* and *never*.

6. There is no pattern of correct answers. Both computer and paper-and-pencil examinations are compiled by a computer and the position of the correct answers is selected at random.

Decrease Anxiety

Your activities on the day of the examination strongly influence your level of anxiety. By carefully planning ahead, you will be able to eliminate some anxiety-provoking situations.

1. Visit the examination site prior to the day of the exam. Evaluate travel time, parking, and time to get to the designated area. Get an early start to allow extra time.

2. If you have to travel some distance to the examination site, try to spend the night in the immediate vicinity.

3. Do something pleasant the evening prior to the examination. This is not the time to "crash study."

CRANIAL NERVE MNEMONIC

S = Sensory	M = Motor	B = Both

O	Olfactory	O	On	S	Some
O	Optic	O	Old	S	Say
O	Oculomotor	O	Olympus'	M	Marry
T	Trochlear	T	Tiny	M	Money
T	Trigeminal	T	Tops	B	But
A	Abducens	A	A	M	My
F	Facial	F	Finn	B	Brother
A	Acoustic	A	And	S	Says
G	Glossopharyngeal	G	German	B	Bad
V	Vagus nerve	V	Viewed	B	Business
S	Spinal	S	Some	M	Marry
H	Hypoglossal	H	Hops	M	Money

© 1994 Nursing Education Consultants

FIGURE 1–6 CRANIAL NERVE MNEMONIC
From Zerwekh J, Claborn J, Miller CJ: Memory Notebook of Nursing, Vol II. Dallas, TX: Nursing Education Consultants Publishing, Inc. 1994, p 91, with permission.

FIGURE 1–7 HYPERTHYROIDISM
From Zerwekh J, Claborn J, Miller CJ: Memory Notebook of Nursing, Vol I. Dallas, TX: Nursing Education Consultants Publishing, Inc, 1994, p 46, with permission.

BLOOD SUGAR MNEMONIC

Hot & Dry = Sugar High

Cold & Clammy = Need Some Candy

FIGURE 1–8 BLOOD SUGAR MNEMONIC
From Zerwekh J, Claborn J, Miller CJ: Memory Notebook of Nursing, Vol I. Dallas, TX: Nursing Education Consultants Publishing, Inc, 1994, p 50, with permission.

4. Anxiety is contagious. If those around you are extremely anxious, avoid contact with them prior to the examination.

5. Make your meal before the test a light, healthy one.

6. Avoid eating highly spiced or different foods. This is not the time for a gastrointestinal upset.

7. Wear comfortable clothes. This is not a good time to wear tight clothing or new shoes.

8. Wear clothing of moderate weight. It is difficult to control the temperature to keep everyone comfortable. Take a sweater or wear layered clothes that can be removed if you get too warm.

9. Wear soft-soled shoes; this decreases the noise in the testing area.

10. Make sure you have the papers that are required to gain admission to the exam site. Do not forget your reading glasses, if you wear them.

11. Do not take study material to the exam site. You cannot take it into the exam area and it is too late to study.

12. Do not panic when you encounter content with which you are unfamiliar in a question. Use good test-taking strategies, select an answer, and continue. Remember, you are not going to know all of the right answers.

13. Reaffirm to yourself that you know the material. It is not time for any self-defeating behavior or negative self-talk. **YOU WILL PASS!!** Build your confidence by visualizing yourself in 6 months working in the area you desire. Create that mental picture of where you want to be and who you want to be—certified nurse practitioner. Use your past successes to bring positive energy and "vibes" to your certification. **WE KNOW YOU CAN DO IT!**

FIGURE 1–9   TOXIC LEVELS OF LITHIUM, DIGOXIN, AND THEOPHYLLINE
From Zerwekh J, Claborn J, Miller CJ: Memory Notebook of Nursing, Vol II. Dallas, TX: Nursing Education
Consultants Publishing, Inc, 1997, p 43, with permission.

Study Habits

Enhancing Study Skills

- Decide on a study schedule—write it down and stick with it.
- Divide the review material into segments—pediatrics, well woman, geriatric, and so forth.
- Prioritize the segments; review first the areas in which you feel you are deficient and/or weak.
- Identify areas that will require additional review.
- Establish a realistic schedule—study in short segments or "bursts." Avoid marathon sessions.
- Plan on achieving your study goal several days prior to the examination.
- Do not study when you are tired or when there are frequent distractions or interruptions.
- Review general concepts of practice from a variety of resources.

Group Study

- Keep the group limited to four or five people.
- Group members should be mature and serious about studying.
- The group should agree on the planned study schedule.
- If the group makes you anxious or you do not feel it meets your study needs, do not continue to participate.

Testing Practice

- Include the testing practice in your schedule.
- Select about 50 questions for a practice testing session of 1 hour. This will allow you to evaluate the pace of the exam (i.e., approximately a question per minute).
- Try to answer the questions as if you were taking the real examination. Do not look up the right answer immediately after answering the question.

- Utilize the testing strategies described in this chapter.
- Evaluate the practice exams for problem areas; testing skills and knowledge base.
- Evaluate the questions you answer incorrectly. Review the rationale for the right answer and understand why you missed it.
- Utilize the questions at a later point to review the information again.

References

Beitz J: Unleashing the power of memory: The mighty mnemonic. *Nurse Educator*, 22(2), 25–28, 1997.

Bloomingfield R: Mnemonics, Rhetorics, and Poetics for Medics. Salem, NC: Harbinger Medical Press, 1982.

Rayfield S, Manning L: Nursing Made Insanely Easy. Shreveport, LA: ICAN, Inc, Publishing, 1997.

Zerwekh J, Claborn J: Test-taking strategies. In NCLEX-RN®: A Comprehensive Study Guide, 3rd ed. Dallas, TX: Nursing Education Consultants Publishing, Inc, 1997.

Zerwekh J, Claborn J, Miller CJ: Memory Notebook of Nursing, Vol I. Dallas, TX: Nursing Education Consultants Publishing, Inc, 1994.

Zerwekh J, Claborn J, Miller CJ: Memory Notebook of Nursing, Vol II. Dallas, TX: Nursing Education Consultants Publishing, Inc, 1997.

2

Growth & Development

Physical Assessment of the Older Adult

1. As an individual ages, which physiologic change would affect responses to pharmacologic agents?

   1. Increased gastric emptying.

   2. Increased glomerular filtration rate.

   3. Decreased percentage of body fat.

   4. Decreased albumin concentration.

2. The number one cause of accidental death in clients older than 65 years of age is:

   1. Motor vehicle accidents.

   2. Poisoning.

   3. Falls.

   4. Drowning.

3. The nurse practitioner selects which assessment tool to evaluate balance and gait problems in the elderly?

   1. Lawton & Brody Balance and Coordination Scale.

   2. Tinetti Balance and Gait Evaluation.

   3. Instrumental Activities of Daily Living Scale.

   4. Index of Independence of Activities of Daily Living.

4. The nurse practitioner is assessing the nutritional status of an elderly client. The nurse practitioner identifies the common physiologic changes in the gastrointestinal system to be:

   1. Increased peristalsis.

   2. Decreased absorption of iron.

   3. Maintenance of normal fat metabolism.

   4. Increased drug metabolism.

5. What are the normal physiologic changes in the thyroid gland that occur with aging?

1. Hypertrophy with a decrease in the triidothyronine (T_3) and thyroxine (T_4) levels.

2. Normal size with an increase in thyroid-stimulating hormone (TSH) and a decrease in T_4.

3. Atrophy of the gland with a decrease in TSH, T_3, and T_4.

4. Increase in nodularity with normal TSH and T_4.

6. The aging process causes what normal physiologic changes in the heart?

1. The heart size stays the same, the valves thicken and become rigid secondary to fibrosis and sclerosis.

2. Cardiomegaly occurs along with prolapse of the mitral valve and regurgitation.

3. Dilatation of the right ventricle occurs with sclerosis of pulmonic and tricuspid valves.

4. Hypertrophy of the right ventricle occurs with decreasing capacity and compromised efficiency of the coronary arteries.

7. Which pulmonary physiologic change is commonly associated with the aging process?

1. Increased cough response.

2. Decreased vital capacity.

3. Decreased anteroposterior (AP) diameter of thorax.

4. Increased residual P_{CO_2}.

8. Which of these clinical findings would indicate a deviation from the normal age-related changes in the neurologic system and may have some diagnostic significance for the older client?

1. Decreased sense of touch.

2. Increased tolerance to pain.

3. Decreased short-term memory.

4. Decreased ability to maintain balance.

9. During a teaching session, the nurse practitioner instructs the client regarding normal skin lesions in the older population. These would include:

1. Seborrheic dermatitis.

2. Senile keratosis.

3. Senile lentigo.

4. Squamous cell.

10. Which assessment is a normal physiologic change of the respiratory system that occurs with aging?

1. Decreased residual lung volume (RV).

2. Hyperresonance.

3. Increased forced vital capacity (FVC).

4. Increased tactile fremitus.

11. This nurse practitioner indicates an understanding of the normal aging process with which documentation of the gastrointestinal system in the physical examination?

1. Increase in the size of the liver (16 cm).

2. Absent bowel sounds.

3. Femoral bruit.

4. Increased adipose tissue.

12. During the physical examination of an older client, the nurse practitioner indicates an understanding of deviations in the neurologic system from the normal aging process with which clinical finding?

1. Decrease in short-term memory.

2. Decrease in deep tendon and superficial reflexes.

3. Decrease in sense of touch.

4. Positive Romberg's sign.

13. Which functional assessment tool should the nurse practitioner use to evaluate the safety for a cerebrovascular accident client planning to return to his home environment?

1. OARS ADL Scale.

2. Bennet Social Isolation Scales.

3. Mini Mental State Examination.

4. Norton Scale.

14. The nurse practitioner understands which factor is most influential in the driving ability of an older adult?

    1. Ability to coordinate the transmissions.

    2. Acuity of vision.

    3. Comprehension of the details of the road rules.

    4. Reaction times.

15. As an individual ages, which physiologic change would affect sleep?

    1. Decreased rapid-eye-movement (REM) sleep.

    2. Increased delta or stage IV sleep.

    3. Decreased nocturnal awakenings.

    4. Decreased sleep latency.

16. When treating an infection in the older adult, the nurse practitioner must consider:

    1. Thymus-derived immunity is increased.

    2. Immune function declines with age.

    3. Immune function increases with age.

    4. Antibody production increases.

17. The diminished immunity of the older adult can be attributed to a decline in:

    1. B-cell function.

    2. T-cell production.

    3. B-cell production.

    4. T-cell function.

18. Which physiologic factor of aging contributes to incontinence in the elderly?

    1. Decreased vascularity of the bladder mucosa.

    2. Increased urethral closing pressure.

    3. Increased ability to concentrate urine.

    4. Decreased bladder capacity.

19. What is the pathophysiologic age-related change that predisposes an older adult to dehydration?

    1. A decrease in body fat along with a significant decrease in lean muscle mass makes the older client more susceptible to minute changes in blood volume.

    2. Thirst is normally experienced when there is a loss of 2% of the client's body weight or when osmolality is increased; this mechanism is significantly diminished in the older adult.

    3. With aging, the glomeruli reduce in number, which leads to a corresponding increase in glomerular filtering surface, which causes the kidney to increase its ability to concentrate urine in the older adult.

    4. Antidiuretic hormone (ADH) increases as the kidney loses function, leading to diminished ability to maintain osmolality.

20. According to the Holmes and Rahe social adjustment scale, the highest degree of adjustment is required after:

    1. Loss of a job.

    2. Death of a spouse.

    3. Marriage.

    4. Divorce.

Answers & Rationales

Physical Assessment of the Older Adult

1. **(4)** Medications are often protein bound (not fat); albumin decreases with age. A low albumin level decreases the number of protein-binding sites, causing an increase in the amount of free drug in the plasma. Drug overdose may occur in the elderly. Gastric emptying and glomerular filtration rate *decrease* with the aging process.

2. **(3)** Falls are the major cause of morbidity and mortality in the elderly. It is often the precipitating event for a cascade of problems leading to death. Complications from falls include fractures, pneumonia, pressure ulcers, pain, and immobility.

3. **(2)** The Tinetti Balance and Gait Evaluation is an activity-based test that asks the client to perform tasks, such as sitting and rising from a chair, turning, and bending it. It requires no more than 15–20 minutes to perform. Another appropriate test for assessment of falls is the timed "Up and Go" test, which assesses balance and gait speed. Lawton and Brody are the authors of the Instrumental Activities of Daily Learning, which assesses complex tasks such as shopping, laundry, food preparation, and so forth. The Index of Independence of Activities of Daily Living helps to identify activities of daily living with which the client needs assistance.

4. **(2)** Decreased hydrochloric acid, which occurs with aging, leads to decreased absorption of iron and vitamin B_{12}. Fat absorption would decrease, as would peristalsis and drug metabolism.

5. **(4)** There is usually adequate secretion of TSH and a normal serum concentration of T_4. Aging may produce fibrosis and increased nodularity, but overall the thyroid function remains within normal limits.

6. **(1)** The heart does not increase in size with normal aging. An enlarged heart is a result of cardiac dysfunction. Dilatation of the left ventricle occurs with myocardial infarctions and altered cardiac functioning secondary to cardiac disease, not normal aging. The aging process does cause fibrosis and sclerosis of the cardiac valves; all valves are equally affected.

7. **(2)** A decrease in the vital capacity, along with a 50% increase in residual volume, occurs during the aging process. Other aging changes include a less effective cough, impaired ciliary action, and weaker respiratory muscles. Increased AP diameter is associated with aging and in chronic obstructive pulmonary disease (COPD) clients. Po_2 usually decreases, but Pco_2 usually remains unchanged.

8. **(4)** This may indicate a cerebellar complication. The first three findings are normal age-related changes.

9. **(3)** The senile lentigine is a gray-brown, irregular, macular lesion on sun-exposed areas of the face, arms, and hands that are normal skin lesions. The other lesions are commonly occurring abnormal skin lesions in the older adult.

10. **(2)** A normal age-related change is an increase in the AP diameter, which results in hyperresonance. Age-related changes result in an increase in the RV and a decrease in the FVC. An increased tactile fremitus is a deviation that is of diagnostic significance.

11. **(4)** Common age-related changes with the gastrointestinal system include increased adipose tissue, decrease in liver size, reduced motility and peristalsis, decrease in acid secretions and motor activity of the stomach, and decrease in the glomerular filtration rate. Absence of bowel sounds after 5 full minutes and bruits are deviations of clinical significance.

12. **(4)** The Romberg's sign indicates the inability to maintain balance, which indicates need for further evaluation. Options #1, #2, and #3 are normal age-related changes. A decrease in short-term memory that affects the functional ability would then be considered a deviation.

13. **(1)** The OARS ADL Scale is the more appropriate screening tool for identifying at-risk populations. The Bennet Social Isolation Scale would be appropriate to evaluate the social interactions and resources. The Mini Mental State Examination is used to evaluate memory, orientation, and attention. The Norton Scale is used to evaluate pressure ulcer risk.

14. **(2)** The most age-dependent driving factor is sensory change, and the elderly driving client being assessed for driving capacity should use any corrective devices for optimal performance. While poor hearing alone is generally not a limiting factor for motor vehicle operation, vision assessment has received the greatest emphasis in assessing older drivers. Documenting the best corrected binocular visual acuity, color perception, and dark vision are basic elements to assessing driving visual acuity. The other factors have not been clearly demonstrated as highly applicable from laboratory performance to on-the-road skills for the elderly driver.

15. **(1)** REM sleep begins approximately 120 minutes from sleep onset and recurs in three to four regularly spaced, 10- to 15-minute cycles. REM sleep is associated with skeletal muscle atonia, rapid eye movements, and dreaming. This is decreased with aging. The delta, or stage IV, sleep is deep sleep and is also decreased with aging. There is an increased nocturnal awakening along with an increased sleep latency. Sleep is generally less efficient in the older client. More time is spent in bed with a decreased time in sleeping.

16. **(2)** Immune function declines with age, making the older adult more susceptible to infection. The older adult has less thymus-derived immunity due to the shrinking of the thymus gland, thus making it more difficult for the older adult to produce antibodies.

17. **(4)** The older adult has a diminished cell-mediated immunity due to a decline in T-cell function. The T cells have a decreased ability to produce cytokines, needed to facilitate B-cell growth and maturation, and a decreased ability to proliferate in response to an antigen.

18. **(4)** A decreased bladder capacity along with the decreased ability to concentrate urine and the decreased urethral closing pressure following menopause lead to incontinence. Other factors are depression, decreased mobility, decreased vision, lack of attention to bladder cues of fullness, and so forth.

19. **(2)** The elderly experience significant hypodipsia and diminished thirst sensations, which leads to problems associated with adequate fluid intake. The older adult has increased body fat and less lean muscle mass. In addition, the quantity of total body water as a proportion of body weight decreases. The functional decline of the aging kidney leads to a gradual loss of glomeruli that results in a diminished filtering surface. The kidney does not concentrate urine effectively, and there is a decreased effect of ADH.

20. **(2)** The Holmes and Rahe social adjustment scale found that death of a spouse was the most stressful life event, followed by divorce, marital separation, and loss of a job.

Health Promotion & Maintenance

1. The current American Cancer Society dietary recommendations for cancer prevention include:

   1. Maintaining a desirable body weight and eating a variety of foods, including fruits and vegetables, and foods that are high in fiber.

   2. Increasing the amount of protein in the diet.

   3. Including a moderate amount of alcohol in the diet.

   4. There are no dietary recommendations for the prevention of cancer.

2. In the presence of dyslipidemia and diabetes, the National Cholesterol Education Program guidelines set the goal for lipid levels as:

   1. LDL <130 mg/dl and triglyceride levels <200 mg/dl.

   2. LDL <160 mg/dl and triglyceride levels <240 mg/dl.

   3. LDL <100 mg/dl and triglyceride levels <180 mg/dl.

   4. LDL <150 mg/dl and triglyceride levels <220 mg/dl.

3. The American Diabetes Association recommends screening adults starting at age 45 with a fasting plasma glucose (FPG) test every:

   1. 1 year.

   2. 3 years.

   3. 5 years.

   4. 10 years.

4. Tertiary prevention activities for an older woman who has had a cerebrovascular accident (CVA) would include:

   1. An annual influenza vaccination.

   2. A physical therapy program.

   3. An annual mammogram.

   4. An annual ophthalmologic examination to evaluate for glaucoma.

5. A client is continuing his recovery at home after an extensive surgery. The practitioner would instruct the client to increase his intake of what foods to promote healing?

   1. Tomatoes, rice, whole bran cereal.

   2. Milk, poultry, yellow vegetables.

   3. Red meat, oranges, green beans.

   4. Liver, corn, eggs.

6. When an older client has an alteration in the sensory/perceptual function of hearing, which plan would be most appropriate for the nurse practitioner to implement during a health promotion session?

   1. Increase the pitch of the voice.

   2. Stand behind the client when speaking.

   3. Speak in a tone that does not include shouting.

   4. Use typical complex sentences to prevent insulting the client.

7. The nurse practitioner demonstrates an understanding of primary prevention of falling among the elderly through which management plan?

   1. Evaluate a need for assistive devices for ambulation after the client has been injured from a fall.

   2. Provide resources to correct hazards contributing to falling in the home environment.

   3. Reinforce the need to use prescribed eyeglasses to prevent further injury from falls.

   4. Provide information about medications, side effects, and interactions.

8. Which of the health promotion screenings should be implemented annually for the elderly client over 65?

   1. Chest x-ray.

   2. Pneumococcal vaccination.

   3. Sigmoidoscopy.

   4. Stool guaiac.

9. While teaching a class to a group of senior citizens, which would be most important for the nurse practitioner to consider during the presentation?

   1. Provide a lot of overhead lighting in order to enhance visualization.

   2. Provide handouts on blue paper with black print.

   3. Review a video narrated by a woman.

   4. Recognize that the clients' past life experiences are beneficial in learning new information.

10. The most common occupationally related disease is:

    1. Repetitive motion injury.

    2. Hearing loss.

    3. Lung disease.

    4. Cancer.

11. The newest recommendations from the American Cancer Society for yearly mammography to begin is at age:

    1. 50.

    2. 45.

    3. 60.

    4. 40.

12. A 48-year-old male presents to the clinic after having his cholesterol checked at a health fair. He states they told him it was >300, and that he needed to see his primary care provider to have further testing. Appropriate interventions for the nurse practitioner include:

    1. Prescribing a cholesterol-lowering agent.

    2. Ordering an electrocardiogram (ECG) and an exercise stress test.

    3. Starting the client on an exercise program.

    4. Performing a thorough history and physical and drawing blood for a lipid profile.

13. In teaching a client who is to have a test for colon-rectal screening, the nurse practitioner should instruct the client to:

    1. Eat at least two servings of rare meat daily prior to collecting samples.

    2. Avoid antibiotics, aspirin, iron, and anti-inflammatory medications.

    3. Take extra vitamin C to avoid a subsequent bladder infection that would make collecting samples difficult.

    4. Eat extra servings of vegetables such as broccoli, cabbage, potatoes, cantaloupe, and turnips to increase the fiber and ensure good samples.

14. The recommended number of servings of the bread/cereal/pasta/rice group is how many servings per day?

    1. 6 to 11 servings.

    2. 2 to 4 servings.

    3. 3 to 5 servings.

    4. 2 to 3 servings.

15. The age at which a *screening* mammogram is recommended as part of a woman's periodic health evaluation, if the woman is not at increased risk for breast cancer, is:

    1. 30 years old.

    2. 35 years old.

    3. Before the age of 40.

    4. Before the age of 50.

16. The history collected on a new client who enters a practice is to include:

    1. Interval history, past medical and surgical history, family medical and surgical histories, psychosocial history, usual dietary habits, physical activity, tobacco and other substance use, sexual practices, and a review of systems.

    2. Interval history, past medical history, family medical history, dietary habits, substance use, and sexual practices.

    3. Past medical and surgical histories, family medical history, psychosocial history, physical activity, tobacco and other substance use, and sexual practices.

    4. The history listed on the form provided to clients for completion prior to the physical examination is sufficient and no interview needs to be done.

17. A 50-year-old female presents to the clinic for a first-visit checkup. She states she is in good health and takes no medications. She does not know her family history, as she was adopted. She is 62 inches tall and weighs 175 lb. She is a secretary and admits to a sedentary lifestyle. She does not smoke, and admits to drinking four to five beers per week, along with an occasional glass of wine. Appropriate interventions for the nurse practitioner to recommend in this client's plan of care include:

    1. Immediately starting on an exercise plan that includes jogging 2 miles a day.

    2. Recommending vitamin supplements and protein shakes to be included in her diet and eliminating or reducing the amount of alcoholic beverages she drinks on a weekly basis.

    3. Changing her job to one that will increase the amount of exercise she gets.

    4. Having her keep a 24-hour record of her usual dietary intake, doing a physical examination to assess her readiness to begin an exercise program, and discussing dietary changes that are necessary for weight loss.

18. Which groups are at greatest risk for an altered immune function related to nutritional status?

    1. Young adults.

    2. Adults.

    3. Premature infants.

    4. Older adults.

19. All of the following are models of worksite health promotion **except**:

    1. Multiphasic health screening.

    2. Health risk appraisal.

    3. Onsite emergent care clinic.

    4. Health fair.

20. The nurse practitioner is discussing lifestyle changes and decreasing risk factors for cardiovascular diseases with a group of geriatric clients. What is most important to include in this discussion?

    1. Decrease smoking, increase vitamin supplements, increase protein intake.

    2. Control hypertension, stop smoking, maintain normal weight, exercise regularly.

    3. Maintain normal levels of serum blood sugar, decrease cholesterol intake.

    4. Get a yearly physical examination, increase fiber in diet, exercise regularly.

21. What lifestyle modifications are most effective in controlling hypertension in the older client?

    1. Maintain normal weight, decreased sodium diet, regular exercise.

    2. Increased dietary protein, decrease weight, stress reduction techniques.

    3. High complex carbohydrate, low-sodium diet, decrease stress.

    4. Weight reduction, vitamin supplements, and exercise.

22. In the preparation of reading and education materials for clients, the nurse practitioner is aware that the reading level of most adults is at the:

    1. Twelfth-grade level.

    2. Tenth-grade level.

    3. Sixth-grade level.

    4. Fourth-grade level.

Immunizations

23. Which statement describing the polyvalent pneumococcal vaccine is **incorrect**?

    1. It is recommended for those with chronic respiratory illness.

    2. It can be given on the same visit as the influenza vaccine.

    3. It should be given yearly.

    4. It is never recommended for children.

24. The influenza vaccination is recommended annually for high-risk groups. The nurse practitioner knows that the greatest need for this vaccination would be for:

    1. Adults with chronic disease.

    2. Residents of long-term care facilities.

    3. Dialysis clients.

    4. Health care employees.

25. The nurse practitioner understands that the only contraindication to hepatitis B vaccination is:

    1. Pregnancy and lactation.

    2. History of poliomyelitis.

    3. Prior anaphylaxis or severe hypersensitivity.

    4. Mild viral illness.

26. Immunizations and chemoprophylaxis offered routinely to clients who are 65 years of age and older are:

    1. Diphtheria, pertussis absorbed, antitetanus toxoid (DTP); influenza; and Pneumovax.

    2. Tetanus-diphtheria toxoid (Td), influenza, and pneumococcal vaccine.

    3. Td and influenza; those with chronic diseases are offered the pneumococcal vaccine.

    4. Influenza and pneumococcal pneumonia and Td to those who have not had one in the last 10 years.

27. In taking the history of a healthy 50-year-old adult, the nurse practitioner determines the client is an avid gardener and spends a great deal of time enjoying the out-of-doors. A health maintenance recommendation for this client is to obtain a:

    1. Pneumococcal vaccine.

    2. Tetanus vaccine.

    3. Hepatitis B vaccine.

    4. Varicella vaccine.

28. The American College of Physicians (ACP) recommends that healthy adults receive a Td booster vaccination:

    1. Every 5 years.

    2. Every 8 years.

    3. At age 60.

    4. Every 10 years.

29. Which statement most correctly describes tetanus toxoid?

    1. Tetanus toxoid (T) induces more persistent antitoxin antibody titers.

    2. DPT and diphtheria and tetanus toxoids, absorbed (DT) are safe to give to adults.

    3. The recommended dose for the adult is 0.75 ml IM.

    4. Tetanus toxoid fluid provides the same antitoxin antibody titers as tetanus toxoid.

30. Immunizations recommended for a healthy 40-year-old adult who has had his childhood series include:

    1. Measles, rubella, varicella, and hepatitis B.

    2. Pneumovax, influenza, and rubella.

    3. Tetanus, influenza, varicella, pneumovax, OPV, and hepatitis B.

    4. Influenza, hepatitis A, hepatitis B, varicella, MMR, and tetanus.

3 Answers & Rationales

1. **(1)** The American Cancer Society does recommend maintaining a desirable body weight; research has shown an association between increased deaths from various cancers and varying degrees of being overweight. Another recommendation is to eat a wide variety of foods, consistent with the Food Guide Pyramid put out by the U.S. Department of Agriculture and the U.S. Department of Health and Human Services. A variety of fruits and vegetables should be included in the daily diet (5 to 9 servings/day), as research has shown that there is an association between lower cancer rates and high fruit and vegetable consumption. High-fiber foods are also recommended; a lower risk of colon cancer is seen in those individuals who consume a high-fiber diet. There are no recommendations to increase the amount of protein in the diet at this time; due to the high consumption of red meat in the American diet, many people are already getting large quantities in their current diets. The American Cancer Society recommends limiting the daily consumption of alcohol to two drinks for males, one drink for females, and no drinks for pregnant females. They also state that, ideally, no alcohol should be consumed; regular alcohol consumption has been shown to increase the risk of various cancers.

2. **(1)** The recommendation is low-density lipoprotein (LDL) <130 mg/dl and triglyceride levels <200 mg/dl. All other choices have inaccuracies of goals.

3. **(2)** The American Diabetes Association recommends screening adults starting at the age of 45 every 3 years.

4. **(2)** The physical therapy program will assist her in restoring her optimum level of functioning after a CVA. Option #1 is a primary prevention activity nonspecific to a CVA. Options #3 and #4 are examples of secondary prevention activities nonspecific to a CVA.

5. **(3)** The client needs an increased intake in protein and vitamin C to promote healing. Red meat, citrus fruits, and green vegetables will give the highest amounts of these elements from the selections offered.

6. **(3)** Shouting increases the pitch of the voice. In presbycusis, which is a hearing loss in the elderly, high-pitched consonant sounds are the first to be affected, and the change may occur gradually. The nurse practitioner should face the client when speaking. If there is a need to stand behind the client, then use touch to get the client's attention. The communication should use simple sentences in order to facilitate understanding.

7. **(4)** This information will prevent complications that may result in a fall. Options #1 and #2 are appropriate for tertiary prevention. Option #3 is appropriate for secondary prevention, which is to prevent the client from experiencing another fall.

8. **(4)** This evaluation will assist in identifying any problems with bleeding. Option #1 is not necessary. Option #2 is not a screening and would not be administered annually. A sigmoidoscopy is recommended every 3–5 years for clients over 50.

9. **(4)** This applies the concept of adult educational principles. Overhead lighting may produce an increase in the glare, which can decrease visualization. There is an alteration of color perception (e.g., blue appears green-blue) as an individual ages. As individuals age the ability to hear women's and children's voices decreases, since these are high-pitched voices. This video would not enhance the program if these clients frequently have presbycusis as a result of the normal aging process.

10. **(3)** All of these disorders can be associated with workplace exposure but, currently, lung disease is still the most common occupationally related disease. Musculoskeletal injuries are on the rise.

11. **(4)** In the summer of 1997, the National Institutes of Health (NIH) and the American Cancer Society changed the recommendation to begin yearly mammography at age 40.

12. **(4)** The client's history and physical will reveal the presence of any coronary heart disease risk factors such as age, family history of coronary heart disease, diabetes, current cigarette smoking, blood pressure, height/weight, and cardiovascular exam. A lipid profile is also recommended to assess the level of risk—it consists of a total cholesterol, high-density lipoprotein (HDL), LDL, and triglycerides. It would be prudent to have a precise cholesterol level done, as the previous result was from a screening health fair, and there is no written record of the result. It is also important to assess the level of HDLs and LDLs to see if they are present in normal amounts. These parameters should be assessed first before a cholesterol-lowering agent, ECG, or stress test is ordered. An exercise program is also important, but should only be done after a history and physical and lipid profile results are known; if the lipid profile results or exam is abnormal, stress testing may be appropriate before undertaking a new exercise program.

13. **(2)** Screening for colon-rectal cancer includes annual fecal occult blood screening for individuals over age 50. Avoiding medications that can cause gastrointestinal irritation and bleeding can help avoid false-positive results. Rare meat and vegetables that are high in peroxidase (like the ones listed) will cause false-positive results, while vitamin C can cause false-negative results.

14. **(1)** The recommended servings for each of the food groups are as follows:

Food Group	Servings
Bread/cereal/rice/pasta	6–11 servings
Fruit	2–4 servings
Vegetable	3–5 servings
Meat/poultry/fish, dry beans, eggs, and nuts	2–3 servings
Fats/oils/sweets	Sparing uses

15. **(3)** A screening mammogram is recommended before the age of 40.

16. **(1)** All of these areas are important to probe in the initial interview of a new client. The history will help determine the necessary components of the physical examination and laboratory or radiologic studies that are ordered and the counseling that is done during the appointment.

17. **(4)** An account of the client's usual intake is necessary, so that problem areas can be identified. Before beginning any exercise program, a physical examination should be done to assess the client's physical condition and to aid in the proper selection of a specific exercise plan. A dietary assessment needs to be completed before recommending vitamin and protein supplements; the client may already be receiving adequate amounts in her diet. A more active job would be ideal; however, most people do not have options regarding their choice of job, so increasing her activity outside of work would be most appropriate.

18. **(4)** The older adult is at greatest risk for altered immune function related to nutrition. For a variety of reasons (e.g., altered taste, eating alone, ability to prepare meals, malabsorption) the older adult often does not get enough nutrition. Adequate nutrition in the older adult has been shown to improve the immune status and improve their antibody response to influenza vaccine.

19. **(3)** Multiphasic health screening is a form of period health surveillance where employees undergo a battery of laboratory or diagnostic tests to determine risk factors and disease detection. A health risk appraisal is often part of a multiphasic health screening and involves a scored questionnaire that determines overall health risks or targets specific risks, such as cardiovascular disease. A health fair or special event may provide basic screening services, have booths or exhibits, and presentations on health-related education. An onsite emergent care clinic is not primarily health promotion and prevention, as employees seek services for emergent care.

20. **(2)** Hypertension, smoking, and hyperlipidemia are the major risk factors in the development of cardiovascular disease. Controlling hyperglycemia, and high dietary fiber intake and vitamin supplements assist in maintaining a healthy lifestyle; however, they are not as important in preventing cardiovascular disease.

21. **(1)** These three modifications are the most effective in maintaining normal blood pressure.

22. **(3)** The reading level of most American adults is at the sixth-grade level.

Immunizations

23. **(3)** The pneumococcal vaccine is not given more often than every 10 years and may be effective for longer periods.

24. **(2)** Influenza outbreaks may affect 60% of those in long-term care and fatality rates are high. All the other groups listed are appropriate for the influenza vaccine but are not as high a priority.

25. **(3)** Prior anaphylaxis and severe hypersensitivity would be considered a contraindication; a mild viral illness would not. The client who is pregnant or lactating may be immunized.

26. **(4)** Pneumococcal and annual influenza immunizations are recommended for those who are 65 years of age and older. Adult Td is offered to those who have not had a booster in the last 10 years.

27. **(2)** Adults who enjoy gardening and outdoor activities should have a tetanus vaccine at least every 10 years due to the high-risk activities. A pneumococcal vaccine is recommended for adults age 65 or older, or for those who have a chronic illness or who are immunosuppressed. Most older adults have had chickenpox as a child and do not require the vaccine.

28. **(4)** The ACP recommends that adults receive a Td booster every 10 years or a single booster at age 50 for clients who have completed a full pediatric series, including teenage and young adult boosters.

29. **(1)** Tetanus toxoid induces more persistent antitoxin antibody titers than tetanus toxoid fluid. DPT and DT are for use in children under the age of 7 years; however, they should *not* be used in adults. The recommended dose of DT for an adult is 0.5 ml IM.

30. **(4)** It would be important to start the hepatitis B series as this was not included as part of his childhood vaccination series considering his age. Hepatitis A is also recommended, especially if the person travels to foreign countries, along with varicella as these immunizations were not available during his childhood. An MMR is required for adults born in 1957 or later who have no laboratory proof of immunity or documentation of either previous vaccination or a physician documented case of measles. Tetanus is recommended every ten years, especially in high risk situations (adults that participate in outdoor sports). Pneumovax is indicated in an adult who has a chronic disease, such as diabetes, chronic pulmonary disease, or chronic cardiovascular disease and it is also indicated for adults who are immunocompromised. If the adult did not receive the OPV series as a child, it is recommended to vaccinate the adult with injectable enhanced-potency inactivated polio virus vaccine (IPV), because the risk of vaccine-associated poliomyelitis (VAPP) is lower.

4 Cardiovascular

Physical Examination & Diagnostic Tests

1. The practitioner is performing a physical examination on a healthy male adult. On auscultation the stethoscope would be placed in what areas to best hear the characteristic sounds of S_1 and S_2?

   1. S_1 is best heard at the apex and S_2 at the base of the heart.

   2. Both are heard equally well on the right side at the midclavicular line.

   3. On the left side, S_1 is at the area of the pulmonic valve and S_2 at the aortic valve.

   4. Both sounds are heard best at Erb's point at the third intercostal space at the sternal margin.

2. On the general assessment of an adult client, the practitioner determines the presence of the apical impulse at the point of maximal impulse (PMI) on the client's chest wall. Where on the chest wall is the PMI normally found?

   1. Second intercostal space at the midclavicular line on the left side.

   2. Right lower sternal border, fifth intercostal space.

   3. Left side at the fifth intercostal space on the midclavicular line.

   4. Left fifth intercostal space, lateral to the midclavicular line.

3. The nurse practitioner is auscultating the carotids for a whooshing sound. The correct procedure is:

   1. Use the diaphragm of the stethoscope.

   2. Use the bell of the stethoscope.

   3. Place the stethoscope 1 inch off the area above the sternocleidomastoid muscle.

   4. Position the client at a 30-degree angle, press firmly with the bell of the stethoscope.

4. When inspecting the precordium, the nurse practitioner is checking for:

   1. Scars and anatomic landmarks.

   2. Pulsations and retractions.

   3. Heaves and cardiac dullness.

   4. Pericardial friction rub and lifts.

5. While examining a client in a left lateral decubitus position, the nurse practitioner auscultates a third heart sound (S_3). The nurse practitioner knows that:

   1. This sound is normally heard in children and young adults and is considered a physiologic S_3.

   2. This rarely is associated with myocardial failure in the older adult.

   3. This client should be immediately referred to a cardiologist for evaluation.

   4. This is considered a normal splitting of the S_2 during inspiration and is accentuated by positioning.

6. The nurse practitioner knows that the correct auscultatory site for the aortic area is:

   1. Midclavicular line, fifth interspace, left side.

   2. Left fourth interspace close to the sternum.

   3. Right second interspace close to the sternum.

   4. Midclavicular line, second interspace, left side.

7. The nurse practitioner should include the following in his/her teaching when ordering a lipid profile on a client:

   1. A normal breakfast should be consumed the morning of the exam.

   2. The client should be fasting for 12 hours prior to the exam, with the client's typical diet being ingested for the 7 days prior to the exam.

   3. There are no alcohol or diet restrictions for this test.

   4. The client may take any current medications with a few sips of water before the test.

8. When auscultating the heart sounds of a 72-year-old client with a history of hypertension, the nurse practitioner notes an S_4. This finding could indicate:

   1. A normal variant in people 65 years or older.

   2. The beginning of ventricular failure.

   3. A decreased resistance to ventricular filling.

   4. A severely failing heart.

9. A 55-year-old client has a blood pressure of 168/100. This is classified as:

   1. Moderate hypertension.

   2. Mild hypertension.

   3. High normal blood pressure.

   4. Severe hypertension.

10. The nurse practitioner is examining a client with a history of rheumatic fever and who is being followed for the development of carditis. During the cardiac auscultation, where on the chest wall is the stethoscope placed to determine the most common murmurs associated with this condition?

    1. At the left sternal border, fourth left intercostal space.

    2. Fifth intercostal space, left side at the midclavicular line.

    3. Second or third intercostal space at the left of the sternal border.

    4. Second intercostal space on the right of the sternal border.

11. A client presents with unusual coolness in the left hand as compared to the right hand. What is the next step in the examination?

    1. Palpate the radial pulse on both hands for a full minute.

    2. Feel the forehead with the backs of the fingers.

    3. Feel the forearms with the backs of the fingers.

    4. Hold the hand in a dependent position and re-examine in 3 minutes.

12. S_1 and S_2 are identified when the nurse practitioner auscultates for cardiac sounds. The physiology responsible for the production of these heart sounds is:

    1. Contraction of the ventricles and closure of the atrioventricular (AV) valves

produces S_1; closure of the semilunar valves forms S_2.

2. Closure of the aortic valve produces S_2; opening of the mitral valve and filling of the left ventricle forms S_1.

3. The opening of the AV valves produces S_1; closure of the semilunar valves produces S_2.

4. Opening of the tricuspid produces S_1; closure of the pulmonic forms S_2.

13. The nurse practitioner is assessing a cardiac client who is experiencing an atrial dysrhythmia. The pulse rate is irregular at 110 beats per minute and there is concern regarding a pulse deficit. How is a pulse deficit determined in this client?

1. A 12-lead electrocardiogram (ECG) is necessary to determine the presence and length of the P-R intervals.

2. The apical pulse is counted and then the radial pulse is counted; the pulse deficit is determined by the difference in the two rates.

3. The apical pulse is counted and an increase or decrease is correlated with the phases of the respiratory cycle.

4. The apical pulse and radial pulse are determined simultaneously; the pulse deficit is established if the apical rate is higher than the radial rate.

14. The nurse practitioner notes a grade V systolic murmur while examining a client's precordium. Which describes this type of murmur?

1. Barely audible, faint with the bell of the stethoscope.

2. Heard only with the diaphragm of the stethoscope.

3. Heard with the stethoscope partly off the chest.

4. Heard without the aid of the stethoscope.

15. Normal physiologic changes in the geriatric population that affect conductivity and contractility of the myocardium include:

1. Increased automaticity and excitability.

2. Increased contractility and conductivity.

3. Decreased excitability and conductivity.

4. Decreased automaticity and contractility.

16. When assessing temperature of an extremity as part of a peripheral vascular assessment on a client, which part of the hand is the most sensitive?

1. Palm.

2. Fingertips.

3. Back of the wrist.

4. Back of the fingers.

17. A 45-year-old male's lipid profile results are sent to the nurse practitioner. They are as follows: total cholesterol = 287 mmol/L; high-density lipoprotein (HDL) = 30 mg/dl; low-density lipoprotein (LDL) = 165 mg/dl; triglycerides = 238 mg/dl. The nurse practitioner interprets these results as:

1. Abnormal; the elevated triglyceride level is of the most concern and should be treated immediately.

2. Borderline; this is considered to be a borderline risk lipid profile.

3. Abnormal; the total cholesterol and LDL levels are elevated, and the HDL is too low.

4. Normal; these results are of no concern; follow-up with client in 1 year.

18. A client returns to the chest pain clinic 3 weeks following myocardial infarction (MI) complaining of pericardial pain and elevated temperature. Physical examination reveals a pericardial friction rub. What diagnostic studies are indicated?

1. 24-hour Holter monitoring.

2. Echocardiogram.

3. Complete blood count (CBC) with differential.

4. Cardiac enzymes with myoglobin.

19. On assessment of a geriatric client, the nurse practitioner notes bilateral pulsations and distention of the jugular veins when the client's head is elevated 45 degrees. What further assessment information needs to be obtained at this time?

    1. Estimate the level of venous pressure by measuring from the sternal angle to the highest level of venous pulsations.

    2. Place the client in supine position and determine effect of position change on distention and pulsations of jugular vein.

    3. Measure carotid pulses due to the increased left ventricular pressure.

    4. Have the client hold his breath to facilitate evaluation for presence of carotid bruits.

20. The nurse practitioner is examining a woman with a known history of mitral valve disease. What type of murmur heard on auscultation supports a history of mitral stenosis?

    1. Diastolic murmur, heard loudest at the apex with the client on her left side.

    2. Mid systolic ejection murmur heard loudest over the left lower sternal border.

    3. Holosystolic murmur, heard loudest over the apex and left axillary area.

    4. Diastolic murmur, heard loudest with her in sitting position leaning forward.

21. The nurse practitioner is doing an assessment on a client who is 2 weeks post-MI of the left ventricle. The nurse practitioner would pay particular attention to what area of the physical assessment?

    1. The lower extremities and the jugular vein for the presence of systemic venous congestion.

    2. The area on the chest where the PMI is heard most clearly.

    3. The presence of dyspnea and auscultation of crackles in the lungs.

    4. The level of dependent edema and fluid intake over the past 24 hours.

22. Which symptoms would indicate to the nurse practitioner that the client is experiencing intermittent claudication?

    1. Petechiae and itching of the lower part of the leg.

    2. Extensive discoloration and edema of the upper leg.

    3. Profuse rash and discoloration from the trunk down to the feet.

    4. Complaints of pain on walking, relieved by sitting down.

23. Stress testing, or the exercise tolerance test, is the most widely used diagnostic test in ischemic heart disease. It is most accurate, up to 98%, in the following type client:

    1. Males under the age of 40 with atypical angina pectoris.

    2. Asymptomatic premenopausal female without risk factors.

    3. Males over the age of 50 with typical angina pectoris.

    4. Males on digitalis with typical angina pectoris.

Disorders

24. The diagnosis of hypertension (HTN) should be established on the basis of:

    1. At least three readings with an average systolic blood pressure (BP) of 140 mm Hg and a diastolic pressure of 90 mm Hg.

    2. At least five readings 1 month apart.

    3. One reading of 140 mm Hg systolic and 90 mm Hg diastolic or above.

    4. One reading taken in three different positions.

25. A client has a 2-year history of hypertensive heart disease. The nurse practitioner expects the major pathophysiologic change to be:

    1. Right ventricular hypertrophy.

    2. Left atrial dilation.

3. Left ventricular hypertrophy.

4. Right atrial dilation.

26. From the following description, what data most clearly describes atrial tachycardia?

   1. Heart rate of 96, P waves present on each QRS complex, T wave every other beat.

   2. P waves present on every other beat, heart rate of 100, and irregular.

   3. Heart rate of 110, P waves present prior to each QRS complex, and regular.

   4. P waves for every third QRS complex, adequate P-R interval, rate of 90.

27. What clinical manifestation of an MI is frequently **not** present in the geriatric cardiac client?

   1. Prolonged severe chest pain.

   2. Diaphoresis, pallor, syncope.

   3. Dyspnea, increasing anxiety.

   4. Gastrointestinal distress, orthopnea.

28. The nurse practitioner is performing an assessment on a client who is having difficulty controlling his left-sided congestive heart failure (CHF). The nurse practitioner understands that the primary symptoms associated with this type of failure are:

   1. Systemic venous congestion.

   2. Dyspnea and pulmonary congestion.

   3. Increased peripheral edema and anorexia.

   4. Atrial fibrillation with a rate around 110.

29. The nurse practitioner is concerned that a post-MI client is developing a problem of constrictive pericarditis. What is one of the characteristic findings and how is it evaluated?

   1. Cardiac tamponade occurs; it is identified by the presence of muffled heart sounds and the presence of a paradoxical pulse.

   2. Pericarditis with a pericardial triphasic friction rub is common; it is best heard at the apical area of the heart.

3. There is a mitral valve prolapse that is characterized by a late systolic murmur heard at the apex and the left sternal borders.

4. There are altered waves on the jugular venous pulse; this is determined with a light that is directed tangentially to illuminate the shadows of the pulsations.

30. A geriatric client has a diagnosis of left-sided congestive heart failure. The nurse practitioner would identify what common condition frequently associated with CHF?

   1. History of peripheral vascular disease.

   2. History of untreated hypertension.

   3. Current treatment for ventricular dysrhythmias.

   4. History of chronic obstructive pulmonary disease.

31. In evaluating the effectiveness of cardiopulmonary resuscitation (CPR) on the older adult client, the nurse practitioner would note:

   1. Dilated pupils.

   2. Palpable carotid pulse.

   3. Capillary refill within 2 seconds.

   4. Pink and warm skin.

32. The nurse practitioner is evaluating an ECG. The client presented at the clinic with complaints of weakness and fainting. His ECG reveals a cardiac rate of 68, absent P waves, regular QRS complex, T-waves are present after each QRS complex. The best interpretation of this information is:

   1. A normal ECG; need to further evaluate client's complaints of weakness.

   2. Third-degree block with junctional rhythm; keep client at rest and transfer to emergency room for cardiology consult.

   3. First-degree block; need to further evaluate possibility of digitalis toxicity and/or levels of cardiac antiarrhythmic medications.

   4. Administer sublingual nitroglycerin and refer the client for a cardiology consult.

33. The nurse practitioner is conducting a follow-up examination on a client with coronary artery disease (CAD) and a history of pericarditis. What is one of the characteristic physical findings in pericarditis and how is it evaluated?

    1. A paradoxical pulse is common; it is identified by evaluating the changes in the amplitude of arterial pulse pressure associated with the respiratory cycle.

    2. There is a pulse deficit, which is determined by counting the radial pulse and the apical pulse at the same time and evaluating the difference.

    3. A pericardial friction rub is present; it is best heard with the diaphragm of the stethoscope and is loudest to the left of the sternum at the fourth or fifth intercostal spaces.

    4. There is an S_4 present; it is commonly heard at the apex with the bell of the stethoscope and the client in a left lateral position.

34. The typical symptoms of an MI usually experienced by the elderly include:

    1. Dyspnea and diaphoresis.

    2. Back pain and muscle cramping.

    3. Numbness and tingling of the left arm.

    4. Epigastric pain and nausea.

35. Cardiovascular risk factors predisposing females for cardiovascular disease include:

    1. Absence of estrogen adversely effects lipoprotein metabolism.

    2. Fat deposited on hips mobilizes, raising serum cholesterol.

    3. Coronary arteries are longer and wider in diameter.

    4. Resting ejection fraction is lower.

36. The nurse practitioner is planning the treatment for a geriatric client who has been newly diagnosed with hypertension. What parameters are most important in determining the appropriate pharmacologic therapy?

    1. Determine medications and dosage based on the client's weight, age, and availability.

    2. Step method utilizing diuretics and β-adrenergic blockers with the utilization of other medications as necessary.

    3. Initiate lifestyle changes prior to beginning the medications to determine if medication is necessary.

    4. Other medical conditions the client is being treated for, side effects, age, and cost of medication.

37. Which statement accurately describes coronary artery disease in geriatric clients?

    1. Cardiovascular disease is increased in the female client who is on estrogen replacement.

    2. A major risk factor for cardiovascular disease in females and males is chronic hypertension.

    3. The majority of geriatric clients with coronary artery disease also have type II diabetes.

    4. Males over 60 years old continue to maintain the highest level of CAD.

38. A client with a history of chronic obstructive pulmonary disease (COPD) comes to the clinic for his annual checkup with complaints of increasing difficulty breathing. Assessment findings include S_3 gallop, early systolic ejection click, and increased P-wave amplitude in leads II, III, and aVF of the ECG. The nurse practitioner would expect to observe which change on the chest x-ray?

    1. Hypertrophy of the left ventricle.

    2. Hypertrophy of the right ventricle.

    3. Hypertrophy of the left atrium and ventricle.

    4. Hypertrophy of the right atrium and ventricle.

39. When cardiac output falls in CHF, the body attempts to compensate. What electrolyte imbalances occur as a result of this response?

    1. Hypernatremia and hyperkalemia.

    2. Hyponatremia and hypokalemia.

3. Hypophosphatemia and hypercalcemia.

4. Hyperphosphatemia and hypocalcemia.

40. When assessing the carotid pulse of a 72-year-old indigent client at a community-based clinic, the nurse practitioner notes a bounding pulse with rapid rise and sudden collapse. The nurse practitioner would include which additional assessment to support this finding?

1. Auscultation for a diastolic murmur.

2. Auscultation for paradoxical pulse.

3. Blood pressure in both arms lying, sitting, and standing.

4. Blood pressure for an auscultatory gap.

41. The nurse practitioner understands that the pain experienced with angina pectoris or an MI is caused by irritation of the myocardial nerve fibers by the increase in:

1. Blood glucose.

2. Lactic acid.

3. Serum potassium.

4. Serum magnesium.

42. During the history and physical examination of a client with suspected early CHF, which is the most prominent finding?

1. Moist crackles in the lung bases bilaterally.

2. Anorexia with weight loss of 3 lb in 1 week.

3. Increased urinary output, peripheral edema.

4. Facial edema and distended neck veins.

43. Chest pain that is sudden and severe, described as tearing, and accompanied by a decrease in peripheral pulses may indicate a diagnosis of:

1. Angina.

2. Acute myocardial infarction.

3. Aortic dissection.

4. Pericarditis.

44. Dietary therapy for hyperlipidemia occurs in two steps, a Step I and a Step II diet. A Step I diet includes, as daily intake:

1. Total fat ≤30% of total calories, <300 mg cholesterol, 8–10% saturated fat.

2. Total fat ≤30% of total calories, <200 mg cholesterol, <7% saturated fat.

3. Total fat ≤40% of total calories, <400 mg cholesterol, <15% saturated fat.

4. Total fat ≤30% of total calories, <2000 total calories, <3 gm sodium.

45. The most frequent life-threatening dysrhythmia experienced by a client with an acute MI is:

1. Atrial fibrillation.

2. Ventricular tachycardia.

3. Third-degree heart block.

4. Ventricular fibrillation.

46. In an overweight, older adult female client with an elevated cholesterol level and abnormal lipoprotein profile, the first step in treatment includes:

1. Prescribing a bile acid sequestrant agent.

2. Initiation of a diet and exercise program.

3. Estrogen replacement therapy.

4. Referral to a cardiologist.

47. The nurse practitioner understands that the most common symptom of CHF in adults is:

1. Anorexia.

2. Dependent edema.

3. Dyspnea.

4. Weakness.

48. The nurse practitioner teaches the cardiac client to avoid foods high in saturated fats, which include:

1. Nuts, legumes, and seeds.

2. Fish, shellfish, and mussels.

3. Palm oil, coconut oil, and butter.

4. Peanut oil, soybean oil, and olive oil.

49. An elderly male client is complaining of chest pain. A parameter to assist the practitioner to differentiate the chest pain of angina from that of an infarction is:

    1. Myocardial pain with an infarction is more severe.

    2. Anginal pain is more substernal and does not radiate to other areas.

    3. Anginal pain is frequently relieved by nitroglycerin.

    4. Pain from an infarction is always associated with other symptoms.

50. The nurse practitioner is evaluating a client in the office who is complaining of chest pain. The ECG shows some signs of ischemia and the client is to be transferred to the emergency department. What drug might the nurse practitioner give the client while awaiting transport to the emergency department?

    1. Furosemide (Lasix) 40 mg IV.

    2. Morphine sulfate 25 mg IV.

    3. Streptokinase IV.

    4. Acetylsalicylic acid (aspirin) 81 mg PO.

51. An elderly client is being evaluated for a complaint of dizziness. The symptom that will make the nurse practitioner consider that this is a life-threatening event as opposed to a disease that is not life-threatening is:

    1. The onset of the dizziness occurs in certain positions.

    2. It is accompanied by tinnitus.

    3. The symptoms worsen when standing and improve when lying down.

    4. It is preceded by rapid breathing.

52. A 58-year-old male presents to the nurse practitioner with a history of chest pain that has been increasing over the past several days. The client states that the pain worsens upon lying down. He denies any shortness of breath, cough, or radiation of the pain. He does give a history of a recent coxsackievirus infection. On exam, it is noted that the client has a cardiac friction rub. One probable diagnosis considered by the nurse practitioner is:

    1. Acute myocardial infarction.

    2. Pleural effusion.

    3. Pericarditis.

    4. Esophageal reflux.

53. The nurse practitioner would most likely suspect which differential diagnosis for an elderly client presenting with atrial fibrillation and functional decline?

    1. Hyperthyroidism.

    2. Hypothyroidism.

    3. Sick sinus syndrome.

    4. Congestive heart failure.

54. Which assessment made by the nurse practitioner with an older client would be a deviation from normal aging changes?

    1. Decreased exercise tolerance, slightly smaller heart.

    2. Grade II/VI systolic ejection murmur.

    3. Slight prolongation of the intervals on the ECG.

    4. Jugular venous pressure (JVP) 4 cm.

55. During the cardiac auscultation with an older adult, a grade II/VI murmur, heard best at the second right intercostal space, is noted. The murmur is auscultated louder with squatting. There is a small carotid pulse with a delayed upstroke. The client's history is benign, and his activity tolerance is within normal limits for his age. The nurse practitioner would interpret this murmur to be indicative of:

    1. Aortic regurgitation.

    2. Aortic stenosis.

    3. Mitral valve prolapse.

    4. Mitral regurgitation.

56. The most frequently diagnosed valvular heart problem in the elderly is:

    1. Aortic stenosis.

2. Mitral stenosis.

3. Mitral regurgitation.

4. Aortic regurgitation.

57. An older male with no known coronary artery risk factors presents with a cholesterol level of 255 mg/dl. The nurse practitioner would:

    1. Start him on an HMG-CoA reductase inhibitor (statins), the most potent lipid-lowering agents.

    2. Start him on a Step I diet, since all clients should be given a trial on a diet.

    3. Repeat cholesterol and obtain HDL and calculated LDL.

    4. Do nothing, since he has no coronary risks other than maleness.

58. A client has a history of mitral valve stenosis and comes to the clinic for an annual checkup. What findings on the physical exam would correlate with the beginning of complications often seen with these clients?

    1. History of chest pain relieved by rest, increase in peripheral edema.

    2. Chest pain with deep inspiration and low-grade fever for 3 weeks.

    3. History of dyspnea on exertion, increasing fatigue, presence of diastolic murmur.

    4. Orthostatic hypotension, tachycardia but regular pulse, 15-point pulse deficit.

Pharmacology

59. A 75-year-old client presents to the office complaining of "not feeling well." He has a history of chronic lung disease and CHF. His vital signs are pulse 78 and irregular, respirations 26, blood pressure 158/100. An electrocardiogram indicates sinus rhythm and confirms the rate. The P-R interval is 0.28 second, P waves are present, and each is followed by a QRS complex. There are frequent premature atrial beats. The client is on digitalis, potassium, theophylline, hydrochlorothiazide, and a calcium channel blocker. What is the next best action to take?

    1. Obtain serum theophylline, digitalis, and potassium levels.

    2. Increase dosage of calcium channel blocker and diuretic to obtain better blood pressure control.

    3. Order pulmonary function studies to determine the progress of pulmonary disease.

    4. Refer the client to a cardiologist for further evaluation and treatment of congestive failure.

60. A 69-year-old female was started on a thiazide diuretic for hypertension 1 month ago. She arrives in the clinic complaining of muscle cramps and dizziness. Physical exam findings are:

    - BP 132/88 mm Hg (previous 186/112)
    - Pulse 112
    - Respirations 24
    - Tenting positive
    - Skin turgor decreased
    - Neck veins flat
    - STAT serum electrolytes
      Sodium 114 mEq/L
      Chloride 92 mEq/L
      Potassium 3.0 mEq/L
    - STAT blood glucose—201 mg/dl

Initial treatment for this client should include fluid replacement:

1. Orally with free water and a potassium supplement.

2. Intravenously with normal saline and regular insulin subcutaneously.

3. Intravenously with 1000 ml of normal saline with 40 mEq KCl at 50 ml/hr.

4. Intravenously with 1000 ml of Ringer's lactate at 250 ml/hr.

61. A client is recovering from an acute episode of thrombophlebitis and is being treated with warfarin (Coumadin) 5 mg PO daily. In reviewing medication information, the nurse practitioner would include what information in her teaching?

    1. Decrease the servings of green leafy vegetables and do not take a multivitamin supplement.

    2. Limit dairy products, since they tend to decrease medication effectiveness.

    3. Do not walk for exercise; aerobic exercises are more effective.

    4. Maintain a daily record of intake and output to evaluate renal function.

62. The nurse practitioner is evaluating a client who is complaining of "not feeling good." He has a history of CAD and CHF. Vital signs are pulse 72, respirations 20, blood pressure 130/88, temperature is normal. There are no complaints of chest pain or difficulty breathing, some nausea but no vomiting over the past 2 days, and lower extremities are negative for edema. The client states he has been able to take his medications. His current medications are digoxin (Lanoxin) 0.25 bid, hydrochlorothiazide (Hydrodiuril) 100 mg bid, potassium (Micro-K) 10 mEq daily, and nitroglycerin transdermal patches. What is the priority of care for this client?

    1. Obtain a STAT electrocardiogram and white blood cell (WBC) count.

    2. Obtain arterial blood gases and oxygen at 4 L/min.

    3. Obtain serum digoxin and potassium levels.

    4. Obtain serial cardiac enzymes now and q6h × 2.

63. The nurse practitioner has prescribed losartan (Cozaar) 50 mg PO qd. This medication promotes vasodilation by:

    1. Inhibiting conversion of angiotensin I to antiotensin II.

    2. Promoting the release of aldosterone.

    3. Promoting the synthesis of prostaglandin.

    4. Inhibiting calcium influx into smooth muscle cells.

64. A client with a history of hypertension is started on Aldactone 50 mg PO qd. The nurse practitioner instructs the client to call the clinic if which symptoms are experienced?

    1. Muscle weakness, fatigue, and paresthesias.

    2. Decreased reflex response, nausea, and vomiting.

    3. Muscle twitching, numbness of the limbs, and depression.

    4. Weight gain, excessive thirst, and fever.

65. A client with a history of unstable angina is seen in the cardiac clinic for a checkup. The assessment reveals increased weight of 10 lb, distended jugular neck veins, and an S_3. What changes in the pharmacologic treatment should be initiated?

    1. Discontinue β-blockers and calcium channel blockers.

    2. Initiate thrombolytic therapy.

    3. Discontinue nitrate and aspirin therapy.

    4. Initiate diuretic and vasoconstrictor therapy.

66. A client arrives at the emergency room of a small rural hospital complaining of "feels like my heart is racing." He is connected to a cardiac monitor that reveals a supraventricular tachycardia rate of 184, a QRS complex <0.10 second, and a BP of 112/62. Which treatment modality is indicated?

    1. Synchronized cardioversion with 50 joules.

    2. Defibrillation with 100 joules.

    3. Adenosine 6 mg IV push.

    4. Lidocaine 1 mg/kg IV push.

67. An 80-year-old client with a history of glaucoma who develops unstable angina is started on diltiazem (Cardizem) 30 mg PO

qid and aspirin 324 mg PO qd in addition to timolol ophthalmic solution (Timoptic) i gtt OD bid. This client would have an increased risk for:

1. Bleeding episodes.

2. Fainting episodes and falls.

3. Rebound supraventricular tachycardia.

4. Blurred vision.

68. A client with a serum cholesterol of 256 mg/dl, HDL of 38 mg/dl, and LDL of 172 mg/dl is instructed on dietary modifications and niacin (nicotinic acid) 1 gm PO tid. Specific instructions include:

1. Limiting fluid intake.

2. Measures to minimize orthostatic hypotension.

3. Administration of the drug an hour after eating.

4. Slight modifications in diet that are required with drug therapy.

69. When monitoring for the therapeutic effects of verapamil (Calan SR), the nurse practitioner would assess for a/an:

1. Increase in heart rate.

2. Decrease in systemic vascular resistance.

3. Increase in blood pressure.

4. Decrease in ventricular premature beats.

70. An adult male client with essential hypertension was treated by the nurse practitioner with enalapril (Vasotec) 5 mg daily. After 6 months of therapy, the blood pressure was measured at 150/100 mm Hg. The nurse practitioner recommended sodium restriction and increased the enalapril to 10 mg daily. The client's blood pressure was unchanged after 3 additional months. At this point, the nurse practitioner should:

1. Double the dose of enalapril (Vasotec).

2. Add 25 mg of hydrochlorothiazide (Hydrodiuril) daily.

3. Double the dose of enalapril and add 25 mg of hydrochlorothiazide daily.

4. Switch to captopril (Capoten) 50 mg tid.

71. When prescribing antihypertensive drug therapy for elderly clients, the nurse practitioner recognizes that elderly clients have decreased receptor sensitivity and a changing baroreceptor response. Which class of antihypertensive agents should be avoided with elderly clients?

1. Calcium entry antagonists.

2. Diuretics.

3. β-Blockers.

4. Angiotensin converting enzyme (ACE) inhibitors

72. Medications used in managing ischemic heart disease include:

1. β-Blockers, sedatives, aspirin.

2. Nitrates, β-blockers, calcium channel blockers, aspirin.

3. Vasoconstrictors, aspirin, anxiolytics.

4. Nitrates, ACE inhibitors, aspirin, lipid-lowering drugs.

73. The nurse practitioner initiates antihypertensive therapy for a nonsmoking male. One week later, the client returns for a follow-up visit and complains of a recurrent dry cough since initiating the medications. This is most likely a side effect of a(an):

1. β-Blocker.

2. Thiazide diuretic.

3. ACE inhibitor.

4. Calcium channel blocker

74. The role of digoxin in the management of CHF is still being defined, but is definitely indicated in CHF:

1. With atrial fibrillation.

2. With mitral stenosis.

3. With normal ejection fraction and sinus rhythm.

4. Due to acute pericardial disease.

75. Which statement accurately describes coronary artery disease in geriatric clients?

    1. Cardiovascular disease is increased in the female client who is on estrogen replacement.

    2. A major risk factor for cardiovascular disease in female and males is chronic hypertension.

    3. The majority of geriatric clients with coronary artery disease also have Type II diabetes.

    4. Males over 60 years old continue to maintain the highest level of coronary artery disease.

76. The nurse practitioner should monitor the elderly client for which of the most common adverse reactions of digoxin?

    1. Blurred vision.

    2. Confusion.

    3. Diarrhea.

    4. Eating disorder.

77. The nurse practitioner has been successfully treating an older client's hypertension with diet, exercise, and hydrodiuril (HCTZ) 25 mg PO qd for 5 months. During today's clinic visit, the client's blood pressure was 154/90 and temperature was 99.9°F. The physical examination revealed clear breath sounds, S_1 and S_2 with no murmurs, gallops, or rubs; and no jugular venous distention. The client denied syncope, headaches, or visual changes; and had a tender and edematous right ankle. Which laboratory values would be most appropriate for evaluation?

    1. Blood urea nitrogen and sodium.

    2. Serum cholesterol and serum calcium.

    3. Serum potassium and blood count.

    4. Serum uric acid and complete blood count.

78. An elderly white male with a long history of COPD has recently developed hypertension. Which class of antihypertensive agents should the nurse practitioner avoid for this client?

    1. ACE inhibitors.

    2. β-Blockers.

    3. Calcium channel blockers.

    4. Diuretics.

79. Which class of pharmacologic agents would the nurse practitioner select for a hypertensive elderly client with a new diagnosis of CHF?

    1. ACE inhibitors.

    2. β-Blockers.

    3. Calcium channel blockers.

    4. Diuretics.

80. A mildly hypertensive male client presents with red, painful swelling of his great toe. In addition to treating the gout, the nurse practitioner also knows he/she must:

    1. Order laboratory studies for diabetes.

    2. Explore for possible alcohol abuse.

    3. Advise him to lose weight.

    4. Change his thiazide antihypertensive.

81. An elderly male with a diagnosis of systolic hypertension for 3 months presents for follow-up care. He is on a no-added-salt diet and has lost 8 lb in 3 months. Weekly BP checks at the senior center average 180s/70s. Health history includes benign prostatic hypertrophy, diet-controlled type II diabetes, and CAD with MI 8 years ago. Chief complaint includes periodic angina, occasional heartburn, slowed urinary stream with some dribbling, and decreasing energy level. BP today is 188/78. Current medications include cimetidine (Tagamet) 200 mg prn, aspirin 325 mg qd, nitroglycerin, and Maalox prn. The client is married and sexually active. Which medication would the nurse practitioner initiate after complete physical including ECG, and all indicated blood work?

    1. ACE inhibitor.

    2. Diuretic.

    3. α_1-Blocker.

    4. β-Blocker.

82. A geriatric client has been on procainamide (Pronestyl) for 4 years to control his cardiac dysrhythmias. The nurse practitioner would evaluate for what side effect in the chronic use of this medication?

    1. Elevated liver functions.

    2. Appearance of antinuclear antibodies.

    3. Shortened AV interval.

    4. Tachycardia.

83. Secondary prophylaxis for acute rheumatic fever (ARF) in a 55-year-old school teacher includes:

    1. Penicillin V 125–250 mg PO bid indefinitely.

    2. Erythromycin 800 mg PO bid.

    3. One-time dose of 2.0 million units benzathine penicillin G combined with penicillin G procaine (Bicillin C-R) IM.

    4. No medication prophylaxis is needed after the client reaches the early twenties.

4 Answers & Rationales

Physical Examination & Diagnostic Tests

1. **(1)** S_1 is heard loudest at the apex, S_2 at the base. Each sound should be carefully assessed as to the intensity of the sound in each area.

2. **(3)** The PMI represents the thrust and contraction of the left ventricle (LV). The LV lies behind the right ventricle (RV) and extends to the left, forming the left border of the heart.

3. **(2)** The correct procedure is to listen for carotid bruits with the bell of the stethoscope, which brings out low-frequency sounds and filters out high-frequency sounds. It should be placed very lightly on the neck with just enough pressure to seal the edge.

4. **(2)** The purpose of inspection and palpation of the precordium is to determine the presence and extent of normal and abnormal pulsations. A slight retraction of the chest wall just medial to the midclavicular line in the fifth interspace is a normal finding, while marked actions or retraction of the rib is abnormal and may indicate pericardial disease. Pericardial friction rubs are heard by auscultation.

5. **(1)** The splitting during inspiration refers to S_1 and S_2. The S_3 is normal in children, young adults, and pregnant women. In the older adult with heart disease this often signifies myocardial failure.

6. **(3)** The right side of the chest close to the sternal border at the second intercostal

space is the correct area to auscultate the aortic valve. The mitral valve is auscultated at the fifth left intercostal space at the midclavicular line. The tricupsid value is auscultated at the fourth left intercostal space at the sternal border. The pulmonic valve is auscultated at the second left intercostal space at the sternal border.

7. **(2)** A 12-hour fast is recommended, due to the influence of intake on cholesterol levels (they may increase). A normal diet for the 7 days prior to the exam is recommended so that an accurate picture of the client's normal life is obtained. Alcohol should not be consumed 48 hours before the test—it may increase cholesterol, HDL, LDL, and triglyceride levels. If possible, all medication should be withheld until the test is over, especially corticosteroids, diuretics, β-blockers, oral contraceptives, and estrogens.

8. **(1)** An S_4 is a normal variant in people 65 years of age or older and may result from increased resistance to ventricular filling atrial contraction.

9. **(1)** According to the classification of hypertension, this is within the moderate range.

10. **(2)** The fifth intercostal space at the midclavicular line on the left side is the best place to auscultate the closure sounds of the mitral valve. Option #1 describes the area of the tricuspid valve, Option #3 describes the area of the pulmonic valve,

and Option #4 describes the aortic valve area.

11. **(3)** It is important to determine if the coolness extends proximally from the hand. Then, palpation of pulses would be appropriate.

12. **(1)** Closure of the AV valves, which allows the filling of both ventricles simultaneously, produces the first heart sound (S_1); closure of the aortic and pulmonic valves produce the second heart sound (S_2).

13. **(4)** The apical and peripheral pulse (radial) must be evaluated simultaneously in order to determine if all of the apical beats are being reflected in the radial pulse. If there is an apical rate of 100 and a radial rate of 90, the client is said to have a pulse deficit of 10 points. This is usually done with two people counting over the same time period.

14. **(3)** A grade V heart murmur is very loud and can be heard with the stethoscope partly off the chest wall. A grade VI murmur is the loudest and is audible with the stethoscope just removed from contact with the chest wall and accompanied by a thrill. A grade I murmur is barely audible or very faint with the bell of the stethoscope.

15. **(4)** The normal aging process impairs automaticity, conductivity, and contractility. Ischemic changes and degeneration decrease sinus node automaticity and conduction velocity, resulting in bradycardic rhythms or atrial fibrillation. The poor myocardium contractility, usually related to hypertension or valvular disease, causes decreased ventricular emptying and increased filling pressures. These changes predispose the elderly to congestive heart failure.

16. **(4)** The most sensitive area on the examiner's hand is the back of the fingers.

17. **(3)** Desired levels for a lipid profile are total cholesterol <200 mg/dl; HDL >35 mg/dl; LDL <130 mg/dl; triglycerides <250 mg/dl. A high total cholesterol, coupled with a low HDL, is a positive risk factor for CHD, and is the most concerning for this client. In addition, this client has an elevated LDL level. These parameters, taken as a whole, would mandate intervention in this client.

18. **(3)** Dressler's syndrome (post-MI syndrome) may develop 1–4 weeks following myocardial infarction and is characterized by pericarditis with effusion and fever. Dressler's syndrome is caused by antigen–antibody reactions. Laboratory findings include elevation of white blood cells and sedimentation rate. Treatment includes corticosteroids.

19. **(1)** Jugular vein distention is common in geriatric clients. When it is present with the client's head elevated at a 45-degree angle, then further examination needs to be conducted regarding the venous pressure, which is reflective of pressure in the right heart chambers. Supine positioning will increase venous pressure and does not provide valid information in this situation. Auscultation for carotid bruits is an important part of assessment, but does not have significant value in evaluating jugular vein distention.

20. **(1)** Mitral valve stenosis is a diastolic murmur of low intensity heard at the apex of the heart. Option #2 describes characteristics of a murmur with aortic stenosis. Option #3, a holosystolic murmur, is characteristic of mitral regurgitation, which allows for backflow of blood from ventricles into the atrium. Option #4 best describes aortic regurgitation.

21. **(3)** The client had a left ventricular MI. One of the most common complications is left-sided failure resulting in congestive failure. This would be first manifested as pulmonary congestion and difficulty breathing.

22. **(4)** Classically, intermittent claudication is described as pain on activity that is relieved by stopping the activity.

23. **(3)** A positive stress test result indicates the likelihood of coronary artery disease is 98% in males over the age of 50. Results are progressively lower in asymptomatic persons, with false positives increased in asymptomatic men under the age of 40, premenopausal women without risk factors, and clients on digitalis.

Disorders

24. **(1)** A diagnosis of HTN from a single measurement of BP elevation should not be done. A minimum of three readings with an average systolic BP of 140 mm Hg and a diastolic BP of 90 mm Hg establishes the diagnosis. An average of two or more readings taken at each of two or more visits should follow an initial screening. The client should be seated with his/her arm at heart level. No caffeine or nicotine ingestion should be allowed 30 minutes prior to the reading. The room should be quiet a minimum of 5 minutes, and an appropriate cuff should be used. One high reading should be confirmed within 2 months.

25. **(3)** In the early stages of hypertensive heart disease, where there is an increased peripheral resistance to blood flow, the most significant change occurring to the heart is the left ventricular hypertrophy with an increase in the size of the myocardial cells without a corresponding increase in cell number (i.e., hyperplasia). After a period of time, all of the other options listed occur in the heart.

26. **(3)** Sinus or atrial tachycardia is characterized by a rate at or above 100, P waves are present for each QRS complex, and P-R interval is below 0.20, the T wave occurs after each QRS complex, and the beat is regular.

27. **(1)** The classic chest pain of an infarction may not be present in the geriatric client due to altered pain perception and diminished pain sensation.

28. **(2)** Respiratory symptoms are predominant in clients with left-sided heart failure. Venous congestion and peripheral edema are associated with right-sided failure.

29. **(1)** Cardiac tamponade occurs as a complication of pericarditis. An excessive accumulation of fluids between the pericardium and the myocardium interferes with effective cardiac contraction. The triphasic friction rub is common to pericarditis, but is not indicative of a complication of constrictive pericarditis. Jugular venous pressure is utilized to determine levels of venous distention.

30. **(2)** Untreated hypertension causes significant increased work on the left ventricle, eventually causing CHF.

31. **(2)** Palpable carotid pulse with each compression is the best sign of effective CPR. The other answers are appropriate but not the best indicator of effective resuscitation efforts.

32. **(2)** This is a description of complete block with hemodynamic consequences. The client should be seen immediately by a cardiologist for the possibility of pacemaker insertion. First-degree block has characteristic P waves, and a long P-R interval. The client should not just be referred for follow-up, he should be seen by a cardiologist as soon as possible.

33. **(3)** A triphasic friction rub or a pericardial rub occurs in the majority of clients with pericarditis. Paradoxical pulse may occur if constrictive pericarditis and cardiac tamponade are present. Pulse deficits and the presence of S_4 are not characteristic of problems with pericarditis.

34. **(1)** Elderly individuals experience atypical symptoms of a myocardial infarction including dyspnea, diaphoresis, vomiting, syncope, confusion, and weakness.

35. **(1)** Cardiovascular risk factors predisposing females to cardiovascular disease include body size is smaller, estrogen level is declining, heart and thoracic cavity is smaller and lighter, coronary arteries are smaller in diameter, P-R interval is shorter, resting ejection fraction is higher, body fat percentage is increased, and fat distributed in the abdomen may be mobilized more easily in response to stress and raise serum cholesterol and blood glucose levels.

36. **(4)** The nurse practitioner must consider the geriatric client's other medical problems and treatment prior to prescribing medications for hypertension. Frequently, geriatric clients cannot take the β-blockers due to chronic pulmonary conditions; the client may already be on diuretics for problems of fluid retention. The step therapy is appropriate if there is no other significant medical history. Lifestyle changes should be initiated and medication adjusted as changes are made.

37. **(2)** Hypertension is considered a major factor in the development of CAD in the geriatric client. Female clients have an increased incidence of CAD after menopause; estrogen replacement appears to have cardioprotective effects on the heart, thus decreasing the incidence of CAD. Diabetics have an increased incidence of CAD; however, the majority of CAD clients are not diabetic.

38. **(4)** Cor pulmonale is characterized by hypertrophy of the right ventricle secondary to pulmonary hypertension (resistance). The increased P wave amplitude (P pulmonale) occurs as the right atrium enlarges.

39. **(2)** Excess secretion of aldosterone predisposes to potassium excretion. Total body sodium content will be above normal, but the excessive secretion of antidiuretic hormone causes greater retention of water, diluting the serum level.

40. **(1)** Waterhammer pulse (bounding with a rapid rise and sudden collapse) is produced by an increase in pulse pressure and may be caused by an increased stroke volume, a decrease in peripheral resistance, or both. Because the nurse practitioner is suspecting either aortic regurgitation or a patent ductus arteriosus (primarily in children), auscultation for a diastolic murmur is indicated.

41. **(2)** Occlusion of the coronary arteries deprives the myocardial cells of glucose needed for aerobic metabolism. Anaerobic metabolism occurs, which causes the accumulation of lactic acid. Lactic acid irritates the myocardial nerve fibers, sending pain messages to the cardiac nerves and upper thoracic posterior roots located in the left shoulder and arm.

42. **(1)** The moist crackles (rales) heard in the bases of the lung are the most prominent physical examination findings of early congestive heart failure. They are caused from transudation of fluid into the alveoli and into the airways. Later findings include distended neck veins, peripheral edema, hepatomegaly, and ascites (rather than weight loss).

43. **(3)** Aortic dissection almost invariably begins with sudden onset of severe chest pain that is tearing or ripping in quality and is accompanied by loss or decrease in peripheral pulses and neurologic deficits. The pain of angina and acute myocardial infarction is usually described as a pressure. Pericarditis produces pain that is more gradual in onset.

44. **(1)** A Step I diet involves daily intake of ≤30% total calorie intake made up of fat, <300 mg/day cholesterol intake, and 8–10% daily saturated fat intake. A decrease to <200 mg/day of cholesterol and 7% saturated fat is a Step II diet, prescribed if Step I is ineffective. The third selection is closer to the current average American's diet. Although watching calorie and sodium intake is important for weight and BP control, it is not part of a Step I diet plan for hyperlipidemia.

45. **(4)** Although the other dysrhythmias may be experienced by the client following a myocardial infarction, the most life-threatening is ventricular fibrillation. The vast majority of deaths due to ventricular fibrillation happen within the first 24 hours, and of these deaths, over half occur in the first hour. The majority of out-of-hospital deaths from myocardial infarction are due to ventricular fibrillation.

46. **(2)** Diet and exercise are the mainstay of any treatment program and would be used initially in all cases. A bile acid sequestrant agent or estrogen replacement therapy may eventually be necessary if no improvement is seen with diet/exercise therapy. Referral to a cardiologist is not necessary, unless the client develops symptoms or shows resistance to treatment.

47. **(3)** Dyspnea is the most common symptom of CHF. Initially, it is present only with moderate exertion, but as severity of CHF increases, the dyspnea may occur with mild exertion or at rest. Fatigue is another common complaint. Right-sided heart failure is associated with weakness, anorexia, nausea, and dependent edema. Chronic left ventricular failure usually leads to right ventricular failure.

48. **(3)** Palm and coconut oils, along with butter, are very high in saturated fats and should be avoided. The other selections are moderately high in fat content, but consist of mostly unsaturated fats.

49. **(3)** Anginal pain is difficult to differentiate from that of an infarction. One of the most characteristic symptoms is the relief of the anginal pain with the administration of sublingual nitroglycerin.

50. **(4)** Aspirin helps prevent the formation of platelet-aggregating substances and may help the occlusion of narrowed coronary arteries. While Lasix, morphine, and streptokinase all have their place in treating acute myocardial infarction, it is unlikely that they are available in the average primary care office.

51. **(3)** Dizziness that improves when lying down and worsens when standing is symptomatic of cardiac involvement and may indicate serious cardiac dysrhythmias. If dizziness occurs in certain positions, it is indicative of benign positional vertigo, which is common in the elderly. Dizziness accompanied by tinnitus is common in acute labyrinthitis and, if proceded by rapid breathing, may be caused by hyperventilation.

52. **(3)** The stated history of a recent coxsackievirus infection, pain that worsens when supine, and a friction rub is classic for viral pericarditis. The client's age makes an acute myocardial infarction unlikely and the pain is not typical for pleural effusion or reflux.

53. **(1)** Signs and symptoms of hyperthyroidism in the older adult include progressive functional decline, atrial fibrillation, MI, tachycardia, weakness, fatigue, weight loss, anorexia, diarrhea, nervousness, tremor, pruritus, memory loss, and heat intolerance. Symptoms of hypothyroidism include arthralgia, weakness, decreased mental function, depression, constipation, weight loss, dry coarse skin and yellowish cast, dry sparse hair, and mask-like, puffy face with periorbital edema. Bradycardia would be assessed with both sick sinus syndrome and congestive heart failure. Sick sinus syndrome is often associated with the "bradycardia-tachycardia" syndrome.

54. **(4)** This is a sign of congestive heart failure. Option #1 is a normal sign of aging. Option #2 is a result of sclerosing of the aorta, which occurs with aging. Option #3 is expected with the aging process.

55. **(2)** This assessment is consistent with aortic stenosis. Aortic regurgitation is a diastolic murmur and secondary from rheumatic heart disease. There is no history given of rheumatic heart disease. Mitral valve disease is one of the most common valvular disorders. A small percentage of mitral valve prolapse clients do suffer from autonomic dysfunction and complain of palpitations, atypical chest pain, orthostatic dizziness, near syncope, cold extremities, throbbing headaches, and neurasthenia and manifest tachyarrhythmias. Mitral regurgitation may remain asymptomatic for many years, because the left ventricle dilates and adjusts well to the increase in volume load. Onset of dyspnea and fatigue may not occur for decades.

56. **(1)** Aortic stenosis is most common and is caused by calcification. The symptoms would include syncope, angina, and dyspnea on exertion.

57. **(3)** The nurse practitioner needs to repeat the cholesterol and obtain HDL and LDL levels before initiating any treatment. The HDL and LDL will help stratify risks and guide aggressiveness of intervention.

58. **(3)** Mitral stenosis most often results in CHF; there is generally no chest pain or fever. Atrial fibrillation is not uncommon; however, it is very irregular, and the irregular pulse may result in a pulse deficit.

Pharmacology

59. **(1)** The client is presenting with symptoms of digitalis toxicity—first-degree block and increasing cardiac irritability. If the potassium level is low, it may be precipitating the toxicity. Also, it is important to determine that serum theophylline levels remain within the therapeutic range. There is no evidence presented to indicate that the pulmonary disease is progressing. The blood pressure

may be adequate control for this client, and further information should be obtained prior to adjusting the medications. Based on the information presented, referral to a cardiologist is not appropriate at this time.

60. **(3)** Thiazide diuretics inhibit sodium reabsorption, promoting the excretion of sodium, chloride, and water. As the extracellular fluid volume decreases, plasma renin activity and aldosterone levels increase, resulting in potassium loss. Treatment is to restore the volume with normal saline and correct the potassium depletion. If the sodium is increased too rapidly, irreversible neurologic damage can occur.

61. **(1)** Vitamin K is an antidote for Coumadin. Increased intake of green leafy vegetables could cause an increase in vitamin K levels and decrease the effectiveness of the medication. Also, multivitamin supplements may contain additional vitamin K.

62. **(3)** The client presents with the classic profile of digitalis toxicity, which is frequently related to hypokalemia, especially since the potassium replacement is rather low for an adult and there is a history of poor eating and nausea. Other options may be done; however, it is important to determine the presence of hypokalemia and digitalis toxicity, so it may be addressed immediately.

63. **(1)** ACE inhibitors, such as losartan (Cozaar), decrease the conversion of angiotensin I to angiotensin II, a potent vasoconstrictor, and inhibit the release of aldosterone.

64. **(1)** Aldactone is a potassium-sparing diuretic. Clients should be instructed on signs of hyperkalemia.

65. **(1)** β-Blockers are myocardial depressants that suppress heart rate and contraction (negative inotropic). Calcium channel blockers decrease AV conduction, which suppresses heart rate. Both drugs are contraindicated with the onset of left ventricular dysfunction.

66. **(3)** The American Heart Association's Advanced Cardiac Life Support (ACLS) Guidelines recommend adenosine as the drug of choice for emergent treatment of supraventricular tachycardia, when a client is hemodynamically stable.

67. **(2)** The combination of calcium channel blockers and β-adrenergic blocking agents, systemic or ophthalmic, may result in excessive hypotension.

68. **(2)** Niacin can cause vasodilatation leading to orthostatic hypotension. Antihyperlipidemic drugs may cause constipation. The effectiveness of antihyperlipidemics is enhanced when taken before or with meals.

69. **(2)** Calcium channel blockers depress the rate of discharge from the sinoatrial node and conduction velocity through the atrioventricular node causing a decrease in heart rate. They also relax the coronary and systemic arteries, producing vasodilation (decrease in afterload and blood pressure) and decreasing myocardial contractility (negative inotropic effect).

70. **(2)** The dose of the client's medication had been doubled by the nurse practitioner according to the recommended protocols. The aim of HTN therapy is to use the drugs alone or in combination to return arterial pressure to normal levels with minimal side effects. Since the therapy had been continued, doubled, the next step is to add a low-dose thiazide diuretic. Therefore, the hydrochlorothiazide addition is the correct choice. Because of reduced side effects, the ACE inhibitors are used alone first, with a slight preference for certain ACE inhibitors (enalapril over captopril and losartan [Cozaar] over both of them).

71. **(3)** Blood pressure should be lowered cautiously using smaller doses of calcium entry antagonists, ACE inhibitors, or diuretics in the elderly. β-Blockers are not appropriate in normal doses for the elderly because of decreased β-receptor sensitivity in these clients. Larger doses also result in depression, impotence, fatigue, and declining mental function. Elderly clients are especially likely to experience CHF and peripheral vascular insufficiency from β-adrenergic blocker toxicity.

72. **(2)** Nitrates are venous and arterial dilators that decrease myocardial oxygen demand. β-Blockers have an antianginal effect and reduce myocardial oxygen demand. Calcium channel blockers relieve myocardial ischemia by reducing myocardial oxygen demand and dilating the coronary arteries. Aspirin is effective for primary and secondary prevention of myocardial infarction. Unless contraindicated, small doses of aspirin (162–325 mg daily) should be prescribed for clients with angina. Clients remaining symptomatic when treated with nitrates, β-blockers, or calcium channel blocking drugs should be treated with a β-blocker plus a combination of another agent. Appropriate combinations are a nitrate or a β-blocker plus a calcium channel blocker other than verapamil. Combination therapy does not include sedatives, vasoconstrictors, ACE inhibitors, or lipid-lowering drugs.

73. **(3)** Adverse side effects of ACE inhibitors include cough (1–30%), headache, and dizziness. Adverse effects of calcium channel blockers include peripheral edema, dizziness, headache, nausea, and tachycardia. Adverse effects of thiazide diuretics include nausea, vomiting, diarrhea, dizziness, and headache. Side effects of β-blockers include fatigue, impotence, depression, and shortness of breath.

74. **(1)** Digoxin, once a first-line drug for all clients with CHF, is now used in clients with atrial fibrillation, other tachycardias, and clients with left ventricular dysfunction. By controlling the ventricular rate in the client with atrial fibrillation or tachycardias, cardiac output increases. In cases of diastolic dysfunction with a sinus rhythm, digitalis is of no benefit. Digoxin is of relatively little value in most forms of cardiomyopathy, myocarditis, mitral stenosis, and chronic constrictive pericarditis.

75. **(2)** Hypertension is considered a major factor in the development of CAD in the geriatric client. Female clients have an increased incidence of CAD after menopause, and estrogen replacement appears to have cardioprotective effects on the heart, thus decreasing the incidence of CAD. Diabetics have an increased incidence

of CAD; however, the majority of CAD clients are not diabetic.

76. **(2)** Noncardiac adverse reactions include a change in the mental status. While visual disturbances; diarrhea; and anorexia, nausea, or vomiting are also adverse reactions, they are not the most common in the elderly.

77. **(4)** The assessments point to gout. A side effect of thiazide is hyperuricemia. Blood for a CBC should be drawn prior to therapy. The other distractors are not addressing the assessment of a tender and edematous right ankle. The cardiac assessments were benign. There are no indications of a concern with hypo- or hypernatremia or hypo- or hyperkalemia.

78. **(2)** β-Blockers do increase the peripheral vascular resistance, a phenomenon that already occurs with normal aging, so these drugs can precipitate or worsen symptoms of asthma, COPD, peripheral vascular disease, sexual dysfunction, or congestive heart failure. The other classes have no effect or decrease the effect on peripheral resistance.

79. **(1)** ACE inhibitors have been shown to prolong life in clients with congestive heart failure by improving overall cardiac function. Options #2 and #3 should be contraindicated in CHF. While Option #4 may be correct, it is not a priority to Option #1.

80. **(4)** The most likely precipitating cause of his gout is the thiazide diuretic used to control his hypertension, since it blocks the excretion of uric acid. Although gout may be more common in the obese, in alcoholics, and in diabetics, they are not indicated here.

81. **(1)** The ACE inhibitor will preserve renal function and have less impact on sexual functioning. The nurse practitioner must monitor potassium and carefully follow renal status for change. The ACE inhibitor has fewer negative side effects or interactions with the other medical conditions of this client.

82. **(2)** Eighty per cent of the clients who chronically use procainamide develop

antinuclear antibodies. Twenty per cent of these clients develop a lupus-like syndrome.

83. **(1)** Secondary prevention or preventing the recurrent attacks of acute rheumatic fever is controversial. Some authorities identify the early twenties and 5 years since last ARF attack as the criteria to stop the use of prophylactic penicillin, unless the client is at increased risk of exposure to streptococcal infections, such as school teachers or health professionals. Other authorities recommend lifelong prophylactic drug therapy. Although erythromycin is an alternative medication for penicillin-sensitive individuals, the dose in Option #2 is for a client having a dental or surgical procedure. The secondary prophylaxis dose for erythromycin is 250 mg PO bid.

5

Respiratory

Physical Examination & Diagnostic Tests

1. The nurse practitioner knows that normal breath sounds that have a low pitch and soft intensity and that are heard better on inspiration are called:

    1. Bronchial.

    2. Vesicular.

    3. Bronchovesicular.

    4. Rhonchi.

2. When auscultating for vocal resonance in a client with possible consolidation of lung tissue, the nurse practitioner hears "a-a-a" when the client says "e-e-e." This is called:

    1. Tactile fremitus.

    2. Bronchophony.

    3. Whispered pectoriloquy.

    4. Egophony.

3. The nurse practitioner understands the following about hyperresonance in percussion of the lungs:

    1. It is a normal finding in the adult client.

    2. It occurs commonly in pediatric clients.

    3. It is characterized by soft intensity, high pitch, short duration, and extreme dullness quality.

    4. It is characterized by loud intensity, high pitch, medium duration, and dull quality.

4. What is the correct procedure when percussing the chest?

    1. Start at the right upper side of the anterior chest and move to the left side.

    2. Begin at the upper left side of the posterior chest and compare to the respective anterior side, moving from front to back.

    3. Percuss systematically and symmetrically the anterior chest, moving from the left to right side, then do the posterior chest.

    4. Percuss the posterior chest and then measure for diaphragmatic excursion on the anterior chest.

5. The nurse practitioner understands that pleural friction rubs are:

   1. Auscultated in the lower anterolateral chest.

   2. Heard best at the end of expiration.

   3. Characterized by a continuous low-pitched snoring sound heard early in inspiration.

   4. Noted when the client says "e-e-e" and the examiner hears through the stethoscope "a-a-a."

6. Normal physiologic changes in the respiratory system of the geriatric client include:

   1. Increased rigidity of the rib cage and an increase in the anteroposterior (AP) diameter of the chest.

   2. Increased ciliary action resulting in a more forceful and recurrent cough.

   3. Increase in number of smaller alveoli with a decrease in residual capacity.

   4. Decrease in AP diameter of the rib cage with a decrease in lung expansion.

7. When assessing for tactile fremitus, the nurse practitioner would place her hands over what area of the client's chest?

   1. On the anterior chest at the level of the sixth intercostal space.

   2. At the level of bifurcation of the bronchi on the posterior chest wall.

   3. At the apex on the anterior chest wall.

   4. At the level of the diaphragm on the posterior chest wall.

8. On assessment of the client's respiratory status, crepitation is felt over the third rib at the midaxillary line on the left side. The interpretation of this finding is:

   1. There is a consolidation of fluid in the left lower lobe of the lung.

   2. Severe inflammation is present on the visceral pleural surfaces of the left lung.

   3. An increase in pressure has occurred in the pleural cavity on the right lung.

   4. Air is present in the subcutaneous tissue from an air leak in the respiratory system.

9. An important anatomic landmark on the anterior thoracic wall is the angle of Louis. Where on the thorax is this landmark present?

   1. The midnipple line on either side of the manubrium.

   2. Bilaterally at the manubriosternal junction.

   3. Midline at the base of the suprasternal notch.

   4. Just below the clavicle, but above the manubrium.

10. During the assessment of a geriatric client's respiratory status, the nurse practitioner determines the presence of coarse tactile fremitus posteriorly at the second intercostal space. The best interpretation of this finding is:

    1. Increased air trapping in the alveoli on the affected side.

    2. Presence of fluid or solid mass within the lungs.

    3. Increased pressure in the bronchial tree.

    4. Presence of hyperactive airway disease.

11. When the lateral diameter of the chest is the same size as the AP diameter, the nurse practitioner correctly documents this finding as a:

    1. Biot deviated chest.

    2. Pigeon chest.

    3. Funnel chest.

    4. Barrel chest.

12. An adult male client comes to the clinic with the chief complaint of "coughing up blood." He has no history of respiratory or cardiac problems. His vital signs are pulse 96, respirations 28, blood pressure 140/92,. temperature of 99°F orally. The initial diagnostic evaluation of this client includes:

    1. Electrocardiogram (ECG), pulmonary function studies, sputum cytology.

2. Purified protein derivative (PPD) skin test, chest x-ray, sputum smear for acid-fast bacillus.

3. Arterial blood-gas (ABG) studies, complete blood count (CBC), chest x-ray.

4. Direct bronchoscopy with biopsy and complement fixation antibody titer.

13. When assessing the pulmonary function studies of a client, which assessment finding is seen in chronic air flow limitation such as emphysema?

1. Decrease in forced vital capacity (FVC) and forced expiratory volume timed (FEV_1).

2. Increase functional residual capacity (FRC) and residual volumes (RV).

3. Decrease residual volume (RV) and increase in total lung capacity (TLC).

4. Increase in forced expiratory volume timed (FEV_1) and total lung capacity (TLC).

14. When interpreting PPD skin tests in clients at a long-term care facility, the nurse practitioner identifies positive results in individuals with:

1. Redness or erythema at the site.

2. An induration reaction of ≥ 5 mm.

3. An induration reaction of ≥ 10 mm.

4. An induration reaction extending to 15 mm.

Disorders

15. A client has received a blunt trauma injury to his chest. An assessment finding that would be most indicative of further respiratory complications would be:

1. Complaints of increased pain over the affected area.

2. Oximetry readings consistently around 90%.

3. Decreased breath sounds on the affected side.

4. Fever of 102°F and increased sputum production.

16. The nurse understands that the following characteristic is more likely to occur when the adult client has pneumonia (due to *S. pneumoniae*) rather than bronchitis:

1. Rusty sputum.

2. Cough.

3. Dyspnea.

4. Wheezing.

17. What would be a priority intervention for a client experiencing a respiratory arrest?

1. Start chest compressions at 15 compressions and two breaths.

2. Open the airway with a head tilt and chin lift.

3. Give oxygen via a rebreathing mask at 10 L/min.

4. Pinch the nose and give two breaths.

18. A client comes to the emergency room complaining of difficulty breathing. What is most important to establish initially on this client?

1. The type of activity that produces the dyspnea.

2. The presence of consolidation via a chest x-ray.

3. Arterial blood-gas levels with respect to oxygen pressures.

4. The presence of bilateral breath sounds over the lower lobes.

19. A client is severely dyspneic and the history strongly suggests the possibility of a foreign body in the bronchi. What observation would contribute to the documentation of this problem?

1. Unilateral retraction of the right chest wall.

2. The presence of crepitation on the anterior chest wall.

3. Retraction of the lower chest wall.

4. A friction rub heard over the area of the bronchi.

20. The nurse practitioner is assessing a client who is complaining of shortness of breath and chest discomfort. His respirations are shallow and at a rate of 26. When evaluating the diaphragmatic excursion, it is determined that the diaphragm on the right is slightly higher than on the left side. The best interpretation of these findings is:

    1. This is normal due to the liver on the right side.

    2. There may be atelectasis in the right lower lobe.

    3. Consolidation is present in the right lower lobe.

    4. This indicates the presence of early stages of chronic obstructive lung disease.

21. The nurse practitioner is planning a community screening program for lung cancer in geriatric clients. Which examination is best to use for this program?

    1. Bronchoscopy with biopsy for cytology.

    2. Arterial blood-gas studies.

    3. Pulmonary function test.

    4. Chest x-ray and compare with previous x-ray.

22. An adult male comes to the office complaining of chest pain and shortness of breath. He states the problems started suddenly after running sprints in basketball practice. He states he has no past history of pulmonary problems. He is about 72 inches tall and weighs approximately 145 lb, his pulse rate is 118, his respiratory rate is 30, there are decreased breath sounds, and there is hyperresonance over the left lung. The best diagnosis for this client is:

    1. Spontaneous pneumothorax.

    2. Exercise-induced asthma.

    3. Pulmonary edema.

    4. Acute bronchiectasis.

23. An adult presents at the clinic with complaints of tingling in her face and hands, sudden shortness of breath, and vague chest discomfort. She appears very anxious and denies any history of respiratory problems. On examination her hands are cool to touch, her vital signs are respirations 34, pulse regular at a rate of 100, blood pressure 110/76, and normal temperature. Respiratory examination reveals bilateral breath sounds with tachypnea, no adventitious sounds, normal percussion, and visual examination of the chest. The best immediate treatment is:

    1. Rebreathing into a paper bag and encouraging controlled diaphragmatic breathing.

    2. Albuterol (Proventil) two puffs with a metered-dose inhaler (MDI).

    3. Oxygen at 4 L and arterial blood gases after 30 minutes.

    4. Establish an IV, infuse 500 ml normal saline for volume depletion.

24. A newly diagnosed COPD client is being discharged from the hospital. The nurse practitioner is discussing home care with the client. What information is important for the nurse practitioner to include in the home care teaching?

    1. Use the bronchodilator prior to exercising.

    2. Maintain bed rest for the first few days at home.

    3. Decrease the amount of fluid intake to prevent fluid overload.

    4. Maintain flow rate on oxygen around 5–7 L.

25. A client is admitted to a rural emergency department by ambulance. Primary assessment reveals:

    • Respirations: 38/min with use of accessory muscles, prolonged expiration and wheezes
    • ECG: Sinus tachycardia rate 140
    • Blood pressure: 192/98
    • Lethargic: Responds to name only by opening eyes
    • Cyanosis of lips

    Therapeutic interventions initiated by emergency medical technicians include:

    • Intravenous therapy of D_5W at 30 ml/hr
    • Oxygen therapy at 48% by venturi mask.

STAT ABGs indicate:

- pH = 7.24
- $Paco_2$ = 82 mm Hg
- HCO_3 = 36
- PaO_2 = 76 mm Hg

Prior to obtaining a second set of ABGs, the nurse practitioner would:

1. Assist respirations with bag-valve mask with 100% oxygen.
2. Administer 1 ampule of sodium bicarbonate.
3. Change oxygen delivery to nasal cannula at 2 L.
4. Disconnect the supplemental oxygen.

26. Instructions to the elderly client with COPD concerning nutritional therapy would include foods that are:

1. High caloric, high protein, low carbohydrate.
2. High caloric, low protein, high carbohydrate.
3. Low caloric, high protein, low carbohydrate.
4. Low caloric, low protein, high carbohydrate.

27. Age-associated changes that increase the risk for pneumonia in the elderly client includes an increase in:

1. Compliance of the chest wall.
2. Diameter of the trachea and bronchi.
3. Lung parenchyma.
4. Cough forcefulness.

28. A client arrives at the clinic complaining of difficulty breathing, a cough, and chest pain. History indicates the client was discharged from the hospital 2 days ago after vascular surgery and has a 15-pack-year smoking history. Diagnostic studies should include:

1. Sputum for culture and sensitivity.
2. Cardiac troponin proteins.
3. Pulse oximetry.
4. Arterial blood gases.

29. The nurse practitioner is aware that the flu or influenza:

1. Can be caused by receiving a flu vaccine when one's resistance is low.
2. Is characterized by a slow, insidious onset of chills, fever, and muscle aches.
3. In older adults may persist for several weeks with symptoms of lack of energy and extreme tiredness.
4. Is primarily contagious in the early autumn and spring.

30. An older adult client presents with complaints of dyspnea, cough, fatigue, and dependent edema that has been worsening over the past few days. In planning the treatment for this client, the nurse practitioner considers:

1. Streptokinase therapy.
2. Hospitalization for evaluation of heart function.
3. Prescription for Lasix 40 mg PO qd.
4. Addition of a calcium channel blocker to the client's medications.

31. An adult client with a history of asthma calls to tell the nurse practitioner that she is "blowing 55%" on the peak flowmeter. What advice would the nurse practitioner give this client?

1. Call an ambulance immediately.
2. Bronchodilator now and evaluation in the office today.
3. Office evaluation this week.
4. Refer to a pulmonary physician.

32. An elderly client is evaluated by the nurse practitioner for a complaint of cough, fever, chest pain, and sputum production. In gathering a history on this client, it is important to know if the client has:

1. Received the pneumococcal vaccine.
2. Traveled out of the country.
3. Pets in the household.
4. Recently started new medications.

33. An elderly client presents with signs and symptoms that make the nurse practitioner suspect the diagnosis of pneumonia. Which assessment would the nurse practitioner most likely evaluate during the examination?

    1. Chest pain with inspiration.

    2. Confusion, with a low-grade temperature.

    3. Congested, productive cough.

    4. Fever with leukocytosis.

34. In developing a plan for an older client with pneumonia, the nurse practitioner understands that 30–40% of community-acquired pneumonia is caused by which organism?

    1. *Haemophilus influenzae.*

    2. *Klebsiella pneumoniae.*

    3. *Mycobacterium tuberculosis.*

    4. *Streptococcus pneumoniae.*

35. Which plan would be most appropriate to include in the health promotion plan for an older client who is at risk for developing pneumonia?

    1. Administer the pneumococcal vaccination annually.

    2. Administer the pneumococcal vaccination and yearly influenza immunization.

    3. Sputum culture annually along with a chest x-ray.

    4. PPD done every 3–5 years.

36. The nurse practitioner evaluates an older client with a current history of alcoholism. The client presents with an elevated temperature, congested cough producing rusty sputum, and occasional chills. The suspected diagnosis is bacterial pneumonia. The Gram-stained sputum smear would most likely reveal which organism?

    1. *Haemophilus influenzae.*

    2. *Klebsiella pneumoniae.*

    3. *Staphylococcus aureus.*

    4. *Streptococcus pneumoniae.*

37. An elderly client residing in a nursing home has recently been exposed to tuberculosis. The nurse practitioner interprets the initial PPD test to be negative. Which plan would be most appropriate at this time?

    1. Evaluate the client in another year.

    2. Repeat the PPD test in 1 week.

    3. Ignore the results and immediately begin ethambutol.

    4. Evaluate the client in 6 months, since he is asymptomatic at this time.

38. The nurse practitioner knows that Horner's syndrome is commonly associated with:

    1. Chronic bronchitis.

    2. Pulmonary tuberculosis.

    3. Pancoast's syndrome of lung cancer.

    4. Pulmonary embolism.

39. An adult client who smokes presents with complaints of breathlessness. The nurse practitioner notes on examination dilated blood vessels on the chest, and mild edema of the head and the supraclavicular area. She recognizes this condition as:

    1. Thyroid abnormality.

    2. Chronic bronchitis with mild congestive failure.

    3. Asthma with fluid retention.

    4. Superior vena cava obstruction.

40. An elderly client presents with postural hypotension and laboratory studies reveal hyponatremia. The most likely cause of this is:

    1. Diabetic ketoacidosis.

    2. Severe trauma.

    3. Bronchogenic carcinoma.

    4. Antacid overuse.

41. The nurse practitioner knows the following about asthma in the elderly:

    1. Subcutaneous epinephrine is standard therapy.

    2. It is usually of the allergic type.

3. Attacks are usually preceded by viral infections.

4. Clinical presentation is usually dyspnea, costal retraction, and fever.

42. Clinical signs and symptoms of late-phase asthma include:

1. Bronchoconstriction refractory to bronchodilator therapy.

2. Sneezing, watery eyes, and cough.

3. Wheezing and increased sputum production.

4. Bronchodilation secondary to release of histamine.

43. The nurse practitioner is assessing a client for asthma. What is a common clinical manifestation of asthma?

1. Pruritis.

2. Diffuse crackles.

3. Nocturnal exacerbation.

4. Chronic hypoxemia.

44. During a routine follow-up visit for a client with asthma, she states that she has been doing fine except when she goes out for dinner, when she notices she has increased bronchospasm and wheezing. Which would be an appropriate response?

1. "Have you been taking your medication?"

2. "Do you usually have wine with dinner?"

3. "I recommend you not go out for dinner."

4. "Does going out to dinner make you stressed?"

Pharmacology

45. The nurse practitioner is following up on a client who is experiencing acute asthmatic problems. Albuterol (Proventil) by MDI has been ordered as treatment. Which client response would indicate to the nurse

practitioner that the client understands how to take his medication?

1. "I will take one puff of the medication and then wait a minute before taking the second puff."

2. "I will take two puffs of the medication every 4 hours, even if I am not short of breath."

3. "It is important for me to take this medication on a regular cycle to prevent future attacks."

4. "I will take two puffs, one right after the other, whenever I begin to get short of breath."

46. A client who was recently diagnosed with tuberculosis calls the clinic because her urine is reddish orange. She is taking isonizid (INH; Laniazid), rifampin (Rifadin), and pyrazinamide. An appropriate response for the nurse practitioner to make would be:

1. "These are urinary tract infection symptoms; drink plenty of fluids."

2. "This is a normal response to the rifampin."

3. "Often this is an indication of liver toxicity. Stop the medications."

4. "This is probably bleeding and you should see a physician immediately."

47. A 55-year-old female comes into the emergency room with complaints of extreme shortness of breath. She is confused and her past medical history is not available. Her vital signs are pulse 124, respirations 32, blood pressure 124/80, temperature normal. Physical examination reveals diffuse expiratory wheezes, hyperresonance on percussion, and a prolonged expiratory phase. The best treatment for this client includes:

1. Aminophylline by mouth.

2. Beclovent (beclomethasone) inhaler.

3. Epinephrine by injection.

4. Proventil (albuterol) metered-dose inhaler.

48. A client with a history of bronchial asthma is seen in the clinic for increased episodes of difficult breathing. The client has been taking theophylline 100 mg PO tid. The client is a 40-year-old obese male with an 18-pack-year history of cigarette smoking and an excessive intake of coffee daily, and he eats a low-carbohydrate, high-protein diet. Which identified factors decrease the therapeutic effects of the theophylline?

    1. Age and gender.

    2. Coffee intake and weight.

    3. Age and weight.

    4. Smoking history and diet.

49. A 70-year-old man comes to the clinic with complaints that he is experiencing increased difficulty breathing over the past few days. He has a history of chronic obstructive lung disease and coronary artery disease. He was recently diagnosed with hypertension. Examination reveals no jugular vein distention, slight increase in the AP diameter of the chest, no productive cough, breath sounds are present but expiratory wheezes are noted bilaterally, denies complaints of chest pain. His vital signs are pulse 72, respirations 34, and blood pressure 170/100. His current medications are ipratropium bromide (Atrovent) inhaler two puffs every 6 hours, nitroglycerin transdermal patches, and propranolol (Inderal) 60 mg bid PO. The best treatment for this client is:

    1. Discontinue the propranolol (Inderal) and begin verapamil (Calan) 80 mg tid PO qd.

    2. Begin theophylline (Theo-Dur) 200 mg q12h PO.

    3. Discontinue the propranolol (Inderal) and begin on atenolol (Tenormin) 50 mg PO qd.

    4. Start beclomethasone (Beclovent) inhaler two puffs three or four times daily.

50. The recommended range for maintaining serum theophylline levels is:

    1. 0.05–2 μg/ml.

    2. 5–15 μg/ml.

    3. 20–25 μg/ml.

    4. 30–40 μg/ml.

51. A client in a long-term facility whose roommate has been diagnosed as having active tuberculosis should be started on chemoprophylaxis:

    1. As soon as possible and initiated at the time of screening skin testing.

    2. In 72 hours after PPD skin test results are obtained.

    3. Only if PPD skin test results are positive.

    4. In 3 months if the repeated skin test is positive.

52. In adults with asthma, the most common reason why outpatient treatment fails and results in hospitalization is:

    1. Exposure to allergens.

    2. Increased use of steroids.

    3. Improper inhaler technique.

    4. Use of cromolyn inhalers.

53. Which can elevate theophylline levels?

    1. Concomitant treatment with cimetidine (Tagamet).

    2. Intravenous ampicillin.

    3. Heavy smoking.

    4. History of seizure disorder.

54. A client with a long history of chronic airflow limitation has noticed a change in sputum over the past few days (e.g., increased amount of thick, yellow-green mucous, congestion). Appropriate therapy is:

    1. Hismanal 10 mg PO qd.

    2. Augmentin 500 mg tid PO × 10 days.

    3. Tylenol with codeine.

    4. Vancenase MDI 2 puffs.

55. Which medication is most effective in promoting a decrease in airway inflammation as well as providing long-term medication coverage in a client with asthma?

1. Isoetharine (Bronkometer).

2. Beclomethasone dipropionate (Vanceril, Beclovent).

3. Albuterol (Proventil, Ventolin).

4. Pirbuterol (Maxair).

56. The nurse practitioner is planning prophylactic treatment for a client with asthma. What is the best medication to use for the asthmatic client who is not currently experiencing an exacerbation?

1. Antibiotics.

2. Inhaled glucocorticoids.

3. β_1-Agonist.

4. Methacholine challenge.

57. Clients with asthma need to be instructed to:

1. Begin their inhaled steroids as soon as symptoms appear.

2. Using the MDI, take two puffs of the β_2-agonist prn.

3. Use their inhaled steroids when they experience bronchospasm.

4. Start their antibiotic regimen when they experience bronchospasm.

58. A client presents in the clinic with a dry, hacking, nonproductive cough that is interfering with her sleep. The nurse practitioner would encourage the client to purchase an over-the-counter preparation that contains:

1. Pseudoephedrine.

2. Phenylpropanolamine.

3. Guaifenesin.

4. Dextromethorphan.

59. A client with a history of Parkinson's disease has a positive TB skin test and INH is ordered as a prophylactic medication. Prior to beginning INH, it is important for the nurse practitioner to determine:

1. Whether the client's Parkinson's condition is being treated with levodopa (Larodopa).

2. How long the client has been diagnosed with Parkinson's disease.

3. How much respiratory compromise the client is currently experiencing.

4. The adequacy of urinary output and renal function.

60. A geriatric client is seen for an upper respiratory infection and the nurse practitioner decides to prescribe erythromycin. On review of the client's history, what current medication would be a contraindication to the administration of erythromycin?

1. Cisapride (Propulsid).

2. Lisinopril (Zestril).

3. Moexipril (Univasc).

4. Atenolol (Tenormin).

61. A client with chronic asthma is seen in the clinic complaining of vomiting and stomach cramps. He is confused and is unsure what medications he is currently taking, vital signs are blood pressure 158/92, pulse 152 and irregular, and respirations 28 and shallow. What stat diagnostic study should be obtained?

1. Serum electrolytes.

2. Digoxin level.

3. Theophylline level.

4. Arterial blood gases.

62. A client is seen in the clinic complaining of increased difficulty breathing and an intermittent productive cough that worsens in the evening. The history reveals that the client has a 20-pack-year history of smoking. Breath sounds are clear to auscultation, there is no evidence of fever, and chest radiography is within normal limits. The nurse practitioner instructs the client concerning the importance of smoking cessation and fluid therapy and prescribes:

1. Erythromycin 500 mg PO qid × 14 days.

2. Albuterol 2 mg PO tid.

3. Mucomyst inhalation 10 ml of 10% solution q4h prn.

4. Tetracycline 100 mg q12h × 14 days.

63. When initiating preventative care to decrease the incidence of pneumonia in clients in an extended-care facility, the nurse practitioner would identify clients receiving immunosuppressive therapy, repeated antibiotic use, sedation, and:

   1. β_1-Adrenergic blocking agents.

   2. Calcium channel blockers.

   3. Diuretics.

   4. Histamine (H_2) antagonists.

Answers & Rationales

Physical Examination & Diagnostic Tests

1. **(2)** The sounds heard over normal lung tissue are called vesicular breath sounds. The inspiratory phase of the vesicular breath sound is heard better than the expiratory phase and is about 2.5 times longer for these low-pitched, soft sounds. Bronchial breath sounds are normally heard over the trachea and usually indicate pathology. Bronchial breath sounds are high-pitched, loud sounds with a shortened inspiratory and lengthened expiratory phase. Bronchovesicular breath sounds have an intermediate pitch and intensity with equal duration of expiratory and inspiratory sounds heard mainly over the second interspace anteriorly and between the scapulae posteriorly. Rhonchi are abnormal breath sounds that are low-pitched, with a snoring quality.

2. **(4)** Tactile fremitus is a palpable vibration of the thoracic wall that is produced when the client speaks. Bronchophony is the increase in loudness and clarity of vocal resonance. Whispered pectoriloquy is exaggerated bronchophony and is heard through a stethoscope when the client whispers a series of words (i.e., "ninety-nine"). In egophony, the spoken voice has a nasal or bleating quality when heard through a stethoscope, and the spoken "e-e-e" sounds like "a-a-a."

3. **(2)** Hyperresonance is an abnormal percussion tone in adults, but normally occurs in a child's lung. It is characterized by very loud intensity, very low pitch, long duration, and a booming quality.

4. **(3)** Both anterior and posterior chest are to be percussed systematically and symmetrically, moving from left to right. Diaphragmatic excursion is usually only measured on the posterior chest.

5. **(1)** Pleural friction rubs are loud, dry, creaking or grating sounds produced by the rubbing together of inflamed and roughened pleural surfaces that are heard best during the latter part of inspiration and the beginning of expiration. They are most often heard in the lower anterolateral thorax. Option #3 is characteristic of sonorous rhonchi.

6. **(1)** There is a decrease in the number of alveoli, and the alveoli become rigid and lose the ability to recoil. The loss of alveolar elasticity affects the ability of the client to exhale effectively and there is an increase in the residual volume. There is also a decrease in basilar inflation and a decrease in the ability to expel foreign matter. The AP diameter of the chest increases as seen in clients with kyphosis.

7. **(2)** The bifurcation of the trachea or bronchi on the posterior chest wall is the best area for assessment of tactile fremitus. Care should be taken to avoid the area over the scapula.

8. **(4)** Crepitation or crepitus (also called subcutaneous emphysema) is air bubbles under the skin from a rupture somewhere in the respiratory system, less common from an infection by a gas-producing organism. Crepitation always requires attention.

9. **(2)** This landmark can be used to determine the position of the second rib and intercostal space and the corresponding spaces below that level. It is a visible and palpable angle of the sternum at the point where the second rib attaches to the sternum.

10. **(2)** Fluid or solid mass transmits the vibrations so that tactile fremitus may be felt on the exterior chest wall. Increased air trapping will cause a decreased or absent fremitus. A reactive airway results in wheezing due to edematous airway.

11. **(4)** The adult chest is somewhat asymmetric and the AP diameter is often one half the transverse diameter.

12. **(2)** The client should be initially evaluated for tuberculosis. Pulmonary function studies, ABG studies, and bronchoscopy are not indicated at this time. Complement fixation studies are done to diagnose atypical pneumonia.

13. **(1)** Hyperinflation due to air trapping causes an increase in FRC, RV, and TLC (which may be twice normal). A corresponding decrease in FVC and FEV_1 occurs. This causes a flattening of the diaphragm, decreased inspiratory efficiency, and increased work of breathing.

14. **(3)** Positive interpretation of PPD skin test results are as follows:

Induration	Positive in:
≥5 mm	Individuals with human immunodeficiency virus (HIV) infection
	Recent close contact with individuals with active TB
	Individuals with chest x-ray indicating healed TB
≥10 mm	Medically underserved individuals
	IV drug users
	Clients in long-term care facilities
≥15 mm	All individuals

Disorders

15. **(3)** The most common respiratory complication after a traumatic injury to the chest is pneumothorax caused from a fractured rib. Oximetry readings at 90% and increased pain are expected at this point and may not be indicative of a problem.

16. **(1)** Pneumococcal pneumonia due to *S. pneumoniae* often presents abruptly with high fever, shaking chills (rigor), productive cough of purulent or rusty sputum, headache, and pleuritic chest pain. In acute bronchitis, cough is the primary symptom and initially is dry and nonproductive. Fever, dyspnea, wheezing, and possible mucoid sputum production are also characteristic of acute bronchitis.

17. **(2)** According to the American Heart Association, the protocol for cardiopulmonary resuscitation (CPR; rescue breathing) due to respiratory arrest would be to open the airway by tilting the head and lifting the chin.

18. **(1)** It is most important to determine what precipitates the dyspnea. Is it present during rest or does it occur with activity? What level of activity precipitates the problem? This is important information necessary in order to determine the severity of the client's complaint.

19. **(1)** The most common area for a foreign body obstruction is the right bronchi; this will produce a unilateral retraction of the right chest wall. Retraction of the lower chest occurs with lower respiratory problems such as asthma. A pleural friction rub is heard when there is inflammation between the visceral and parietal pleura. Crepitation is present when air is leaking into the subcutaneous tissue.

20. **(1)** This is a normal finding due to the bulk of the liver. Atelectasis and consolidation will present with normal diaphragmatic movement but with dullness to percussion over the affected area. Obstructive lung disease will result in hyperresonance and limited diaphragmatic excursion but it will be bilateral.

21. **(4)** For preliminary screening, the chest x-ray is the best, since it is less expensive and less invasive. It is even more beneficial if it can be compared to previous chest x-rays. All of the other options are beneficial in diagnosing the malignancy, but the x-ray is best for a screening program.

22. **(1)** Spontaneous pneumothorax often occurs after strenuous exercise; predominant symptoms include sudden pain and dyspnea. The clinical hallmark of asthma is wheezing; with pulmonary edema there is frequently coughing, frothy sputum, and crackles heard on auscultation. Bronchiectasis is most often chronic and is characterized by moist crackles and wheezing on auscultation; cough is usually present.

23. **(1)** The situation described is hyperventilation. By slowing the breathing and breathing into a paper bag, the carbon dioxide levels will be restored and the acid-base problem resolved. Albuterol, oxygen, ABGs, and IV fluids are not appropriate initial treatment.

24. **(1)** In order to prevent dyspnea on activity, the bronchodilator should be used prior to walking or increased physical activity. The client should not stay in bed but should be encouraged to gradually increase activity. Fluid intake of 2–3 L/day should be encouraged, unless there are cardiac problems. The oxygen level should not exceed 3 to 4-L flow.

25. **(3)** Elevated bicarbonate levels of blood are expected in clients with chronic hypercapnia. Hypoventilation and acidemia can result when too much oxygen is delivered. Supplemental oxygen should not be discontinued because the PaO_2 levels decrease faster than the stimulus to breathe returns to eliminate the accumulated store of carbon dioxide (CO_2). Discontinuing supplemental oxygen, even for a short period of time, could cause serious complications.

26. **(1)** Nutritional needs are met by high-caloric, high-protein foods. High-carbohydrate foods need to be avoided in clients who retain CO_2 because carbohydrates metabolize into CO_2 as a waste product.

27. **(2)** Age-associated physiologic changes include a decreased compliance of the chest wall, making deep inspiration difficult; the trachea and bronchi increase in diameter, increasing dead space, resulting in a decrease of volume of air reaching the alveoli; the lung parenchyma become less elastic, which decreases the function of the alveoli; and breathing becomes more shallow and cough forcefulness decreases due to respiratory muscles weakening.

28. **(4)** This client is at risk for a pulmonary embolism due to hypercoagulation related to smoking and vascular injury (recent surgery). Assessment reveals common symptoms of pulmonary embolism: dyspnea, cough, and pleuritic pain. Diagnostic tests include ABGs, 12-lead ECG, chest x-ray, and echocardiogram.

29. **(3)** The flu or influenza is a highly contagious respiratory infection that occurs epidemically during the winter cold months. It is characterized by a sudden onset of chills, elevated temperature (101°–104°F), headache, fatigue, muscle pain, dry cough, laryngitis, rhinorrhea, and red eyes following a waiting period of 24–48 hours from time of exposure via respiratory droplets from an infected person or indirectly by drinking from a contaminated glass. Flu vaccines do not cause the flu; they are made with a killed virus.

30. **(2)** Worsening dyspnea and fatigue with increasing cough may be indicative of early pulmonary edema. Clients with pulmonary edema require hospitalization with oxygen therapy, IV furosemide (Lasix), and morphine. Clients who are suspected to be in pulmonary edema **should not** be treated on an outpatient basis. Calcium channel blockers are of little benefit in heart failure.

31. **(2)** This client is considered to be in the "yellow" zone of personal best peak flow but is close to the "red" zone (50% or less of personal best). The client should use her bronchodilator immediately and, if not improved, may need emergency intervention by the nurse practitioner.

32. **(1)** The pneumococcal vaccine is recommended for elderly clients, since their immune systems are less efficient. The symptoms of fever, chest pain, and sputum production are suggestive of pneumonia.

33. **(2)** Confusion may be the first sign that the elderly client is septic. The client may not have a temperature or leukocytosis. The client may not experience any discomfort or a cough.

34. **(4)** *Streptococcus pneumoniae* is the most common cause of community- and nursing home–acquired pneumonia. *Haemophilus influenzae* is common in elderly clients with underlying chronic diseases (e.g., COPD, diabetes). *Klebsiella pneumoniae* and other gram-negative bacteria are pathogens in alcoholics, immunocompromised hosts, and hospitalized clients. *Mycobacterium tuberculosis* is an infrequent cause of pneumonia.

35. **(2)** This will decrease complications and hospitalizations for the older client. The pneumococcal vaccination is not administered annually. Options #3 and #4 are not recommended. The PPD should be done annually for high-risk clients.

36. **(2)** *Klebsiella pneumoniae* and other gram-negative bacteria are important pathogens in alcoholics, immunocompromised hosts, and hospitalized clients. *Haemophilus influenzae* is common in elderly clients with underlying chronic diseases (e.g., COPD, diabetes mellitus). *Staphylococcus aureus* generally affects elderly clients recovering from influenza; also frequent in hospitalized clients and diabetics. *Streptococcus pneumoniae* is the most common bacterial pathogen (30–40% of pneumonia cases), and is the most common cause of community- and nursing home–acquired pneumonia.

37. **(2)** Up to 25% of elderly clients with newly diagnosed TB have a negative tuberculin skin test due to waning cellular immunity with senescence. If the initial PPD test is negative, a repeat PPD test 1 week later is recommended in elderly clients. The repeat test is useful to stimulate a booster phenomenon in clients whose initial infection occurred many years in the past. The other options contain incorrect information.

38. **(3)** Horner's syndrome, which is paralysis of the cervical sympathetic nerves resulting in ptosis, loss of sweating, constriction of the pupil, and sinking of the eyeball on one side, is very commonly associated with malignant tumors in the upper lung, leading to nerve compression.

39. **(4)** Superior vena cava obstruction is a complication of malignancy involving the mediastinum and rapidly progresses into an oncologic emergency.

40. **(3)** Hyponatremia results from an overproduction of antidiuretic hormone caused by an ectopic production from the bronchogenic tumor. Ketoacidosis and trauma result in fluid loss causing hypernatremia as does overuse of sodium-containing antacids.

41. **(3)** In older individuals the asthma is usually accompanied by infection. It is rarely allergic and costal retraction and fever are not usually seen. Subcutaneous epinephrine is not standard treatment but is sometimes indicated in emergent situations.

42. **(1)** Late-phase asthma occurs at 6–12 hours after the initial or acute bronchoconstrictive phase. The inflammatory response is the result of mast cell degranulation and release of histamine. Histamine acts on the lung by causing bronchoconstriction, vascular permeability, and vasodilatation. In late-phase asthma, bronchoconstriction is refractory to most bronchodilator therapy.

43. **(93)** Nocturnal exacerbation of asthma is a common clinical sign. It is linked to the variation in circulating catecholamines and vagal tone. Chronic hypoxemia and diffuse crackles are seen in the client with chronic bronchitis. Pruritus is often seen in contact allergic reactions.

44. **(2)** Asking the client about the consumption of wine with dinner is the most appropriate response. Many wines, especially white wines, contain sulfites that can trigger a mild allergic response.

Pharmacology

45. **(1)** In order for the medication to be most effective, there needs to be a 1-minute lapse time between the two puffs of medication. The first puff will open the upper airways. This will allow more effective penetration of the lower tract with the second puff of medication.

46. **(2)** The client would not stop taking the medications, as this is a common side effect of rifampin. Also, soft contact lenses may become discolored.

47. **(4)** β-Agonist (albuterol) MDI is the first line of treatment to decrease airflow obstruction. Aminophylline by mouth would take too long to be effective. Epinephrine is used predominantly for anaphylactic reaction. Beclovent is a steroid inhaler that is most effective when used prophylactically rather than in acute episodes.

48. **(4)** The use of tobacco increases the metabolism of theophylline, causing a need for greater dosage than required in nonsmokers. A high-protein, low-carbohydrate diet increases the metabolism of theophylline and decreases serum concentrations. Coffee (and other xanthine-containing beverages) may increase the central nervous system effects of xanthine derivatives.

49. **(1)** β-Blockers (Inderal and Tenormin) are known to cause exacerbation of chronic respiratory problems. Another antihypertensive, such as a calcium channel blocker, should be considered. The client's pulse is at 74, and his blood pressure remains elevated, which indicates the β-blocker is probably not effective in decreasing the blood pressure in this client. Theophylline derivatives are not indicated unless other medications are not effective. Drug interactions and increased levels of toxicity present problems in the elderly client.

50. **(2)** Therapeutic plasma levels range from 5–15 μg/ml. Drug levels of 20 μg/ml or greater are associated with toxicity.

51. **(1)** Chemoprophylaxis is initiated at the time of the screening skin testing. Skin testing should be repeated in 3 months, if initial test results are negative. If the second skin testing is negative, chemoprophylaxis can be stopped.

52. **(3)** One of the most common causes of outpatient treatment failure is improper inhaler technique. While exposure to allergens may trigger an asthma attack, the proper use of inhalers will control those attacks. Use of both steroids and cromolyn inhalers has decreased the severity of asthma attacks.

53. **(1)** Theophylline is used in the treatment of chronic lung disease and can accumulate in toxic levels. Cimetidine decreases the hepatic clearance of theophylline. Nicotine and some antiseizure drugs may actually increase clearance and ampicillin does not change the clearance.

54. **(2)** Antibiotic therapy is indicated when there is a change in color, consistency, or amount of sputum. Cough suppressants and antihistamines should be avoided.

55. **(2)** Beclomethasone dipropionate is a long-acting corticosteroid that stabilizes mast cells and greatly reduces mast cell degranulation when exposed to allergens. All of the other medications are bronchodilators used for rapid reversal of bronchospasm.

56. **(2)** Treatment of the client with asthma includes inhaled glucocorticoids for their anti-inflammatory effects. Antibiotics are indicated if there is a concurrent infection such as acute bronchitis. β$_2$-agonists are used for their bronchodilator effects and rapid onset of action. Methacholine challenge is used in the diagnosis of asthma.

57. **(2)** The client with asthma should be instructed to keep their inhaled β$_2$-agonist with them at all times in case of bronchospasm and use them prn. The β$_2$-agonists are effective in reversing bronchospasm. Inhaled steroids are long acting and will not give immediate relief; therefore, the client should be instructed to use them regularly as prescribed and use their inhaled β$_2$-agonist prn. Beginning antibiotics is not indicated for acute bronchospasm.

58. **(4)** Dextromethorphan is specific for control of coughing. Guaifenesin is an expectorant, and Options #1 and #2 are decongestants to decrease nasal and upper respiratory congestion.

59. **(1)** INH requires concurrent administration of vitamin B_6 to prevent problems of optic neuritis. Vitamin B_6 will decrease the effectiveness of levodopa. If the client is to receive the INH, his antiparkinson medication needs to be re-evaluated.

60. **(1)** The combination of cisapride (Propulsid) and erythromycin-based antibiotics can precipitate fatal dysrrhythmias. Another antibiotic should be considered (*Testing tip: three of the distractors are antihypertensive medications; only one is different, and it is the correct answer.*)

61. **(3)** The drug therapy regimen for chronic asthma usually includes theophylline.

Symptoms of toxicity include anorexia, nausea, vomiting, confusion, restlessness, tachycardia, dysrrhythmias, and seizures.

62. **(2)** The hallmark clinical presentation of acute bronchitis is a productive cough. The nurse practitioner should rule out pneumonia. This was accomplished with this client through the normal chest x-ray and breath sounds. Bronchodilators (albuterol) have been found to eliminate the cough of acute bronchitis. Antibiotic therapy (erythromycin and tetracycline) is not recommended. Research has demonstrated that antibiotic-susceptible organisms rarely cause acute bronchitis.

63. **(4)** Histamine antagonists neutralize the normal gastric acid barrier, allowing for an increased colonization of gram-negative bacilli and *Staphylococcus aureus*.

6

Immune & Allergy

Physical Examination & Diagnostic Tests

1. When taking the history of a client with known allergies, what is the most important information to determine?

   1. Reaction associated with each allergen.

   2. Drug allergies.

   3. Food allergies.

   4. Environmental exposure.

2. Which test is used to test determine the concentration of gamma globulins that contain most of the immunoglobulins?

   1. Immunofixation electrophoresis.

   2. Complement fixation.

   3. Protein electrophoresis.

   4. Antinulcear antibody.

3. Diagnostic studies used in the differential diagnosis of systemic lupus erythematosus (SLE) include:

   1. CBC, SMA-12, and ESR.

2. Chest radiograph and coagulation profile.

3. Antinuclear antibody (ANA), ESR, and C-reactive protein.

4. CBC, urinalysis, and chest radiograph.

4. Which tests are appropriate for the nurse practitioner to order in an initial work-up for asymptomatic clients at risk for human immunodeficiency virus (HIV)?

   1. CD4 count, HIV enzyme-linked immunosorbent assay (ELISA).

   2. Serology for cytomegalovirus, herpes simplex virus, and Epstein-Barr virus.

   3. HIV ELISA and Western blot.

   4. Hepatitis screen and Western blot.

5. The nurse practitioner would anticipate which laboratory finding in a client with joint pain, "butterfly rash," photosensitivity, weight loss, and fever?

   1. Presence of antinuclear antibodies.

   2. Negative serum complement level.

   3. Increased red blood cell (RBC) and white blood cell (WBC) count.

   4. Glycosuria.

6. When assessing a client for angioedema, the nurse practitioner would examine the:

   1. Neck and ears.

   2. Heart sounds.

   3. Abdomen.

   4. Eyes and mouth.

7. Clients who believe they have been exposed to HIV should have an HIV antibody test how soon after the exposure.

   1. The next day and 2 months later.

   2. 6 months after exposure and again at 12 months.

   3. 6–12 weeks after exposure and again at 6 months.

   4. 4 weeks and 12 weeks after exposure.

8. The most reliable test for the presence of specific immunoglobulin E (IgE) antibody is:

   1. Skin testing.

   2. Radioallergosorbent testing (RAST).

   3. Smears for eosinophils.

   4. Complete blood count.

9. To diagnose allergic rhinitis in the primary care office setting, the nurse practitioner would consider performing:

   1. A nasal smear for eosinophils.

   2. A total serum IgE.

   3. Skin testing.

   4. Radioallergosorbent testing.

Disorders

10. Client education regarding common antigens of anaphylaxis includes:

    1. Extreme weather.

    2. Egg albumin.

    3. Pungent odors.

    4. Animal dandruff.

11. The nurse practitioner understands that an HIV infection results in a reduction of:

    1. Helper T cells.

    2. Suppressor T cells.

    3. Killer T cells.

    4. Suppressor B cells.

12. Which assessment finding is commonly associated with a diagnosis of systemic lupus erythematosus?

    1. Excitability, diarrhea, vomiting.

    2. High fever, measle-like rash on limbs, weight gain.

    3. Joint pain, malar rash, photosensitivity.

    4. Weight loss, diarrhea, epigastric pain.

13. After a repeat HIV antibody test, a client continues to test positive but is asymptomatic. The nurse understands which of the following about possible transmission of the virus by the client?

    1. The client is infectious when symptoms are active.

    2. The client is infectious for life.

    3. The dormant virus is not infectious while the client is asymptomatic and the T-cell count is high.

    4. Laboratory tests should be done monthly to identify the infectious periods of the disease process.

14. The nurse practitioner has been assigned a new client. Problem list indicates this client has CREST syndrome. The nurse practitioner will be following this client for:

    1. Scleroderma.

2. Dental caries.

3. Systemic lupus erythematosus.

4. Rheumatoid arthritis.

15. A client presenting with complaint of fatigue, malaise, arthralgias, oral ulcers, malar rash, and a positive ANA would most likely be diagnosed as having:

    1. Rheumatoid arthritis.

    2. Fibromyalgia.

    3. Scleroderma.

    4. Systemic lupus erythematosus.

16. The most common clinical manifestations of Sjögren's syndrome are:

    1. Corneal dryness and lack of saliva.

    2. Increased urination and hunger.

    3. Abdominal discomfort and headaches.

    4. Joint destruction and alopecia.

17. An elderly female client presents to the nurse practitioner with a low-grade temperature and a unilateral throbbing headache. She also reports scalp sensitivity and some visual disturbances. Lab results show a markedly elevated ESR and anemia. She has been relatively healthy except for a recent history of polymyalgia rheumatica (PMR). Symptoms indicate a clinical presentation of:

    1. Bacterial meningitis.

    2. Acute migraine headache.

    3. Temporal (giant cell) arteritis.

    4. Subdural hematoma.

18. A middle-aged female client presents with weight loss, heart burn, dysphagia, dry cough, pain, stiffness of the fingers and knees, and Raynaud's phenomenon. The nurse practitioner recognizes these as the symptoms of:

    1. Rheumatoid arthritis.

    2. Lupus erythematosus.

    3. Graft-versus-host disease.

    4. Scleroderma.

19. The erythematous confluent macular eruption of the face known as the butterfly rash is characteristic of:

    1. Allergic drug eruption.

    2. Systemic lupus erythematosus.

    3. Rosacea.

    4. Seborrheic dermatitis.

20. The nurse practitioner is discussing general health care with a female client who is in remission for SLE. Important points to include are:

    1. Avoid getting pregnant.

    2. Decrease physical and psychological stress.

    3. Avoid isometric and aerobic exercise.

    4. Maintain diet low in fat and carbohydrates.

21. A 50-year-old male client presents with complaints of frequent sinus infections, a decrease in the ability to hear, and arthralgias. Laboratory findings are: RBC—mild normochromic and normocytic anemia, elevated ESR, mild hypergammaglobulinemia (elevated IgA), proteinuria, and hematuria with granular or cellular casts. Physical examination findings include mild conjunctivitis, vasculitic dermatitis, chronic cough, chest pain, dyspnea, paranasal sinus pain, occasional epistaxis, and imbalance of intake and output. A tentative diagnosis is:

    1. Connective tissue disease.

    2. Wegener's granulomatosis.

    3. Pulmonary neoplasm.

    4. Infectious granulomatous disease.

22. A client presents with sneezing, watery eyes, postnasal drip, full head, and sore throat. The best diagnosis for this client is:

    1. Acute bronchitis.

    2. Allergic rhinitis.

    3. Asthma exacerbation.

    4. Influenza.

23. A 70-year-old woman presents with complaints of morning headache, malaise, and anorexia. The nurse practitioner suspects.

    1. Pneumonia.

    2. Temporal arteritis.

    3. Herpes zoster.

    4. Postmenopausal symptoms.

24. Signs and symptoms that alert the nurse practitioner to identify a client who is at an increased risk for HIV infection include:

    1. Night sweats.

    2. Malaise and fatigue.

    3. Frequent sexually transmitted diseases.

    4. Swollen glands and diarrhea.

25. The human immunodeficiency virus is classified as a:

    1. Cytomegalovirus.

    2. Herpetic virus.

    3. Papillomavirus

    4. Retrovirus.

26. The most frequently occurring symptoms of SLE are:

    1. Splenomegaly and Raynaud's phenomenon.

    2. Pulmonary effusions and hepatomegaly.

    3. Butterfly rash on the face and lymphadenopathy.

    4. Fever, arthritis, arthralgia, and weight loss.

27. A systemic IgE-mediated antigen–antibody response resulting in a life-threatening massive release of mediators is:

    1. Generalized seizures.

    2. Allergic rhinitis.

    3. Anaphylaxis.

    4. Status asthmaticus.

28. The release of histamine results in:

    1. Bronchospasm, vasodilatation and vascular permeability.

    2. Bronchodilatation, vasodilatation, and vascular permeability.

    3. Smooth muscle contraction, decreased vascular permeability, and vasoconstriction.

    4. Pain, increased vascular permeability, and bronchodilatation.

29. Following a bone marrow transplant (BMT), the nurse practitioner can expect the peak onset of an acute graft-versus-host disease (GVHD) to occur:

    1. Between 10 and 15 days after transplant.

    2. Between 30 and 50 days after transplant.

    3. Between 1 and 5 days after transplant.

    4. At 100 days after transplant.

30. A client has a history of recent BMT. The nurse practitioner identifies sign and symptoms of GVHD to include:

    1. Fever, headache, and mental status changes.

    2. Chills, fever, and urticaria over flank area.

    3. Increased serum bilirubin, maculopapular rash, and green, watery diarrhea.

    4. Decreased RBC, hematocrit, hemoglobin, and petechiae; and increased bleeding tendencies.

31. The pathogenesis of SLE is characterized by autoantibody development. This results in:

    1. Increased T suppressor cells.

    2. B-cell decrease.

    3. Polyconal hypogammaglobulinemia.

    4. Decreased T suppressor cells and inhibited cell activity.

32. The cell responsible for the activation of the immune response is:

    1. Band neutrophil.

    2. T4 lymphocyte.

    3. Segmented neutrophil.

    4. B lymphocytes.

33. An adult is brought into the clinic and the family states he has a history of anaphylactic reactions. What signs and symptoms indicate to the nurse practitioner the client is experiencing another reaction?

    1. Cough, wheezing, and hives.

    2. Severe malaise, pallor, stridor, and dyspnea.

    3. Anxiety, nasal congestion, and tachycardia.

    4. Rhinorrhea, nausea, and gastrointestinal (GI) cramping.

34. A nurse at the clinic experiences a needle stick from a client with known hepatitis. What should be administered to provide passive immunity?

    1. IgE.

    2. IgA.

    3. IgG.

    4. IgC.

35. Which sign and/or symptom is indicative of a type I hypersensitivity reaction?

    1. Contact dermatitis.

    2. Immediate wheal-and-flare reaction.

    3. Hematuria.

    4. High fever.

36. Cardiovascular effects of anaphylaxis include:

    1. ST-segment and T-wave changes.

    2. Hypertension.

    3. Prolonged P-R intervals with elevated QT segment.

    4. Elevated serum enzymes.

37. When assessing a client for SLE, what ophthalmologic findings would the nurse practitioner determine to be consistent with this condition?

    1. Retinal hemorrhages.

    2. Conjunctivitis.

    3. Cotton-wool spots.

    4. Arteriovenous (AV) nicking.

38. What information does the nurse practitioner include in the education for the client with allergic rhinitis?

    1. Monitor air quality and the allergy index.

    2. Use a surgical-type mask when going outdoors.

    3. Remain inside during allergy season.

    4. Avoid working in the garden or yard.

39. Which statement is true regarding latex allergy?

    1. It usually only produces symptoms of contact dermatitis and allergic rhinorrhea.

    2. It is a progressive disease that worsens with continued exposure.

    3. It only affects <5% of the health care population.

    4. It is an autoimmune response.

Pharmacology

40. Drugs that have been associated with a lupus-like syndrome include:

    1. Sulfonamides (Septra DS), penicillin (Pen-Vee K, Penicillin G).

    2. Progestin/estrogen combination of oral contraceptives.

    3. Nonsteroidal anti-inflammatory drugs (Motrin).

    4. Procainamide (Pronestyl), hydralazine (Apresoline).

41. A client newly presenting with signs and symptoms of SLE would have their medication profile reviewed to determine if they are on any medication that may have caused a drug-induced lupus. Which drug would be most suspect?

    1. Digoxin (Lanoxin).

    2. Procainamide (Pronestyl).

    3. Trimethoprim-sulfamethoxazole (Bactrim)

    4. Cimetidine (Tagamet).

42. A client is diagnosed with temporal (giant cell) arteritis. The medication of choice is:

    1. Prednisone (Deltasone).

    2. Ibuprofen (Motrin).

    3. Indomethacin (Indocin).

    4. Azathioprine (Imuran).

43. The clinic is notified that an elderly client is being brought in with a bee sting and that she is having difficulty breathing. Which medication should the nurse practitioner have available for her initial care?

    1. Lidocaine topical ointment.

    2. Epinephrine.

    3. Prednisone.

    4. Benadryl elixir.

44. The standard drug used for malaria prophylaxis is:

    1. Ampicillin (Polycillin, Omnipen).

    2. Doxycycline (Vibramycin).

    3. Ceftriaxone (Rocephin).

    4. Chloroquine phosphate (Aralen).

45. Treatment for allergic rhinitis includes:

    1. Antihistamines, corticosteroids and environmental control.

    2. Antibiotics, antihistamines, analgesics, and allergen control.

    3. Cholinergic agents, antibiotics, and analgesics.

    4. Nasal saline, corticosteroids, and antibiotics.

46. Development of an adverse drug reaction is dependent on which factors?

    1. Client age, prior drug reactions, genetic factors, and degree of exposure.

    2. Client gender, oral route of administration, and history of atrophic disease.

    3. Client age, gender, and genetic factors.

    4. Genetic factors, prior drug reactions, and client gender.

47. A medication frequently used for the prophylaxis as well as initial treatment of *Pneumocystis carinii* pneumonia (PCP) is:

    1. Fluconazole (Diflucan).

    2. Amphotericin B (Fungizone).

    3. Trimethoprim-sulfamethoxazole (Septra, Bactrim).

    4. Acyclovir (Zovirax).

48. When instructing the client with allergic rhinitis about the use of nasal decongestants, it is important for them to understand that:

    1. The condition is self-limiting and will resolve in a matter of weeks whether or not the client is re-exposed to the allergen.

    2. A nasal decongestant used continuous for greater than 3 days can result in a worsening of the symptoms.

    3. It is not necessary to avoid exposure to the allergen once therapy has been initiated.

    4. Since allergic rhinitis is only seen in the spring and fall, the condition only requires treatment during these seasons.

49. The major advantage to use of second-generation antihistamines such as astemizole (Hismanal) and loratadine (Claritin) is:

    1. Decreased cost.

    2. Increased anticholinergic activity.

    3. Delayed absorption.

    4. Does not cross the blood-brain barrier.

50. What is the desired action of sympathomimetics (adrenergics) when used in the treatment of allergic rhinitis?

    1. Promote vasoconstriction in nasal mucosa.

    2. Block mast cell degranulation.

    3. Decrease the effect of histamines.

    4. Increase degranulation and end-organ response.

51. The nurse practitioner is prescribing astemizole (Hismanal) for a geriatric client's allergy problems. When considering the client's current medications, which medication would be a contraindication to the administration of astemizole?

    1. Erythromycin ethylsuccinate (E.E.S.).

    2. Verapamil (Calan).

    3. Propranolol (Inderal).

    4. Captopril (Captoten).

52. Cromolyn sodium is used to:

    1. Reduce the histamine load.

    2. Antagonize the effects of histamine.

    3. Stabilize the mast cell membrane.

    4. Reduce antiemetic activity.

53. In the elderly client, histamine$_1$ (H$_1$) blockers may cause which side effects?

    1. Ataxia.

    2. Nausea.

    3. Diarrhea.

    4. GI upset.

54. What information is important for the nurse practitioner to include when teaching a client about the use of antihistamines?

    1. Use of topical antihistamines is safe and has relatively few side effects.

    2. Do not use over-the-counter (OTC) medications without consulting the health care provider.

    3. Constipation and urinary retention are expected side effects and do not need to be reported.

    4. Once the antihistamine therapy has been taken for 3 days, avoidance of allergens is not necessary.

55. A primary advantage of using loratadine (Claritin) in treating a client with seasonal allergies is that it:

    1. Is supplied as an enteric-coated pill.

    2. May be prescribed on once-a-day dosing.

    3. Costs considerably less than other medications.

    4. Effectively decreases nasal secretions.

56. What medications are the choice of treatment in the secondary therapy for the client with an anaphylactic reaction?

    1. Antibiotics and anticholinergics.

    2. Nonsteroidal anti-inflammatory drugs (NSAIDs).

    3. Decongestants and expectorants.

    4. Antihistamines and corticosteroids.

6 Answers & Rationales

Physical Examination & Diagnostic Tests

1. **(1)** The reaction to each allergen is important to know. Often, clients will indicate they have an allergy to a particular food or medication, such as nausea, stomach pain, or diarrhea, and consider it an allergy. The signs and symptoms of the reaction, the speed of onset, how long it lasts, and what successful treatment has been used in the past are important information. Both drug and food allergies should be explored.

2. **(3)** In a protein electrophoresis, proteins are electrically separated on a strip. It is a screening test to measure various proteins in body fluids, usually serum or urine. It assists in screening for diseases that are characterized by an increase or decrease in immunoglobulins. Complement fixation and antinuclear antibody are diagnostic studies for rheumatoid problems.

3. **(3)** Although all of the options listed may be included in a complete physical examination, laboratory tests specific to the diagnosis of SLE include the ANA, ESR, and C-reactive protein. During flares, the ESR and C-reactive protein are elevated. The ANA titer in a client with SLE is positive at a 1:80 ratio.

4. **(3)** The initial screening test for HIV is the ELISA. If the test is positive, confirmation of antibodies is done with a Western blot. Although serology and hepatitis screening along with a CBC and tuberculosis (TB) test are routinely performed, the initial work-up starts with an ELISA test. The CD4 count is performed during the active disease process.

5. **(1)** The majority of clients with SLE have antinuclear antibodies in their blood. There is leukopenia, thrombocytopenia, lymphopenia, and a positive LE cell prep. Proteinuria with cellular casts is often noted.

6. **(4)** Angioedema is most easily seen in the eyes and mouth. It is edema of the mucous membrane tissue. It can also be observed on the tongue, feet, hands, and genitalia. Diffuse erythema may be seen in the upper body parts. Gastrointestinal symptoms, vomiting, cramping, and diarrhea may also be seen.

7. **(3)** The HIV antibody develops between 6 and 12 weeks after exposure. Because of the variability of antibody development, it is recommended that the test be repeated in 6 months to confirm the findings.

8. **(1)** The most reliable test for the presence of the specific IgE antibody is the skin test. RAST is less sensitive than skin testing and is difficult to standardize and reproduce results. The smear for eosinophils and CBC are not specific for IgE antibody testing.

9. **(1)** The nasal smear for eosinophils is a simple office procedure. Many clients who have uncomplicated allergic rhinitis have a normal serum IgE. Skin testing should be performed by allergy-trained providers only.

RAST testing is higher in cost and lower in sensitivity.

Disorders

10. **(2)** Egg albumin is just one of many identified common antigens that may result in an anaphylactic reaction. Others include vaccines, allergen extracts, sulfonamides, penicillins, hormones, legumes (especially peanuts), berries, nuts, seafoods, and venom bites (bee, wasp, yellow jacket bites). Changes in weather, strong scents, and odors are triggers that may precipitate an asthma attack, resulting in bronchospasm and wheezing.

11. **(1)** There is a severe, life-threatening reduction of helper T cells, along with an increase in suppressor T cells. The helper T cells help amplify or increase the production of antibody-forming cells from the B lymphocytes after an encounter with an antigen. Killer T cells are produced after mature helper T cells interact with an antigen. Suppressor T cells suppress the formation of antibody-forming cells from the B lymphocytes which, when their numbers are increased, have a detrimental effect on the immunity and ability of the HIV client to make antibody-forming cells.

12. **(3)** The symptoms most commonly experienced are joint pain, fatigue, Raynaud's phenomenon, chronic or low-grade or recurrent fever, sun sensitivity, hair loss, weakness, butterfly (malar) facial rash, and weight loss. Typically, the pulmonary, cardiac, renal, and central nervous systems are involved.

13. **(2)** HIV infection creates a chronic infectious state in the body that is transmitted via blood or body fluids and transplacentally.

14. **(1)** CREST (**C**alcinosis, **R**aynaud's phenomenon, **E**sophageal dysfunction, **S**clerodactyly, **T**elangiectasia) is associated with a slow progressive form of scleroderma.

15. **(4)** This client is presenting with four of the eleven criteria necessary for diagnosing SLE. There is no singular test for SLE, but the presence of these characteristics plus lab results can differentiate the diagnosis.

16. **(1)** These are the most common clinical manifestations of Sjögren's syndrome. Clients may also have joint inflammation, but this rarely leads to destruction.

17. **(3)** About 40% of temporal (giant cell) arteritis clients have a history of PMR. The other diagnoses may have some of these symptoms but only arteritis has all of the symptoms listed in the situation. It is especially critical to note visual disturbances, as these clients can develop sudden blindness.

18. **(4)** The symptom of Raynaud's phenomenon differentiates this as scleroderma. The esophageal dysfunction is often an initial complaint in this disease, which is four times more common in females.

19. **(2)** The butterfly rash is one of the characteristic symptoms of SLE.

20. **(2)** Psychological and physical stress can exacerbate SLE. A balanced diet helps to limit the side effects of some of the medications, while regular exercise helps to reduce arthralgia and myalgia. Barrier contraception is recommended for the female with SLE. Pregnancy is usually allowed during periods of remission.

21. **(2)** Wegener's granulomatosis is a multisystem disorder that occurs equally in both sexes. Peak occurrence is between 40 and 60 years of age. The disease usually targets the upper respiratory tract and the kidney. Connective tissue disease, pulmonary neoplasm, and infectious granulomatous disease would be considered in the differential.

22. **(2)** The signs and symptoms presented are classic for allergic rhinitis. Acute bronchitis would present with cough and yellow or green sputum production. An asthma exacerbation would present with wheezing, chest tightness, decreased forced vital capacity, and history of exposure to an allergen. Influenza presents with fever, chills, and general malaise.

23. **(2)** The nurse practitioner should rule out temporal arteritis, an inflammatory disorder of unknown etiology, affecting large- and medium-sized arteries. It occurs two times more frequently in women, occurs most frequently in the elderly, and occurs rarely in the African-American population.

24. **(3)** The client with frequent sexually transmitted diseases would alert the nurse practitioner to the client's lack of protected sex and the possibility of multiple partners. Night sweats, malaise, fatigue, swollen glands, and diarrhea can be associated with many other illnesses.

25. **(4)** The HIV virus is a retrovirus. It contains an enzyme, reverse transcriptase, that copies RNA into DNA. When the virus binds to a CD4 receptor, it inserts its RNA and enzymes into the cell where a copy of the virus's RNA is made and enters the nucleus of the cell. As the infected host cell reproduces, the HIV DNA is duplicated and passed on.

26. **(4)** Although any of the above-mentioned clinical symptoms can occur in clients with SLE, fever, weight loss, and arthritis and arthralagias occur most often. Butterfly rash of the face and lymphadenopathy occur <50% of the time. Pulmonary effusion, hepatomegaly, splenomegaly, and Raynaud's phenomenon occur in less than one third of the cases.

27. **(3)** The massive release of mediators triggers a series of events in target organs. Prior sensitization to the antigen must have occurred to trigger an anaphylactic reaction. Anaphylaxis may result from injection of an antigen, ingested food or drugs, or inhaled antigens.

28. **(1)** The release of histamine results in bronchospasm, vasodilatation, and vascular permeability, leading to wheezing, increased mucus production in the lung, and edema of the airway.

29. **(2)** The onset of acute GVHD occurs between 30 and 50 days following BMT. It results from immunocompetent donor T lymphocytes attacking the host tissues.

30. **(3)** The signs and symptoms of GVHD include maculopapular rash, generalized erythroderma with desquamation, increased bilirubin, increased serum glutamic-oxaloacetic transaminase (SGOT) and/or increased alkaline phosphatase, abdominal cramping, and diarrhea. Infection is characterized by fever, mental status changes, and headaches. Decreased RBC, hemoglobin and hematocrit, and petechiae are signs of anemia. Fever, chills, and urticaria are indications of a reaction to white cells in the marrow.

31. **(4)** T lymphocytes are the white cells responsible for control of the immune response. In SLE, T suppressor cells are decreased and cell activity is inhibited. This results in hypergammaglobulinemia and B-cell proliferation.

32. **(2)** The T4 lymphocyte is known as the T helper cell. They are responsible for the proliferation of lymphocytes and macrophages causing activation of the cells in response to an antigen. The B lymphocytes are effector cells that mediate humoral responses by production of antibodies. The band neutrophil and segmented neutrophil are slightly mature and fully mature neutrophils. Neutrophils are the most abundant cells in the bone marrow and blood.

33. **(2)** Severe malaise, pallor, stridor, and dyspnea are signs and symptoms associated with a severe anaphylactic reaction. Symptoms may occur immediately or up to 2 hours after exposure. Severe reactions require immediate intervention.

34. **(3)** IgG is the major antibody against viruses and bacterias and is the principal mediator of the secondary immune response requiring repeated response to the same antigen. There is no IgC antibody. IgA is the secretory immunoglobulin found in tears, saliva, and mucous secretions of the lung and GI tract. IgE mediates allergic reactions.

35. **(2)** A type I hypersensitivity reaction causes an immediate wheal-and-flare reaction. Contact dermatitis is seen in a type IV (delayed) reaction. Hematuria is seen in a type II reaction caused by the presence of preformed circulating cytoxic antibodies, such as in a blood transfusion reaction or autoimmune hemolytic anemia. High fever

can be seen in the type III hypersensitivity reaction when large quantities of antigen–antibody complexes are released in the body.

36. **(1)** Changes in the electrocardiogram (ECG) are associated with coronary ischemia and myocardial ischemia. Although the ECG changes suggest myocardial injury, there is no change in the serum enzymes. Other signs and symptoms include hypotension and tachycardia.

37. **(3)** Cotton-wool spots are the most common ophthalmologic problem associated with SLE. Retinal hemorrhages and AV nicking can be seen in the client with hypertension. Conjunctivitis is an infection of the conjunctiva.

38. **(1)** The client with allergic rhinitis should monitor the air quality and allergy index in their area. A surgical-type mast will not filter out small allergens. Remaining inside during allergy season is an unrealistic expectation and can lead to depression and isolation for the client. The client can enjoy a summer garden if they are careful about the types of plants and flowers they plant. For example, the client with an allergy to ragweed should avoid daisies, dahlias, and chrysanthemums.

39. **(2)** Latex allergy is a progressive disease that worsens with continual exposure. The symptoms range from contact dermatitis to anaphylaxis. Currently latex allergy affects 17% of health care workers and 39% of dental professionals. Latex allergy is an acquired immune response to the latex protein allergen. Currently there is no vaccine and the only defense is to avoid contact with latex.

Pharmacology

40. **(4)** Procainamide (Pronestyl), hydralazine (Apresoline) and isoniazid (INH) have been shown to induce a lupus-like syndrome. Discontinuation of the medication results in disappearance of the clinical signs and symptoms. Antibiotics such as sulfonamides (Septra DS) and penicillin (Pen-Vee K, Penicillin G) have been associated with anaphylactic reactions in some clients. Oral

contraceptives may cause increased blood pressure and increase the risk for development of thromboemboli. NSAIDs such as Motrin have been associated with gastrointestinal upset and gastric pain, especially when taken on an empty stomach.

41. **(2)** Procainamide (Pronestyl) is one of the most common offenders. Twenty per cent of clients receiving this drug develop clinical drug-induced SLE. The other drugs listed have not been associated with SLE.

42. **(1)** This condition, seen primarily in the elderly, can lead to blindness if not treated immediately with corticosteroids. The usual daily dose of prednisone is 60 mg; divided dose initially, then single morning dose (never use every-other-day steroids). Begin a *slow taper* after 4 weeks if asymptomatic and ESR is decreased. Tapering dose is very individualized and the client may be on medications for several months to years. Average time for disease remission is 3–4 years (range 1–10 years).

43. **(2)** Epinephrine would be the first-line drug to be injected for the treatment of the respiratory distress associated with an anaphylactic reaction. The dosage for epinephrine (1:1000 SC) is 0.01 ml/kg for a child and 0.3–0.5 ml/kg for an adult.

44. **(4)** Chloroquine phosphate is the standard drug used for malaria prophylaxis. The dosage is 5 mg/kg body weight up to 300 mg for an adult. Doxycycline (Vibramycin) is often used to treat diarrhea associated with traveling to areas where diarrhea is common from drinking the water; it is also used to treat chlamydia and pelvic inflammatory disease. Ceftriaxone (Rocephin) is used in bacterial septicemia or problems of the respiratory and urinary tracts. Ampicillin (Polycillin, Omnipen) is used to treat a variety of organisms and as prophylaxis for bacterial endocarditis.

45. **(1)** Unless there is a secondary bacterial infection, antibiotics are not indicated. Antihistamines and reduction of exposure to the allergen will help to reduce the symptoms. For continued control and stabilization of the mast cell, corticosteroids are indicated.

46. **(1)** Adults are at greater risk for development of adverse drug reactions, probably due to the increased number of medications used and the amount of exposures. Clients with prior drug reactions are more likely to develop reactions to new drugs. The risk of an adverse drug reaction occurs in the first 2–3 weeks of therapy. Prolonged course of drug use, high dosage, and intermittent therapy increase the risk of an adverse reaction. Genetic factors may contribute to increased mediators and influencing metabolic pathways. Gender has no effect except in muscle relaxants and chymopapain, where women are at greater risk of developing an adverse drug reaction. Route of drug administration contributes to the risk, with IV, IM, SC, PO, and topical in the order of greatest to least risk.

47. **(3)** Trimethoprim-sulfamethoxazole (Septra, Bactrim) is used to treat as well as prevent *Pneumocystis carinii* pneumonia. Usually, a 21-day course of the drug is indicated. It may take 7–10 days to see a clinical response. Fluconazole (Diflucan) and amphotericin B are antifungal drugs; acyclovir (Zovirax) is an antiviral used primarily to treat herpes simplex virus types 1 and 2 and herpes zoster (shingles).

48. **(2)** The chronic use of nasal decongestants for greater than 3 days can result in a rebound effect when discontinued, which will lead to increased nasal congestion. The nasal congestion is the result of reflex vasodilatation. The condition may take as long as 2–3 weeks to resolve. Allergic rhinitis is not a self-limiting illness associated only with the spring and fall. Even though therapy is initiated, the client should be instructed to avoid exposure to the allergen as much as possible.

49. **(4)** The second-generation antihistamines do not cross the blood-brain barrier; therefore, they do not cause sedation and/or psychomotor dysfunction. There is little anticholinergic activity and less dry mouth and constipation. The cost of these antihistamines is 15–30 times greater than the first-generation antihistamines. The medications are rapidly absorbed within 1–2 hours of oral administration on an empty stomach.

50. **(1)** Sympathomimetics (adrenergics) cause vasoconstriction, reducing edema and secretions. Inhaled corticosteroids stabilize mast cells and block degranulation.

51. **(1)** Macrolides (erythromycin) and Hismanal should not be administered concurrently. Fatal dysrhythmias may be precipitated by this combination.

52. **(3)** Chromolyn sodium is used to stabilize the mast cell membrane to prevent release of histamine when the cell comes in contact with an antigen. It does not affect the amount of histamine released from the cell, antagonize the effects of histamine, or reduce antiemetic activity.

53. **(1)** The use of H_1 blockers can cause paradoxical central nervous system stimulation, resulting in ataxia in the elderly. Antihistamines can cause many simultaneous side effects in the elderly that can interfere with their daily living: dry mouth, constipation, as well as impaired vision, gait, and thinking.

54. **(2)** The client should be instructed not to use OTC medications without consulting the nurse practitioner or pharmacist. The client should be cautioned on the extended use of topical antihistamines. Antihistamines do not affect circulating histamine; therefore, it is important for the client to avoid exposure to a known allergen. Constipation and urinary retention are adverse effects that should be reported to the nurse practitioner.

55. **(2)** An advantage of using loratadine (Claritin) is the once-a-day dosing, which helps with client compliance. The cost is greater than some of the other first-generation antihistamines. Loratadine/pseudoephedrine (Claritin D) is available in an antihistamine/decongestant either with twice a day dosing or (Claritin D 24 Hour) loratadine/pseudoephedrine extended release for once-a-day dosing.

56. **(4)** Medications such as antihistamines and corticosteroids are used to counter mediator release and block release of additional mediators. NSAIDs, antibiotics, and decongestants are not indicated in the treatment of anaphylaxis.

Head, Eyes, Ears, Nose, & Throat (HEENT)

Physical Examination & Diagnostic Tests

Head

1. The nurse practitioner is examining lymph nodes in the neck. What is palpated in the anterior triangle of the neck?

   1. Posterior cervical chain.

   2. Anterior superficial chain.

   3. Periauricular lymph nodes.

   4. Supraclavicular lymph nodes.

Eyes

2. When using an ophthalmoscope, the nurse practitioner:

   1. Holds the ophthalmoscope in the right hand (uses right eye) while examining the client's left eye.

   2. Starts the examination with the lens set at zero.

   3. Begins in a position 1 inch from the eye to check the red light reflex.

   4. Examines the anterior chamber in a well-lighted room and asks the client to focus on an object.

3. The nurse practitioner observes lid lag in a client with:

   1. Myasthenia gravis.

   2. Hyperthyroidism.

   3. Hordeolum.

   4. Chalazion.

4. The nurse practitioner is examining an elderly woman. There is a glossy white circle around the pupils of her eyes, and the pupil has a decreased reaction to the direct light reflex. There is a history of presbyopia. Correct interpretation of these findings is:

   1. Beginning development of cataracts with a significant decrease in visual acuity.

   2. Normal changes in the eyes as a result of the aging process.

   3. A decrease in depth perception and the early eye changes associated with glaucoma.

   4. Visual changes secondary to long-term treatment with digitoxin and corticosteroids.

5. The nurse practitioner is preparing to examine the eyes of an adult client. In order to examine the optic disc and retinal vessels, the nurse practitioner uses what aperture on the ophthalmoscope?

   1. Small aperture.

   2. Red-free filter.

   3. Slit.

   4. Grid.

6. When testing the eyes for the presence of a normal consensual response, the nurse practitioner will:

   1. Shine the light into the client's pupil and observe the rate of pupillary constriction.

   2. Direct the light into one pupil, and observe for the constriction or response of the other pupil.

   3. Hold a card in front of one eye and have the client focus on a fixed object, then remove the card and observe movement of the newly uncovered eye.

   4. Ask the client to focus on an object, then direct a light source to the bridge of the nose while observing for symmetrical reflection in both eyes.

7. On ophthalmic examination, there appears to be a narrowing or blocking of the vein at the point where an arteriole crosses over it. The significance of this finding is:

   1. The client needs to be evaluated for chronic hypertension.

   2. This may be indicative of increased ocular pressure associated with glaucoma.

   3. The finding is associated with papilledema causing decreased venous drainage.

   4. This may represent a small embolus in the retinal vessels.

8. When examining the eyes, the nurse practitioner determines that the pupils change in size when the client focuses from a close object to a distant object. This is interpreted as:

   1. Normal visual accommodation.

   2. Extraocular motor nerves are intact.

   3. Consensual response is appropriate.

   4. Visual acuity is within normal limits.

Ears

9. When examining the ears of an adult client, the nurse practitioner determines that the tympanic membrane is gray and translucent. This is interpreted as:

   1. Scarring from previous infections.

   2. Decreased circulation to the membrane.

   3. Presence of serous fluid behind the membrane.

   4. Normal characteristics of the adult ear.

10. The purpose of conducting the Rinne test is to determine conduction of sound through the bone and through the auditory canal. A normal Rinne test is described as:

    1. Equal conduction through the mastoid bone and the ear canal.

    2. Air conduction twice as long as bone conduction.

    3. Bone conduction twice as long as air conduction.

    4. Sound is clearer with bone conduction than air conduction.

11. When assessing the tympanic membrane, specific landmarks are determined and

described according to the face of a clock. Normal landmarks for the right tympanic membrane are located:

1. Direct light reflex at the 5- to 6-o'clock position, malleus at the 1- to 2-o'clock position with umbo in center.

2. Manubrium slanted to the left with malleus at the 10-o'clock position.

3. Direct light reflex in the center of membrane with malleus at the 9-o'clock position.

4. Umbo to the left with anterior malleolar folds at the 10-o'clock position.

Nose

12. The nurse practitioner understands that nasal mucosa:

    1. Is redder than oral mucosa.

    2. Is pale and translucent in appearance.

    3. Appears pink and boggy, without exudate.

    4. Appears dark pink with watery secretion.

Throat

13. Throat cultures are indicated for the following suspects of pharyngitis:

    1. Rhinovirus and coronavirus infection.

    2. Group A β-hemolytic streptococci.

    3. Mononucleosis.

    4. *Candida albicans*.

14. An adult client arrives at the nurse practitioner's clinic with a complaint of low-grade fever, sore throat, a slight headache, and fatigue. On physical examination, the nurse practitioner found exudative tonsils bilaterally, red pharynx with white patches, and enlarged posterior cervical neck nodes. Upon testing, the nurse practitioner would expect to find:

    1. Positive rapid strep test.

    2. Positive mono spot test.

    3. Decreased white blood cell (WBC) count.

    4. Positive viral throat cultures.

Disorders

Head

15. An adult client presents to the nurse practitioner's office with a white plaque near the base of the tongue. The nurse practitioner notes that the plaque does not wipe off and assesses it as:

    1. Hemangioma.

    2. Leukoplakia.

    3. Papilloma.

    4. Erythroplasia.

16. Which of the following are predominant risk factors for oral carcinoma?

    1. History of dental infections, age <40.

    2. Tobacco use, alcohol use.

    3. Herpes simplex virus type 1, tobacco use.

    4. Alcohol use, history of dental abscess.

17. The hallmark of early oral cancer is:

    1. Tissue retraction.

    2. Thickening oral tissues.

    3. Persistent (>14 days) local inflammation.

    4. Halitosis and cough.

18. An adult male client is being evaluated for a complaint of a sore throat. He states that he has difficulty swallowing and has some mouth pain. On exam, the nurse practitioner finds that the client's mouth, tongue, and pharynx are coated with white curd-like plaques that are difficult to remove with a tongue blade. The course of treatment for this client should include:

    1. Referral to an ear, nose, and throat specialist for evaluation.

    2. Amoxicillin 500 mg PO tid × 10 days.

    3. Encourage the client to have human immunodeficiency virus (HIV) screening.

    4. Clear liquids only for the next few days.

19. The nurse practitioner knows that the most common site for head and neck cancer to occur is the:

    1. Sinuses.

    2. Oral cavity.

    3. Larynx.

    4. Nasal cavity.

Eyes

20. An older client who was working in his hobby shop complains of something in his right eye since this morning. Before beginning treatment, the nurse practitioner should:

    1. Instill local anesthetic.

    2. Check the visual acuity.

    3. Flush the eye with tap water for 30 minutes.

    4. Stain the eye with fluorescein.

21. An adult reports awakening with redness and a swollen eyelid. The nurse practitioner notes that the adult is afebrile and the eyelid is nontender and uniformly swollen. The most likely diagnosis is:

    1. Blepharitis.

    2. Hordeolum.

    3. Insect bite.

    4. Dacryocystitis.

22. A client is being prepared for cataract surgery. What information is important for the nurse practitioner to explain to the client?

    1. The procedure is short and the client usually goes home the morning after the surgery.

    2. Both eyes will be patched for the first 24 hours and it is important for the client to stay in bed.

    3. There may be problems with headache and eye pain for the first 24 hours; take the pain medication provided.

    4. Clients usually go home 2–3 hours after the surgery; there will be increased tearing, but it should not be painful.

23. A 60-year-old client works as a welder. He finished work about 8 hours ago and discovered that the protective glass on his welding hood was cracked. He is complaining of agonizing pain and photophobia. The correct diagnosis and action are:

    1. Chemical keratitis; dilate with atropine twice daily.

    2. Viral conjunctivitis; sulfonamide drops four times daily.

    3. Corneal abrasion; binocular patching with polymycin ointment.

    4. Ultraviolet keratitis; binocular patching and 1% cyclopentolate (Cyclogyl) drops.

24. A geriatric client presents at the clinic with complaints of blurred vision that has been getting increasingly worse over the past 2 years. There is also a problem with glare, but no problems with pain. The nurse practitioner would first evaluate for the presence of:

    1. Glaucoma.

    2. Retinal detachment.

    3. Degeneration of macula.

    4. Cataracts.

25. An adult client presents to the nurse practitioner for evaluation of a red, itchy eye for 1 day. The client states that when he awoke the eye was matted shut. The client can recall no trauma to the eye. The pupils are equal and reactive and the client denies any pain to the eye. The nurse practitioner treats this client for:

    1. Conjunctivitis.

    2. Corneal abrasion.

    3. Glaucoma.

    4. Iritis.

26. Which assessment of the eye is a deviation from the commonly occurring age-related changes?

    1. Arcus senilis.

    2. Presbyopia.

3. Sensitivity to glare.

4. Sustained nystagmus.

27. During a routine physical examination on a 55-year-old client, the nurse practitioner identifies arcus cornealis. The significance of this disorder is:

1. High potential for future blindness.

2. None; normal variant of aging process.

3. Abnormal lipid metabolism requiring medical management.

4. Hereditary variant of no consequence.

28. A 70-year-old client comes to the clinic complaining of an increased sensitivity to glare, difficulty adapting to darkness, and altered depth perception. The nurse practitioner should suspect:

1. Cataract.

2. Macular degeneration.

3. Glaucoma.

4. Normal age-related changes.

29. In assessing an adult with bacterial conjunctivitis, the nurse practitioner finds:

1. Minimal tearing, moderate itching, and profuse exudate.

2. Severe itching, moderate tearing, and minimal discharge.

3. Minimal itching, moderate tearing, and mucoid exudate.

4. Minimal itching, moderate tearing, and profuse exudate.

Ears

30. In teaching clients how to avoid acoustic trauma due to noise in the very loud range, the nurse practitioner knows that noise is loudest from a:

1. Vacuum cleaner.

2. Power mower.

3. Clothes washer.

4. Food blender.

31. A geriatric client is complaining of difficulty hearing. He relates that the problem seems to be getting worse over the past few years. What finding would support a diagnosis of presbycusis?

1. Unable to hear a watch tick at 1–2 inches from the ear.

2. Rinne test indicates air conduction greater than bone conduction.

3. History of long-term tetracycline antibiotics for chronic infections.

4. Long-term family history of chronic hearing loss.

32. An adult is seen by the nurse practitioner for ear pain. The adult is afebrile and reports swimming frequently for daily exercise. The left ear canal is markedly edematous and moderately inflamed with thick, yellowish drainage at the external meatus. The most likely diagnosis is:

1. Acute otitis media.

2. Serous otitis media.

3. Sinusitis.

4. Otitis externa.

33. Which of the following organisms is least likely to cause otitis media?

1. *Moraxella catarrhalis.*

2. *Streptococcus pneumoniae.*

3. *Chlamydia trachomatis.*

4. *Haemophilus influenzae.*

34. Which assessment of the ear would indicate a deviation from the normal aging process?

1. A dull, retracted, white tympanic membrane.

2. An elongated lobule.

3. A sensorineural hearing loss.

4. A bulging tympanic membrane with a distorted cone of light.

35. The nurse practitioner indicates an understanding of conductive hearing loss in the older client with which statement?

   1. "This has occurred due to damage of the eighth cranial nerve from gentamicin."

   2. "This is a result of an inner ear infection."

   3. "This is a normal part of aging and is referred to as presbycusis."

   4. "This may be reversible after the cerumen is removed from the ear canal."

36. Sensory hearing loss is common in industrial settings and preventable with the use of adequate hearing protection. This type of hearing loss is usually first noted with changes at what level?

   1. 500 Hz.

   2. 200 Hz.

   3. 3000–4000 Hz.

   4. Above 4000 Hz.

Nose

37. An adult client presents to the nurse practitioner's office with fever and complaints of right facial pain, copious yellow nasal discharge, and acute pain and headache when bending over for 5 days. There is no transillumination of the right maxillary sinus and that area is very tender to palpation. The client's diagnosis is:

   1. Chronic sinusitis.

   2. Acute sinusitis.

   3. Dental abscess.

   4. Temporal arteritis.

38. The nurse practitioner teaches an adult client the following as the most effective preventive measure against the common cold:

   1. Judicious use of vitamin C during cold season.

   2. Ensuring adequate sleep and fluids.

   3. Meticulous handwashing, preferably with an antibacterial soap.

   4. Avoiding contact with children and adults who have a runny nose, cough, and sore throat.

Throat

39. An adult client presents to the nurse practitioner's office with a chief complaint of "severe sore throat" for 3 days. The client states he also ran a fever, but doesn't know how high it got, and that he has been very tired with the sore throat. The physical exam revealed enlarged tonsils with large patchy exudate, inflamed pharynx, and nontender posterior cervical lymphadenopathy. The rest of the exam is nonremarkable. The nurse practitioner would make the diagnosis of:

   1. Infectious mononucleosis.

   2. Leukemia.

   3. Scarlet fever.

   4. Oral candidiasis.

40. Which of the following clinical findings are associated with bacterial streptococcal pharyngitis?

   1. Rhinorrhea.

   2. Cough.

   3. Enlarged tonsils with exudate.

   4. Small oral vesicles.

Pharmacology

41. The antibiotic(s) of choice for acute sinusitis in the adult is(are):

   1. Amoxicillin (Amoxil) 500 mg tid PO × 14 days; trimethoprim-sulfamethoxazole (Bactrim DS) 1 tab q12h PO × 14 days; penicillin V potassium (Pen-Vee K) 500 mg PO bid × 14 days.

   2. Trimethoprim-sulfamethoxazole DS 1 tab q12h PO × 14 days; Pen-Vee K 500 mg PO bid × 14 days.

   3. Penicillin G 150,000 units IM × 1; amoxicillin 500 mg PO tid × 14 days.

   4. Amoxicillin 500 mg PO tid × 14 days; trimethoprim-sulfamethoxazole DS 1 tab q12h PO × 14 days.

42. A geriatric client is diagnosed with chronic open-angle glaucoma. She has a past history of bradycardia and first-degree atrioventricular (AV) block. In consideration of her treatment, what medication is to be avoided?

    1. Pilocarpine (Isopto Carpine).

    2. Timolol (Timoptic).

    3. Hydrochlorothiazide (Diuril).

    4. Acetazolamide (Diamox).

43. Which antibiotic would be appropriate for the nurse practitioner to prescribe for β-lactamase production by strains of *Haemophilus influenzae* and *Moraxella catarrhalis* in an adult with acute otitis media?

    1. Amoxicillin (Amoxil).

    2. Trimethoprim-sulfamethoxazole (Bactrim).

    3. Pen-Vee K.

    4. Metronidazole (Flagyl).

44. The treatment plan for a client diagnosed with infectious mononucleosis includes which of the following?

    1. Rest during acute phase.

    2. Avoid exercise during acute phase.

    3. Take corticosteroids during acute phase.

    4. Take ampicillin orally for 10 days.

45. A client has had yellowish green nasal drainage and frontal headache for a week. The client's temperature has gone up to 101.2°F on most afternoons and she has a cough that worsens when she lies down. The physical exam is within normal limits except for the drainage and a slightly erythematous pharynx. She does not have any drug allergies and has not been on any medications in the last few months. Which medication would be best to prescribe for her?

    1. Diphenhydramine hydrochloride (Benadryl).

    2. Erythromycin (E-mycin).

    3. Pseudoephedrine hydrochloride (Sudafed).

    4. Amoxicillin (Amoxil).

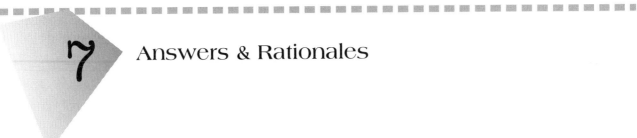

7   Answers & Rationales

Physical Examination & Diagnostic Tests

Head

1. **(2)** The conceptualization of triangles is useful in determining the location of palpable lymph nodes in the neck. The sternocleidomastoid muscle is the division between the anterior (containing the anterior superficial cervical chain) and the posterior (containing the posterior cervical chain) triangles. The trapezius muscle marks the posterior border of the posterior triangle. The supraclavicular or scale nodes are palpated in the angle formed by the clavicle and the sternocleidomastoid muscle.

Eyes

2. **(2)** The correct use of the ophthalmoscope involves using the right hand and right eye to examine the client's right eye. The room should be semidarkened for best visualization. The examiner initially inspects the lens and vitreous body from a distance of about 12 inches (at zero setting) and moves closer to the eye, usually rotating the lenses to the positive numbers (+15 to +20), which assists in focusing on near objects.

3. **(2)** If the lid margin falls above the limbus (junction line where the sclera and cornea meet) so that some sclera is visible, hyperthryroidism may be present. The lid may lag behind the limbus as the gaze moves from an upward to a downward position. Ptosis is a drooping lid margin that falls at the pupil or below and may

indicate an oculomotor lesion or myasthenia gravis. A chalazion is an inflammation or cyst of the meibomian glands that lie within the posterior portion of the eyelid. A localized infection of the small glands around the eyelashes in the hair follicle at the lid margin is called a hordeolum.

4. **(2)** With cataracts there is a clouding of the lens, not a circle around the pupil. The circle around the pupil is arcus senilis, which is normal in the geriatric client. The visual acuity of the client cannot be determined from the information provided. There are no observable pupillary changes in the beginning stages of glaucoma, which is identified by checking the intraocular pressure.

5. **(2)** The red-free filter is used to examine the optic disc for pallor and vascular changes as well as to assess for retinal hemorrhages. The small aperture is used for small pupils, the slit is for the anterior eye, and the grid is for estimating the size of lesions found in the fundal area.

6. **(2)** Consensual response is pupillary constriction of one eye when there is a direct light stimulus to the pupil of the other eye.

7. **(1)** Arteriovenous nicking is associated with longstanding hypertension. Intraocular pressure cannot be determined from an ophthalmic examination. Papilledema is associated with swelling around the optic

disc, and small emboli are represented by an abrupt impediment or severe narrowing of an arteriole not associated with where the retinal veins and arteries cross.

8. **(1)** Changes in pupil size when focusing from near to distant objects is normal accommodation. Extraocular eye movements are the ability to move the eye. Consensual response is constriction of the eye in response to light being shone in the opposite eye. The Snellen eye chart is used to determine the visual acuity.

Ears

9. **(4)** This describes the normal characteristics of the tympanic membrane. There is no evidence of scarring or fluid.

10. **(2)** The normal Rinne test is air conduction is twice as long as bone conduction.

11. **(1)** This describes the correct position for these landmarks on the right ear. In Option #2 the manubrium slants to the right with the malleus at the 1- to 2-o'clock position for the right ear. Option #3 describes the correct position for the left ear. In Option #4, the umbo is in the center with the anterior folds at the 1- to 2-o'clock position for the right ear.

Nose

12. **(1)** The nasal mucosa is redder than the oral mucosa. Increased redness of the nasal mucosa usually indicates infection. Pale, boggy turbinates along with watery secretion often occurs with allergic rhinitis. The normal secretion is mucoid. Purulent, crusty, or bloody secretions are abnormal.

Throat

13. **(2)** Rapid screening for strep can be done from throat swab with antigen agglutination kits, but there is a 5–10% false-negative rate; therefore, it is suggested that culture be performed. The heterophile antibody test (monospot test), which rapidly detects heterophile antibodies, compares with the sensitivity and specificity (95% specific and 90% sensitive) of older heterophile antibody tests to diagnose mononucleosis. *Candida*

albicans and rhinovirus are not diagnosed by bacterial cultures. Oral candidiasis can be diagnosed with a potassium hydroxide (KOH) smear.

14. **(2)** The client in this situation had risk factors (age) and symptoms of mononucleosis; therefore, the monospot, or heterophile antibody test, should be conducted. The classical triad of mononucleosis symptoms include sore throat, fever, posterior cervical lymphadenopathy with or without mild tenderness. Rapid screening for strep can be done from throat swab with antigen agglutination kits and would be obtained first, however, would probably be negative. A WBC count would be ordered for bacterial pharyngitis, in that WBC elevation is found with bacterial infection and a decrease is associated with viral agents.

Disorders

Head

15. **(2)** Leukoplakia is a white patch present on the oral mucosa that cannot be rubbed off. A hemangioma is a benign blood vessel proliferation of the lips, tongue, or buccal mucosa. Erythroplasia is an asymptomatic red, velvety lesion of the mouth. Papillomas are benign verrucous lesions that are manifestations of human papillomavirus infection.

16. **(2)** The high risk factors for oral cancer are tobacco and alcohol use. The risk increases with the number of cigarettes smoked per day. The disease is age related, occurring in those over 40 years of age, and increasing with age. The male-to-female ratio is 3:1. Other risk factors are use of cigars, pipes, and smokeless tobacco. Human papillomavirus has been considered in the etiology for squamous cell carcinoma in the upper head and neck.

17. **(3)** Erythroplasia is accompanied by an inflammatory reaction in a client with suspected oral cancer. If the erythematous lesion persists over 14 days, a high suspicion of early oral cancer exists. Tissue retraction and thickening of the oral tissues are later signs of oral cancer. Halitosis (odor) may be associated with dysfunction within the oral cavity, nasal cavity, sinuses, or esophageal disorders. Cough is the primary symptom of respiratory disorders such as acute bronchitis or pneumonia.

18. **(3)** Adults who present with thrush (oral candidiasis) may be immunologically impaired. It is important to make the diagnosis of HIV early so that treatment modalities may be started. Treatment with amoxicillin may actually worsen the condition.

19. **(2)** The nurse practitioner knows that the risk factors for head and neck cancer include tobacco and alcohol use; poor oral hygiene; and occupational exposure to asbestos, coke, nickel, wood, or leather. The most common site is in the oral cavity, accounting for 48% of the head and neck cancer diagnoses.

Eyes

20. **(2)** Check the visual acuity before treatment as a basis for comparison in the event of complications. Local anesthetic will be helpful for the exam; flushing at this point is unlikely to be helpful, and staining the eye should come later when preparing to examine for abrasion under ultraviolet light.

21. **(3)** Generalized, diffuse swelling and erythema of the eyelid is associated with an insect bite. Blepharitis is a chronic inflammatory condition that is characterized by erythema and scaling of the lid margins. Hordeolum or stye is acute, purulent inflammation of the sebaceous glands (usually the meibomian or zeisian) of the eyelids and usually does not involve the entire eyelid. It may be painful, especially over the gland. Dacryocystitis is an inflammation of the lacrimal sac characterized by erythema and swelling over the lacrimal duct.

22. **(4)** Clients go home almost immediately after the procedure. Eye patches may be worn for the first 24 hours. Care should be taken to protect the operative eye from injury. There is some discomfort, but pain should not be a problem. The client can be up and around as tolerated.

23. **(4)** Ultraviolet burns of the cornea are caused by a welding arc and treated with binocular patching.

24. **(4)** Cataracts are characterized by painless loss of visual acuity over a period of time. Retinal detachment most often occurs suddenly with partial loss of the field of vision. Glaucoma results in the loss of peripheral vision, and macular degeneration primarily involves the central vision field.

25. **(1)** In corneal abrasion, glaucoma, and iritis the chief complaint is pain. Conjunctivitis presents with no pain and with a history of purulent discharge.

26. **(4)** Sustained nystagmus is indicative of a neurologic complication. The other options include normal age-related changes.

27. **(3)** Arcus cornealis is the deposit of lipids at the junction of the cornea and sclera that is present in many people over age 50. When identified in younger individuals, it points to a disorder of lipid metabolism.

28. **(4)** These assessments are normal age-related changes. Signs and symptoms of cataracts include reduced visual acuity; painless, progressive loss of vision; and sensitivity to light, especially on night driving. Reduced color discrimination and double vision may also be seen. Macular degeneration will present with a loss of the central vision. Primary open-angle glaucoma will present with occasional headaches, occasionally halos around lights, and may be asymptomatic in early stages. Primary angle-closure glaucoma will present with episodes of blurred vision, halos around lights at night, and redness with congestion.

29. **(4)** Classic signs of bacterial conjunctivitis include those symptoms listed along with complaints of eyelids being "glued shut" upon arising in the morning. Option #2 is indicative of allergic conjunctivitis. Option #3 is indicative of viral conjunctivitis.

Ears

30. **(2)** Although all of these household appliances are noisy, the client should wear ear plugs or muffs when using a power lawn mower regularly for long periods of time.

31. **(1)** Inability to hear a watch tick at 1–2 inches from the ear is a classic sign of hearing loss characteristic of advancing age. The Rinne test will indicate bone conduction is two times greater than air conduction. Tetracyclines are not ototoxic and the family history may or may not contribute to the problem.

32. **(4)** The adult has the clinical findings of otitis externa. Otitis externa is an inflammation and/or infection of the external ear canal predisposed by excessive wetness such as swimming. Common organisms responsible for otitis externa include *Pseudomonas aeruginosa*, *Proteus mirabilis*, and *Enterobacter aerogenes*. Sinusitis clinical findings focus on sinus tenderness, and a purulent nasal discharge. Clinical findings of otitis media include ear pain, full or bulging tympanic membrane, decreased or negative mobility, and possible erythema. Findings associated with serous otitis media include opaque or translucent tympanic membrane with presence of air bubbles; landmarks may be absent and the light reflex may be diffuse or absent.

33. **(3)** The most frequent bacterial organisms that infect the middle ear are similar to those of the nasopharynx: *Strepococcus pneumoniae*, *Haemophilus influenzae*, and *Moraxella catarrhalis*. Viruses may also cause acute otitis media. *Chlamydia trachomatis* is not a frequent causative agent.

34. **(4)** This would be indicative of an inflammation of the middle ear (acute otitis media). The other options include normal changes that occur with aging.

35. **(4)** Conductive hearing loss may result from acute otitis media, perforation of the eardrum, or obstruction of the ear canal, as by cerumen. The other distractors result in sensorineural hearing loss.

36. **(4)** This type of hearing loss presents with high-frequency loss, above the 4000-Hz level, and then progresses into voice frequencies at 2000–3000 Hz.

Nose

37. **(2)** The client is experiencing the classic characteristics of acute sinusitis. Chronic sinusitis has nasal discharge, congestion, headache, or cough for over 30 days. A dental abscess has severe tooth-associated pain, and jaw tenderness. Temporal arteritis causes pain in the jaw, tongue, and face, but no nasal discharge.

38. **(3)** Transmission of cold viruses is indirect (e.g., self-innoculation from virus being on surfaces of inanimate objects, to mucous membranes of the nose and mouth). It is less likely to be spread by the aerosol route. The client should avoid touching the nose and mouth unless the hands have been thoroughly washed. It is impractical to avoid contact, as cold viruses are found everywhere. Although many individuals believe vitamin C prevents colds, there is little research to support the claim.

Throat

39. **(1)** Mononucleosis is commonly seen in adolescents and young adults. It often presents with fever, exudate on the tonsils, generalized lymphadenopathy, malaise, posterior cervical adenopathy, and palatine petechiae. Leukemia presents with anorexia, irritability, lethargy, and bone pain. The peak incidence is 3- to 5-year-olds. Scarlet fever presents in children 2–10 years, with fever, abdominal pain, headache, sore throat, and strawberry tongue. Oral candidiasis presents with white curd-like plaques on an erythematous mucosa. The tongue is red with a white coat.

40. **(3)** Characteristics of bacterial pharyngitis include headache, mild to severe erythema of the tonsils with white or yellow exudate, dysphagia, positive anterior cervical nodes, sore throat with dysphagia, fever 101°–102.5° F, and nausea. Viral organisms that cause herpangina present with small oral vesicles. Cough is the primary symptom of acute bronchitis. Rhinorrhea is associated with allergic rhinitis.

Pharmacology

41. **(4)** Amoxicillin (Amoxil) is the first-line antibiotic for acute uncomplicated sinusitis in the adult because of cost-effectiveness, efficacy, and cure rates ranging from 67–100%. Even though 35% of *H. influenzae* and 75% of *M. catarrhalis* produce β-lactamase, cure rates when using amoxicillin have not been significantly different. Therefore, several other drugs may be utilized that have a clinical response similar to that of amoxicillin. These include ampicillin, trimethoprim-sulfamethoxazole (Bactrim), cefaclor (Ceclor), cefuroxime axetil (Ceftin), loracarbef (Lorabid), and amoxicillin-clavulanate potassium (Augmentin).

42. **(2)** β-Adrenergic blockers cause problems with bradycardia. Timolol (Timoptic) can be absorbed systemically from the eye and should not be used.

43. **(2)** Amoxicillin is ineffective against β-lactamase production. Erythromycin/sulfa, trimethoprim/sulfa, and cephalosporins are effective against β-lactamase production by strains of *H. influenzae* and *M. catarrhalis*.

Pen-Vee K and metronidazole are not effective in this group. Cephalexin, cefuroxime, or cefixime can be used as alternatives.

44. **(1)** The treatment of mononucleosis includes bed rest while the client has fever and myalgia (10–14 days), supportive acetaminophen or ibuprofen, warm saline gargles, and throat lozenges or spray. The client must avoid strenuous exercise and contact sports the first 2–3 weeks. Corticosteroids are recommended only in clients with impending airway obstruction. Ampicillin is not recommended due to allergic reaction and rash reaction. About 95% of clients with mononucleosis recover uneventfully with supportive treatment.

45. **(4)** The client is experiencing symptoms of acute sinusitis. The first-line antibiotic to prescribe for this condition is amoxicillin due to safety and efficacy. Oral antihistamines such as diphenhydramine should not be used unless the client has allergies. Oral decongestants (pseudoephedrine hydrochloride) are not as effective as topical agents in clients with sinusitis. Erythromycin is not a first-line antibiotic for sinusitis.

Integumentary

Physical Examination & Diagnostic Tests

1. The nurse practitioner describes an annular skin lesion as usually arranged in:

    1. Groups of vesicles erupting unilaterally.

    2. A line.

    3. A pattern of merging together, not discrete.

    4. A circle, or ring-shaped.

2. A client has pitting of the nails. The nurse practitioner understands this is associated with:

    1. Psoriasis.

    2. Iron deficiency anemia.

    3. Malnutrition.

    4. Hyperthyroidism.

3. The nurse practitioner is inspecting a dark-skinned individual for signs of jaundice. The best place to observe is the:

    1. Sclera of the opened eye.

    2. Palms and soles of the hands and feet.

    3. Oral mucosa.

    4. Nail beds.

4. When assessing the hydration status of a client, the best place to evaluate skin turgor on an adult is:

    1. Just below the clavicle.

    2. Below the scapula on the back.

    3. On the inside of the forearm.

    4. Back of the hand.

5. The Wood's lamp is used to evaluate skin lesions. When the light is shone on the client's skin, a green-yellow fluorescence indicates:

    1. Presence of fungi.

    2. Lichenification.

    3. Keratinized cells.

    4. Bacterial colonies.

6. On examination of a client's skin, the nurse practitioner finds a lesion that is about 0.75 cm in diameter, brown, circumscribed, flat, and nonpalpable. The correct term for this lesion is:

   1. Macule.

   2. Papule.

   3. Nodule.

   4. Wheal.

7. The history and physical of a client indicates past occurrences of lichenification. The nurse practitioner identifies the characteristics of this lesion as:

   1. Dried, crusty exudate, slightly elevated.

   2. Rough thickened epidermis, accentuated skin markings.

   3. Keratinized cells shaped in an irregular pattern with exfoliation.

   4. Loss of epidermis with hollowed-out area and dermis exposed.

8. Clubbing of the nails occurs in clients with chronic respiratory conditions. The nurse practitioner assesses for this condition by:

   1. Evaluating the nail for transverse depressions and ridges.

   2. Placing both of the client's hands together with palms inward and index fingers aligned.

   3. Placing nail beds of each index finger together to determine angle of nail plate.

   4. Determining if there is diffuse discoloration of the nail bed from decreased oxygenation.

9. A circumscribed, elevated lesion >1 cm in diameter and containing clear serous fluid is best described as a:

   1. Papule.

   2. Vesicle.

   3. Bulla.

   4. Pustule.

10. In performing a skin assessment, the nurse practitioner understands that the following characteristic of a mole would necessitate immediate intervention:

    1. A 5-mm, symmetrical, uniformly brown mole on the thigh that has been present and has not changed in appearance for over 5 years.

    2. Multiple small (1- to 3-mm) flat moles across the upper back that are dark brown in color, round, and have smooth edges.

    3. A 3-cm waxy papule, with a "stuck-on" appearance, noted on the face.

    4. A new 2-mm mole that is brown with a red, irregular border, and is occasionally pruritic.

11. Dermatophyte skin infections can be diagnosed from skin scrapings and prepped with which solution for microscopic exam:

    1. Hydrochloric acid.

    2. 20% potassium hydroxide (KOH) solution.

    3. Gram's stain.

    4. Distilled water.

12. When administering skin tests to an immunocompromised client, the nurse practitioner must consider:

    1. The importance of not applying more than one skin test at a time.

    2. The skin test may react more aggressively than expected.

    3. Identify a known allergen for the client and utilize it as a control.

    4. The immunocompromised client should not be skin tested.

Skin Disorders

13. A client complains of intolerable itching in the pubic hair. On examination the nurse practitioner notes erythematous papules and tiny white specks in the pubic hair. The differential diagnosis includes all **except**:

    1. Pediculosis pubis.

    2. Scabies.

3. Impetigo.

4. Atopic dermatitis.

14. An elderly lady has an area of vesicles in clusters with an erythematous base that extend from her spine, around and under her arm and breast, to the sternum on her left side. She says the area was very tender last week and the vesicles started erupting yesterday. She is complaining of severe pain in the area. The diagnosis for this condition is:

1. Psoriasis.

2. Herpes zoster.

3. Contact dermatitis.

4. Cellulitis.

15. A chronic skin condition sometimes associated with arthritis is:

1. Eczema.

2. Psoriasis.

3. Neurodermatitis.

4. Pityriasis rosea.

16. Which is a true statement about psoriasis?

1. It usually is worse in the summer.

2. It is highly contagious.

3. It can be aggravated by stress.

4. All clients have accompanying pruritis.

17. A client with actinic keratosis should be told:

1. These lesions are a normal part of aging and are benign.

2. These lesions can develop into squamous cell carcinomas.

3. This is part of an allergic reaction and the offending allergen need to be identified.

4. This skin condition responds well to sunlight, which will help alleviate the symptoms.

18. The following are all true statements regarding urticaria **except** for:

1. Most cases of acute urticaria are mediated by immunoglobulin E (IgE) mast cell degranulation after exposure to certain substances.

2. Chronic urticaria may be related to occult infections.

3. Urticaria is characterized by itchy red swellings of a few millimeters to a few centimeters in size.

4. Laboratory studies are necessary to identify the causative agent.

19. A client who is known to be human immunodeficiency virus (HIV)-positive presents with several painless, persistent, raised purple lesions on the face. The most likely cause is:

1. Seborrheic dermatitis.

2. Molluscum contagiosum.

3. Kaposi's sarcoma.

4. Fungal infection.

20. In making a differential diagnosis between nummular eczema (dermatitis) and dyshidrotic eczematous dermatitis, the nurse practitioner knows that:

1. Nummular eczema is characterized by flushing and clusters of papulopustules on the cheek and forehead.

2. Dyshidrotic eczematous dermatitis is a chronic vesicular type of hand and foot eczema characterized by vesicles (tapioca-like), scaling, lichenification, and pruritius.

3. Nummular eczema is a hereditary disorder characterized by chronic scaling plaques that are usually bilateral, appearing on exposed areas (knees, elbows).

4. Dyshidrotic eczematous dermatitis affects primarily young adults, is contagious, and is characterized by firm papules with a clefted surface and multiple conical vegetations.

21. A middle-aged male client presents to the clinic with a complaint of being bitten last night by another individual during a fight. He has a bite mark on his forearm and the skin has been broken. He reports he has had a tetanus shot about 8 years ago. Recommended treatment by the family nurse practitioner should include all **except**:

    1. Administration of 0.5 ml of tetanus toxoid IM.

    2. Instruct client to watch for signs of infection.

    3. Initiate treatment with penicillin plus a penicillinase-resistant penicillin.

    4. Close wound with sutures or steri-strips.

22. Nail involvement, secondary to primary foot and hand tinea, which is characterized by accumulation of subungual keratin that produces thickened distorted crumbling nails, is termed:

    1. Hippocratic nails.

    2. Onychomycosis.

    3. Koilonychia.

    4. Anonychia.

23. A client complaining of hyperhidrosis should be counseled that:

    1. This is a normal occurrence.

    2. There are no therapies for this complaint.

    3. Bathing in a 20% alcoholic solution of aluminum chloride hexahydrate (Drysol) on a nightly basis may be beneficial.

    4. A history and physical exam need to be completed so that any medical etiologies can be ruled out.

24. During the physical examination, the nurse practitioner assesses a macular-papular skin lesion on a client's back that is warty, scaly, greasy in appearance, and light tan in color. The nurse practitioner would make the diagnosis of:

    1. Actinic keratosis.

    2. Basal cell carcinoma.

    3. Seborrheic keratosis.

    4. Senile lentigo.

25. The nurse practitioner would expect to make which assessment with an older client diagnosed with herpes zoster (shingles) during the prodromal stage?

    1. Erythematous lesions present over four different parts of the body.

    2. A red, pinpoint, painless rash.

    3. A burning pain in a line on only half of the client's chest that does not cross the midline.

    4. Painless purulent lesions for 2 days followed by complaints of itching, burning, and nausea.

26. An elderly retired farmer presents with a dome-shaped pearly firm nodule with telangiectasia on his nose. In making a differential diagnosis, the nurse practitioner recognizes this to be:

    1. Compound nevus.

    2. Melanoma.

    3. Bullous pemphigoid.

    4. Basal cell carcinoma.

27. An adult female presents with an irregular variegated nevus on her lower left back that has doubled in size in the past 3 months. The nurse practitioner should:

    1. Do a punch biopsy to confirm the diagnosis.

    2. Take a photograph of the lesion and recheck it in 1 month.

    3. Refer immediately to a dermatologist.

    4. Reassure the client that these are normal changes related to hormone variations.

28. A client presents with pain in his right chest wall for the past 48 hours. Upon examination, the nurse practitioner notices a vesicular eruption along the dermatome and identifies this as herpes zoster. The nurse practitioner informs the client that:

    1. All symptoms will disappear in 3 days.

2. Oral medication can dramatically reduce the duration and intensity of symptoms.

3. He has chickenpox and can be contagious to his grandchildren.

4. The eruptions will recur at regular intervals.

29. An older adult male client presents to the nurse practitioner's office complaining of flu-like symptoms, a large red spot in the right groin, headaches, and generalized muscle pain. These symptoms have persisted for approximately 4–5 weeks. In taking the client's history, it would be most important to determine whether the client:

1. Was using new skin care products, detergents, and so forth.

2. Was taking any new medications, vitamins, herbal therapies, and the like.

3. Has had a recent insect bite, or potentially exposed to insects, such as ticks (e.g., camping trips, travel to heavily wooded areas).

4. Has been exposed to anyone who has tuberculosis.

Pharmacology

30. An elderly obese woman presents to the clinic with complaints of tenderness and irritation under both of her breasts. The examination reveals a very irritated, moist, inflamed area with macules and papules present. The best treatment for this woman is:

1. Nystatin cream two or three times a day for 10 days; encourage thorough drying of the area and exposure to light and air.

2. Systemic anti-staphylococcal antibiotics (dicloxacillin) and soaking with moist pads of normal saline three times a day.

3. Gentle washing of the area and removal of crusts, then application of antibiotic ointment.

4. Antiviral treatment (acyclovir) and topical ointment to prevent secondary infection.

31. Which classification of drugs have the potential to aggravate psoriasis?

1. β-Blockers.

2. Thiazide diuretics.

3. Vasodilators.

4. Monoamine oxidase (MAO) inhibitors.

32. All of the following is true of postherpetic neuralgia **except** for:

1. Capsaicin (Zostrix) cream may alleviate some of the discomfort.

2. The majority of clients who have postherpatic pain lose it gradually, day by day, week by week.

3. Acyclovir (Zovirax) 200 mg, 5 capsules a day PO in divided doses is an effective therapy.

4. It is more common in clients over age 60.

33. What is the recommended treatment of rosacea?

1. Oral hydrocortisone.

2. Oral ketoconazole.

3. Low-dose tetracycline.

4. Topical 5-fluorouracil.

34. When using lidocaine with epinephrine 1–2% as a local anesthetic in the repair of an injury, it is essential to keep in mind that the maximum allowable dose is:

1. 7 mg/kg.

2. 2 mg/kg.

3. 10 mg/kg.

4. 5 mg/kg.

35. An elderly client presents to the nurse practitioner complaining of a painful, tingling rash across the right side of his abdomen. Exam reveals vesicles with erythematous bases; some of the vesicles are draining cloudy fluid, while others are crusted. The nurse practitioner makes the diagnosis of herpes zoster infection, and places the patient on antiviral therapy. The patient states that the painful rash has kept him from sleeping for the past 4 nights. Appropriate therapy for this client's pain would include:

    1. Amitriptyline (Elavil) 10 mg PO qhs, nonsteroidal anti-inflammatory drugs (NSAIDs) prn as directed, along with application of cool compresses to the lesions for 30 minutes, several times a day.

    2. High-dose corticosteroid therapy.

    3. Application of heat directly to the area involved.

    4. There is no appropriate therapy currently available to treat neuropathic pain.

36. On a return visit to the clinic, a client who is receiving sulfonamide therapy exhibits the following symptoms: generalized rash, mucous membrane lesions, sloughing of the skin of the palms and feet, high fever, and generalized malaise. These findings would alert the nurse practitioner to consider:

    1. Hepatitis B.

    2. Stevens-Johnson syndrome.

    3. HIV infection/acquired immunodeficiency syndrome (AIDS).

    4. *Pneumocystis carinii* pneumonia.

37. An older adult client presents for an office visit with a complaint of a measles-like rash on his trunk and spreading to extremities. He was seen several days ago for bronchitis and started on trimethoprim-sulfamethoxazole (Bactrim DS) 1 tab PO bid. The recommended action for the family nurse practitioner is to:

    1. Instruct the client to continue Bactrim and see if any change occurs in the rash.

    2. Discontinue Bactrim.

    3. Take client off Bactrim for 3 days and restart the medication.

    4. Decrease Bactrim to half dose.

38. What would be the appropriate management for a client with herpes zoster (shingles)?

    1. Acyclovir (Zovirax).

    2. Miconazole (Monistat-Derm).

    3. Clotrimazole (Lotrimin).

    4. Corticosteroid (prednisone).

8   Answers & Rationales

Physical Examination & Diagnostic Tests

1. **(4)** Annular skin lesions may be arranged in a circular manner or in an arciform (arc-shaped) pattern (i.e., tinea corporis). Multiple groups of vesicles erupting unilaterally following the course of cutaneous nerves is herpetiform or zosteriform (i.e., herpes zoster). Linear lesions are arranged in a line (i.e., allergic contact dermatitis to poison ivy). Confluent lesions become merged together and are not discrete (i.e., scarlet fever rash).

2. **(1)** Psoriasis, peripheral vascular disease, diabetes, tuberculosis, and other infectious diseases such as syphilis are associated with pitting deformities of the nail that may vary from pinpoint size to pinhead size and may be linear or irregular in distribution. Iron deficiency anemia, eczema, malnutrition, and pellagra are associated with koilonychia (spoon nails). Hyperthyroidism and hypothyroidism are associated with onycholysis, which is a separation of the nail from the nail bed, originating at the free edge and progressing proximally.

3. **(1)** The place to inspect is in that portion of the sclera that is observed when the eye is open. If jaundice is suspected, the posterior portion of the hard palate should be examined for a yellowish cast. Pallor and cyanosis can be noted in the nail bed, palms, and soles.

4. **(1)** Just below the clavicle or on the abdomen for an adult and on the abdomen for infants and children are the most reliable areas for indication of hydration status.

5. **(1)** Fungal lesions will be visualized as a green-yellow flurorescence when viewed with the Wood's lamp in a dim room.

6. **(1)** A macule is <1 cm in diameter; nonpalpable; and brown, red, purple, or tan (freckles, flat moles, rubella). A papule is elevated and palpable (warts, pigmented nevi). A nodule is 1–2 cm diameter, elevated, and deeper (lipoma). A wheal is elevated, irregular, and has a variable diameter (insect bites, urticaria).

7. **(2)** Lichenification occurs with chronic irritation, often of an exposed extremity (chronic dermatitis). Crusts are dried exudate; scales are heaps of keratinized cells from exfoliation (psoriasis); and loss of epidermis is excoriation as seen in an abrasion.

8. **(3)** The angle of the nail beds should form a diamond when the nail beds are approximated. Transverse ridges and grooves may occur from trauma. Placing the palms together provides no assessment data, and diffuse discoloration may be from a fungal infection or an injury.

9. **(3)** Bulla is the correct term. A papule is solid, a vesicle is <1 cm in diameter, and a pustule contains a purulent exudate.

10. **(4)** The appearance of a new mole with high-risk features including irregular border, color changes, and changes in sensation (i.e., pruritis) would necessitate immediate biopsy to rule out melanoma, and/or referral to a dermatologist. Uniform moles, those that are symmetrical and have smooth borders, and those that are not showing signs of change are those that can be followed with annual skin assessments. Seborrheic keratosis is a benign skin growth that usually presents on sun-exposed areas, and appears waxy or "stuck-on," requiring no treatment.

11. **(2)** Under microscope exam, fungal scrapings in KOH solution, will appear as thread-like hyphae crossing cell walls. The other solutions are not indicated for use to identify dermatophytes.

12. **(3)** It is important to remember to apply controls when skin testing the immunocompromised client. Ask the client what diseases they believe they have immunity to, such as measles. Apply the "known" allergen and the skin test to be tested. If the client is unable to mount an immune response at all, the known allergen will not react. By not applying the controls, the nurse practitioner may assume a skin test is negative, when in fact the client's immune system is unable to respond.

Skin Disorders

13. **(3)** Intense itching is characteristic of pediculosis pubis, scabies, and atopic dermatitis. Impetigo starts out as a tender erythematous papule and progresses through a vesicular to a honey-crusted stage with no itching.

14. **(2)** Herpes zoster typically presents with a history of tenderness followed by eruptions and vesicles that follow a dermatome on one side of the body. This is very painful. Other symptoms may include fever, headaches, and malaise.

15. **(2)** Approximately 10–30% of people with psoriasis develop an accompanying form of arthritis called psoriatic arthritis. The other options are dermatologic conditions but are not directly associated with arthritis.

16. **(3)** Stress can aggravate psoriasis. Sunlight helps psoriasis, so it is usually better in the summer. It is not contagious and only about 30% of clients with psoriasis itch.

17. **(2)** These are potentially precancerous lesions and are found in areas of skin exposed to sunlight. Due to the increasing popularity of sunbathing, they can even be seen in persons in the 30- to 50-year-old age group.

18. **(4)** Laboratory studies are not likely to be helpful in evaluation of urticaria. Identification of causes is usually based on history and physical findings. The other statements are true of urticaria.

19. **(3)** Although any one of these skin conditions can affect the skin, particularly of an HIV-positive client, the description relates most closely to Kaposi's sarcoma and warrants a biopsy.

20. **(2)** Option #2 is correct. Despite the name, dyshidrotic eczematous dermatitis (bullous form is called pompholyx), there is no evidence of sweating. Most clients have an atopic history and emotional stress is often a precipitating factor to the appearance of the vesicles. Nummular (discoid) eczema is a chronic, pruritic, inflammatory dermatitis that occurs in the form of coin-shaped plaques composed of grouped small papules and vesicles on an erythematous base. Option #1 describes rosacea. Option #3 describes psoriasis. Option #4 describes a verruca or common wart.

21. **(4)** Delay wound closure until determination of no infection in approximately 24–48 hours. Mouth flora of humans is abundant, and with a bite there is the possibility for heavy bacterial inoculum and potential severe infection. Tetanus is indicated, since there has been no booster in the last 5 years.

22. **(2)** Onychomycosis is the correct term. Hippocratic nails are clubbed nails and fingers associated with chronic heart and lung disorders; koilonychia is a concavity of the nail plate often associated with iron deficiency anemia; and anonychia is a total congenital absence of the nail.

23. **(4)** Excessive sweating can be normal, but the client needs to have a history and physical exam completed to rule out any underlying causes. There are therapies that can be offered. The Drysol is only for use on feet and axilla. Full bathing is not recommended with this solution.

24. **(3)** The assessment describes a seborrheic keratosis. The actinic keratosis is an irregular, rough, scaly, white to erythematous malular lesion found most commonly on the dorsal surface of the hands, arms, neck, and face. It has malignant potential. The basal cell carcinoma is a smooth, round nodule with a pearly gray border and central induration. The senile lentigo are gray-brown, irregular, macular lesions on sun-exposed areas of the face, arms, and hand.

25. **(3)** Herpes zoster (shingles) is a vesicular dermatomal eruption related to a reactivation of latent varicella virus. It increases with advanced age and is characterized by burning pain and paresthesia along one or two dermatomes. This will not cross the midline. This discomfort may be accompanied by fever, malaise, or headache. The vesicular stage lasts 2–3 weeks. The vesicles are very painful and grouped along one or two dermatomes. They are initially clear or blood-filled and become purulent. The area along the dermatome is erythematous, and the vesicles crust and then scab, which may leave hypopigmented scars. The other options discuss painless lesions and are not specific to this prodromal stage.

26. **(4)** These are classic signs of a basal cell carcinoma, also supported by the employment history of the client. Melanoma would be pigmented, compound nevus would not be firm or have telangiectasia, and bullous pemphigoid results in bullous lesions.

27. **(3)** Refer immediately to a dermatologist, since these are highly suspicious findings of a melanoma. Biopsy should never be done on a melanoma and any delay in time could be detrimental to the outcome.

28. **(2)** Oral acyclovir is very effective in reducing intensity and duration of symptoms if started early in the course of the disease. Herpes zoster does not usually recur at regular intervals, but it frequently lasts for several weeks.

29. **(3)** The signs and symptoms presented are classic for Lyme disease, which is transmitted by ticks. Therefore, it would be important to inquire about potential exposure to ticks in the time period prior to the development of signs and symptoms. Exposure to new skin care products would be important if the nurse practitioner suspected an allergic reaction, which is not consistent with the signs and symptoms presented. While a thorough medication history should always be done, it is most likely not going to reveal the cause of the signs and symptoms in this case. Tuberculosis does not present in this manner.

Pharmacology

30. **(1)** The description is consistent with candidiasis intertriginous, which is treated with an antifungal ointment or oral medication. It is not a staphylococcal infection; the area does not need to be kept moist but needs to be kept dry. An antibiotic ointment will not relieve the problem. Herpes zoster is treated with antiviral medications; this is not described as particularly painful, and it is bilateral.

31. **(1)** β-Blockers can exacerbate psoriasis. They are believed to decrease cyclic-AMP–dependent protein kinase (an inhibitor of cell proliferation). There is no known effect with the other stated classifications.

32. **(3)** Acyclovir offers no benefit for postherpetic pain, since this is a treatment for the acute phase during initial eruption of vesicular lesions.

33. **(3)** Systemic treatment with low-dose tetracycline is very effective for rosacea; topical treatment with metronidazole or low-dose hydrocortisone may also be useful. Oral cortisone and antifungal agents are not known to be effective. Topical 5-fluorouracil is used in the treatment of actinic keratosis, a precancerous skin condition.

34. **(1)** The correct answer is 7 mg/kg of lidocaine with epinephrine for adults and 5 mg/kg for lidocaine without epinephrine. Although local anesthetics are commonly used, the maximum allowable doses are rarely emphasized and overdose can result in anaphylactic shock.

35. **(1)** Amitriptyline in low doses has been shown to be effective in treating neuropathic pain. NSAIDs can also be effective in treating the inflammatory component of herpes zoster pain. The most effective nonpharmacologic method of treating pain from shingles is the application of cool compresses. Heat has been shown to exacerbate neuropathic pain in some cases. Antidepressants and anticonvulsants have been shown to be effective adjuvant therapy in the treatment of neuropathic pain.

36. **(2)** Stevens-Johnson syndrome is a severe form of erythema multiforme that can be fatal. The clinical picture of this syndrome is mucous membrane lesions, conjunctival and corneal lesions, fever, malaise, arthralgia, and sloughing of the skin of the hands and feet. The characteristics that differentiate this condition are the eruption of vesicles and ulcerations of the mucosa and the sloughing skin.

37. **(2)** In case of suspected drug reactions, it is recommended the drug be eliminated and documented in the client's record so it is not reintroduced.

38. **(1)** Antiviral therapy with acyclovir 800 mg five times per day for 7 days may speed healing if started within 2–3 days of onset, especially in immunocompromised individuals. Miconazole and clotrimazole are antifungal creams, and the prednisone would only be used to decrease the incidence of postherpetic neuralgia. Prednisone may increase the incidence of disseminated infection.

Endocrine

9

Physical Examination & Diagnostic Tests

1. What is the correct procedure for palpation of a client's thyroid gland?

   1. Stand behind the client, hyperextend the head, and palpate both sides simultaneously.

   2. Have the client lower his chin and lean his head slightly toward the side being evaluated.

   3. Hyperextend the head and have the client lean away from the side being evaluated.

   4. Have the client lean away from the side being examined and take a swallow of water.

2. When a client sips water and swallows, the thyroid gland:

   1. Moves downward and slightly posterior and feels smooth on palpation.

   2. Elongates and enlarges during the swallow and immediately returns to a resting position at the end of palpation.

   3. Moves slightly out during the sipping and backward during the swallowing.

   4. Moves upward during the swallow and feels symmetrical and smooth to palpation.

3. Which question is **not** part of the Carville Diabetic Food Screen?

   1. Has there been a change in the foot since the last evaluation?

   2. What was the last fasting blood glucose and HgbA$_{1c}$?

   3. Does the foot have an abnormal shape?

   4. Are the nails thick, too long, or overgrown?

4. While conducting the interview for a physical examination, the nurse practitioner identifies what finding in the client's history as being commonly associated with thyroid carcinoma?

   1. Family history of thyroid cancer.

   2. History of hyperthyroidism.

   3. Irradiation of the neck.

   4. Smoking for 15 years.

101

5. When doing a physical examination on a client with hyperthyroidism, a common neurologic finding is:

   1. Memory, attention, and problem-solving deficits.

   2. Diminished deep tendon reflexes.

   3. Severe cognitive impairment.

   4. Delusions and psychosis.

6. The treatment goal for glycemic control in a type II diabetic is to achieve and maintain a glycosylated hemoglobin (HgbA$_{1c}$) of:

   1. <10%.

   2. Between 6% and 9%.

   3. <7%.

   4. >8%.

7. Which finding would alert the nurse practitioner that a client might be experiencing a problem with the endocrine system?

   1. Coagulation abnormalities and fatigue.

   2. Growth abnormalities and glucose intolerance.

   3. Hypoxia and jaundice.

   4. Steatorrhea and abdominal distention.

8. The nurse practitioner notes a solitary thyroid nodule on a client during a routine physical examination. The preferred diagnostic test of choice is:

   1. Thyroid scan and antibody level.

   2. Thyroid-stimulating hormone (TSH) and ultrasound.

   3. X-ray of the thyroid.

   4. Fine-needle aspiration biopsy.

9. An adult female client presents to the nurse practitioner's office complaining of fatigue, weakness, and weight gain over the past 4 months. Physical examination reveals an elevated blood pressure, facial and supraclavicular fullness, hirsutism noted on the face, proximal muscle weakness, and facial and truncal distribution of acne.

Appropriate laboratory tests the nurse practitioner should order include:

   1. Antinuclear antibody test (ANA) and rheumatoid factor (RF).

   2. 3-hour glucose tolerance test and lipid profile.

   3. Red blood cell count and a calcium level.

   4. Desamethasone suppression test, a urine free cortisol level and TSH and thyroxine (T$_4$).

10. In evaluating the laboratory values taken from a client with Graves' disease, one should expect:

    1. TSH levels to be increased.

    2. TSH levels to be decreased.

    3. TSH levels to be within normal limits.

    4. T$_4$ levels to be decreased.

11. What information is correct regarding foot screening using a nylon filament (5.07 Semmes-Weinstein)?

    1. Use a 25-gm filament and apply along perimeter of any scar or ulcer tissue.

    2. Apply the filament at a 45-degree angle to the skin surface.

    3. Apply sufficient force for approximately 1.5 seconds to cause the filament to bend.

    4. Slide the filament across the skin and make repetitive contact to each of the ten sites.

Disorders

12. The etiology of type I diabetes can be best described as:

    1. An autosomal dominant genetic disorder.

    2. Autoimmune destruction of the β cells.

    3. Overnutrition and resulting obesity as the major risk factor.

    4. Prevented by exercise, which increases the concentration of insulin receptors.

13. The nurse practitioner should do an annual referral for the client who has had diabetes for over 5 years to:

    1. A cardiologist.

    2. A dietitian.

    3. A vascular surgeon.

    4. An ophthalmologist.

14. Hirsutism presenting in an adult female with normal menstruation and normal plasma androgens is most likely:

    1. An ovarian tumor.

    2. Cushing's syndrome.

    3. Idiopathic.

    4. Polycystic ovary disease.

15. Pathophysiologic reasons for decreased testosterone level develop in the:

    1. Hypothalamus, posterior pituitary, adrenals.

    2. Anterior pituitary, adrenals, testes.

    3. Testes, adrenals, posterior pituitary.

    4. Hypothalamus, anterior pituitary, testes.

16. When counseling a diabetic client on foot care, it is important to emphasize:

    1. Daily foot soaks in warm, soapy water.

    2. Careful daily foot inspections.

    3. Trim corns and calluses regularly.

    4. Trim toenails as close to the bed of the nail as possible and round nails to avoid scratching other toes.

17. An adult client presents to the nurse practitioner for evaluation of polyuria, polydypsia, and weight loss. Which lab result would require immediate intervention by the nurse practitioner?

    1. An HgbA$_{1c}$ of 14%.

    2. A serum glucose of 150 mg/dl.

    3. An HgbA$_{1c}$ of 6.0%.

    4. A serum glucose of 65 mg/dl.

18. An adult client is being evaluated for hypoglycemia due to a blood sugar of 58 mg/dl on a screening SMAC-20. The nurse practitioner can begin his/her differential diagnosis by:

    1. Deciding if the hypoglycemia is fasting or postprandial.

    2. Ascertaining if it is related to alcohol use.

    3. Deciding if the client has other medical problems.

    4. Reassuring the client that it is a benign problem.

19. An older adult male client complains of lethargy, cold intolerance, weight gain, and yellowing of the palms. The most important laboratory study ordered by the nurse practitioner in diagnosing this condition is:

    1. Complete blood count (CBC).

    2. Liver enzymes.

    3. Thyroid panel.

    4. Cardiac enzymes.

20. A middle-aged normally healthy female presents for evaluation of intermittent palpitations. She originally thought it was related to job stress. She also reports mood variability, tremulousness, difficulty falling asleep, and a 10-lb weight loss despite a normal appetite. She feels warm most of the time and wonders if she is perimenopausal. She has no history of heart disease. The objective data that would yield the most useful information would be:

    1. Electrocardiogram (ECG).

    2. TSH, free T$_4$.

    3. Electrolytes.

    4. Holter monitor.

21. An adult client presents to the clinic complaining of fatigue, weakness, weight gain in spite of lack of appetite, and feelings of depression. Her physical examination reveals that she is an obese, alert female with thinning hair, bilateral chest puffiness, increased facial hair, supraclavicular fat pad, thin arms and legs, purple striae on abdomen, and multiple ecchymotic areas on extremities. Vital signs are blood pressure (BP) 158/96, pulse 88, respirations 22. Laboratory studies are fasting blood sugar (FBS) 200 mg/dl, electrolyte panel within normal limits (WNL) except for potassium (3.0 mEq/L), hemoglobin 11.8 gm, and hematocrit 34%. The nurse practitioner suspects:

    1. Addison's disease.

    2. Pheochromocytoma.

    3. Cushing's syndrome.

    4. Hypoaldosteronism.

22. Clinical findings in a client with hypothyroidism includes:

    1. Hyperactive bowel sounds.

    2. Oily skin and acne.

    3. Postural tremors of the hands.

    4. Edema of face and eye lids.

23. An adult male reports anxiety, tremulousness, headaches, palpitations, and sweating 2–4 hours after eating. Physical exam is normal. No labs are currently available. No history of any medical conditions is noted. The most likely diagnosis is:

    1. Dumping syndrome.

    2. Hypoglycemia.

    3. Alcohol abuse.

    4. Hyperthyroidism.

24. Which of the following is the most likely etiology for hypercalcemia in the medically well asymptomatic adult?

    1. Hyperthyroidism.

    2. Hyperparathyroidism.

    3. Hyperpituitarism.

    4. Hypothryoidism.

25. A middle-aged male with no previous medical history presents with a 30-lb weight gain in 2.5 months. He denies any medication use or allergies. He was currently laid off of a very active job and has been sedentary. Physical exam shows BP 172/111, central obesity, and FBS 200 mg/dl. The most likely cause of client's weight gain is:

    1. Cushing's disease.

    2. Hypothyroidism.

    3. Depression.

    4. Diabetes.

26. A middle-aged female accompanied by her daughter to the clinic presents with agitation, confusion, fever, tachycardia, and diaphoresis. The daughter states these symptoms were preceded by nausea, vomiting, and abdominal pain. There is no history of cardiac disease, diabetes, or substance abuse. She was started on some "anti drug" 2 weeks ago and is scheduled for some kind of throat surgery next week (per daughter). Based upon this history, the nurse practitioner immediately orders:

    1. TSH and T$_4$.

    2. Urinalysis.

    3. Spinal tap.

    4. Computed tomography of head.

27. A 45-year-old female client presents to the nurse practitioner's office complaining of a 6-month history of fatigue, 15-lb weight gain, lethargy, an inability to tolerate cold temperatures, forgetfulness, hair loss, and constipation. Physical findings include dry coarse skin, periorbital edema and puffy facies, bradycardia, hyporeflexia and muscle weakness, and a smooth goitrous thyroid. The nurse practitioner would make the diagnosis of:

    1. Congestive heart failure (CHF).

    2. Diabetes mellitus (DM).

    3. Hypothyroidism.

    4. Thyroid cancer.

28. A diabetic client has been taking 6 U of regular insulin and 12 U of Lente insulin in the morning. In the evening she has been taking 3 U of regular insulin and 8 U of Lente insulin. The client has been monitoring her blood glucose levels and she shows the nurse practitioner the following chart.

	7 AM	Noon	5 PM	Bedtime
Monday	100	76	98	109
Tuesday	119	75	88	110
Wednesday	119	66	86	100
Thursday	123	70	111	122
Friday	128	60	99	110

The nurse practitioner adjusts the client's insulin by:

1. Increasing the regular insulin.
2. Decreasing the regular insulin.
3. Decreasing the Lente insulin.
4. Increasing both insulins.

29. The role of the nurse practitioner in the initial management of a client with a thyroid nodule involves:

1. Referring the client to an endocrinologist for further evaluation.
2. Obtaining a fine-needle aspiration (FNA) of the nodule and sending to cytology.
3. Ordering an ultrasound and thyroid scan.
4. Ordering levothyroxine (Synthroid) to reduce the size of the nodule.

30. When teaching a diabetic client about "sick day" guidelines, the nurse practitioner explains:

1. Stop measuring blood glucose and only check urine for ketones.
2. Do not take your usual dose of insulin at the usual time.
3. Be sure to take metformin (Glucophage) and acarbose (Precose), even if nausea and vomiting are present.
4. Administer extra doses of regular insulin according to instructions for blood glucose levels >240 mg/dl.

31. An adult female client presents to the clinic with complaints of nervousness, tremulousness, palpitations, heat intolerance, fatigue, weight loss, and polyphagia. After a complete history and physical examination, along with thyroid function tests, the nurse practitioner makes the diagnosis of hyperthyroidism, recognizing that the most common cause of this condition is:

1. Thyroid cancer.
2. Graves' disease.
3. Pituitary adenoma.
4. Postpartum thyroiditis.

32. A older adult male client presents to the nurse practitioner's office stating that he found a lump in his neck while shaving. Physical examination reveals a firm, 2-cm nodule that is fixed and nontender located on the right lobe of the thyroid gland. Right posterior cervical lymphadenopathy is also noted. The nurse practitioner should:

1. Order a TSH level to determine thyroid function, and refer the client to a surgeon for a fine-needle biopsy of the nodule.
2. No intervention is necessary at this time—schedule a follow-up visit in 6 months.
3. Prescribe levothyroxine (Synthroid) 0.1 mg PO daily and schedule a 6-week follow-up visit.
4. The client's thyroid should immediately be ablated with radioactive iodine, and the patient should be referred to an endocrinologist.

33. A client with Graves' disease is placed on radioactive I^{131} therapy. When teaching about this treatment, it is important for the nurse practitioner to include what information?

    1. Clients are highly radioactive for approximately 7 days following treatment and need to be isolated.

    2. Clients should not become pregnant during or after receiving this therapy because of the teratogenic effects to the fetus that occur due to chromosomal abnormalities.

    3. Clients may become hypothyroid after this treatment, and will therefore need to have regular TSH and T$_4$ levels drawn, with the potential for thyroid hormone replacement therapy.

    4. This therapy is contraindicated in clients with cardiac disease.

Pharmacology

34. The nurse practitioner has ordered a client with type II diabetes to take glipizide (Glucotrol) 10 mg PO bid. In evaluating the medication's effectiveness, it is thought to reduce blood glucose by:

    1. Delaying the cellular uptake of potassium and insulin.

    2. Stimulating insulin release from the pancreas.

    3. Decreasing the body's need for and utilization of insulin at the cellular level.

    4. Interfering with the absorption and metabolism of fats and carbohydrates.

35. The nurse practitioner would expect which symptom to be a side effect of metformin (Glucophage)?

    1. Gastrointestinal upset.

    2. Photophobia.

    3. Hyperglycemia.

    4. Skin eruptions.

36. A client is receiving antithyroid medication. The nurse practitioner understands that:

    1. Lifelong daily treatment is necessary to keep TSH levels within the normal range.

    2. Antithyroid medications do not cross the placenta.

    3. The medications are somewhat expensive and have serious cardiac and hematologic side effects.

    4. Clients remain on the medications for 1–2 years and then the medication is gradually withdrawn.

37. When prescribing an antihypertensive medication for a type II diabetic client with hypertension, the drug classifications that would tend to reduce insulin sensitivity are:

    1. Diuretics and calcium channel blockers.

    2. Diuretics and β-blockers.

    3. Calcium channel blockers and angiotensin converting enzyme (ACE) inhibitors.

    4. α-Blockers and ACE inhibitors.

38. An adult female sees the nurse practitioner with a complaint of cold intolerance, fatigue, dry skin, weight gain, and heavy menstrual periods. Upon physical exam, she is found to have a pulse of 58 bpm, a "waxy" sallow complexion, and a firm goiter. The TSH level is checked and found to be 176 mU/L. The best treatment choice for this client is:

    1. Begin levothyroxine (Synthroid) at 0.025 mg PO qd and repeat TSH test in 2 weeks.

    2. Administer a "loading dose" of oral levothyroxine (Synthroid), as well as starting a full replacement dose of levothyroxine (Synthroid).

    3. Administer a "loading dose" of IV levothyroxine (Synthroid), and start on a half replacement dose of levothyroxine (Synthroid).

    4. Begin levothyroxine (Synthroid) at a dose of 0.1 mg PO qd and recheck TSH level in 6 weeks.

39. The nurse practitioner is seeing a 64-year-old man for a preoperative evaluation and exam. He is hospitalized with severe coronary artery disease and scheduled to undergo coronary artery bypass grafting. Physical exam finds the client to have mild facial puffiness, hoarse voice, and dry skin. Thyroid function tests were done and the client was found to have a TSH level of 34 mU/L. The recommended treatment for this client is:

1. Give a loading IV bolus of levothyroxine (Synthroid), 0.5 mg, and proceed with surgery.

2. Cancel surgery and send him home to begin a dose of oral levothyroxine (Synthroid), 0.1 mg. Instruct him that surgery will be rescheduled as soon as he is euthyroid.

3. Begin oral levothyroxine (Synthroid) and monitor in the hospital until euthyroid.

4. Proceed with surgery and treat hypothyroidism postoperatively.

40. The nurse practitioner is seeing an obese, middle-aged female client for a follow-up visit. She was diagnosed as a type II diabetic 3 months ago and started on a regimen of diet and exercise. Today her fasting plasma glucose is 200 mg/dl and HgbA$_{1c}$ is 10%. She has lost 2 lb. She reports her home monitoring glucose has ranged from 180–300 mg/dl. The rest of her chemistry profile is WNL. The best treatment choice for this client is:

1. Review her diet and exercise plan, increase exercise regimen, and reduce caloric intake. Schedule her for another follow-up in 3 months.

2. Start her on sliding-scale insulin and instruct her on recording glucose and insulin requirements. Schedule her to return in 1 week to be re-evaluated for long-acting insulin.

3. Initiate treatment with metformin (Glucophage).

4. Initiate treatment with an oral sulfonylurea agent (i.e., glyburide).

41. What is associated with chronic overtreatment with levothyroxine (Synthroid)?

1. Tachycardia.

2. Severe osteoporosis.

3. Insomnia.

4. Sweating.

42. A middle-aged male presents for a diabetes follow-up exam. He has been in food health without identified complications of diabetes. His FBS is 100 and his personal records indicate that he is taking insulin in the prescribed amounts and times. Vital signs are BP 142/98, pulse 80, respirations 20. Today's plan would include:

1. Begin diuretics and a β-blocker.

2. Begin ACE inhibitor and consider a diuretic.

3. Get an ECG and chest x-ray.

4. Return for BP check in 5–7 days.

43. An adult male has recently been started on insulin. His regimen is two daily injections with two thirds of total daily insulin in morning and one third in the evening. He is using the 70/30 mixture of intermediate- and short-acting insulin in both injections. He presents for a follow-up visit with his log of blood glucose. The nurse practitioner notes that his recorded glucose levels before the evening meal have been in the 60–70 mg/dl range. Other checks during the day are in the 100–120 mg/dl range. What adjustments need to be made?

1. Intermediate insulin, change 70/30 combination to self-mix, and reduce AM intermediate dose.

2. Regular insulin, reduce AM dose of 70/30.

3. Intermediate insulin, reduce AM dose of 70/30.

4. Regular insulin, change 70/30 to self-mix, and reduce AM regular dose.

44. A client on antithyroid drug therapy for hyperthyroidism presents with complaints of palpitations and dry mouth for the past 2 days. He has had a cough and cold symptoms for the past 3 days that he has been treating with over-the-counter medications. Which medication would the nurse practitioner encourage the client to avoid?

    1. Benzocaine (Chloraseptic) lozenge.

    2. Guaifenesin (Robitussin).

    3. Ibuprofen (Advil).

    4. Pseudoephedrine (Sudafed).

45. What is the most frequent complaint of clients who use insulin pumps?

    1. Problems with elevated glucose after changing the catheter-type (nonneedle) infusion set.

    2. Skin and site problems related to dressing adhesive not sticking, redness and pain at infusion site, and allergic response to tape.

    3. Mechanical problems with the pump's digital readout.

    4. Understanding "sick day" management modifications.

46. The nurse practitioner understands that troglitazone (Rezulin) is indicated for:

    1. Prenatal clients with gestational diabetes.

    2. Brittle type I clients.

    3. Type II clients who require insulin who have poor glycemic control and insulin resistance.

    4. Type II clients to prevent the rapid postprandial blood glucose surges by delaying carbohydrate absorption.

47. An older client with a history of hypertension and coronary bypass surgery has been diagnosed with hypothyroidism. Appropriate medication management is:

    1. Levothyroxine (Synthroid) 0.1 mg daily and return in 6 weeks for follow-up.

    2. Desiccated thyroid extract 2 grains daily and return in 6 weeks for follow-up.

    3. Levothyroxine (Synthroid) 0.025 mg daily for 6 weeks with slow gradual increase in dosage every 4—6 weeks until therapeutic level is obtained.

    4. Methimazole (Tapazole) 15 mg daily in three divided doses, gradually increasing dose every 4 weeks until a therapeutic level is obtained.

48. An adult is newly diagnosed as being hypothyroid and is placed on levothyroxine (Synthroid) 0.1 mg PO daily. Follow-up by the nurse practitioner should include:

    1. No follow-up visits are necessary.

    2. The client should return to the clinic in 4–6 weeks to evaluate the response to treatment, including a TSH level, and to determine if there has been symptomatic improvement.

    3. The client should have weekly levothyroxine levels drawn.

    4. The client should have monthly CBCs while on levothyroxine (Synthroid), because the medication has been found to be myelosuppressive.

49. Classes of medications commonly used to treat hyperthyroid conditions include:

    1. Antibiotics and corticosteroids.

    2. ACE inhibitors, anxiolytics, and antithyroid medications.

    3. β-Blockers, nonsteroidal anti-inflammatory drugs (NSAIDs), and antithyroid medications.

    4. Calcium channel blockers and corticosteroids.

50. A client with hypothyroidism has been receiving daily levothyroxine (Synthroid) for 3 weeks. The client now presents with complaints of chest pain. The nurse practitioner should:

    1. Discontinue the levothyroxine (Synthroid), as this is a contraindication to continuing this medication.

    2. Schedule the client for a stress test.

    3. Decrease the dose of levothyroxine (Synthroid), order an ECG, and consult with a collaborating physician.

4. Prescribe an anxiolytic agent for the client.

51. Clients started on metformin (Glucophage) need to be monitored closely for the following potential side effect:

    1. Significant increase in weight.

    2. Elevation of low-density lipoprotein (LDL) cholesterol level.

    3. Lactic acidosis.

    4. Increase in insulin requirements.

52. The nurse practitioner understands that lispro insulin (Humalog):

    1. Can be injected just prior to eating.

    2. Is less costly than regular insulin.

    3. Increases the likelihood of late postprandial hypoglycemia due to its length of action.

    4. Has a long-term safety profile and does not cause any teratogenic effects.

9 Answers & Rationales

Physical Examination & Diagnostic Tests

1. **(2)** When examining the thyroid, it is important to have the client relax the sternocleidomastoid muscles. This can be done by having the client lean toward the side being evaluated.

2. **(4)** The thyroid gland is fixed to the trachea and thus ascends during swallowing. This assists the nurse practitioner to distinguish thyroid structures from other neck masses. The gland's size, degree of enlargement, consistency, surface characteristics, and presence of nodules or bruits are noted during the examination.

3. **(2)** There are five questions to the Carville Diabetic Foot Screen. They are as follows: Has there been a change in the foot since the last evaluation? Is there a foot ulcer now or history of foot ulcer? Does the foot have an abnormal shape? Is there weakness in the ankle or foot? Are the nails thick, too long, or overgrown?

4. **(3)** Papillary carcinoma is the most common form of thyroid cancer. It is associated with a history of exposure to radiation. Family history, history of hyperthyroidism, and smoking are not considered significant risk factors for this malignancy.

5. **(1)** The high level of thyroid hormone affects the nervous system, causing sympathomimetic symptoms such as brisk deep tendon reflexes, fine, rapid tremor of the hands, restlessness, irritability, insomnia, dreams, nightmares, and rarely severe cognitive impairment and psychosis.

6. **(3)** The American Diabetes Association (ADA) recommends <7% as an important treatment goal to decrease risk of long-term complications. A lab result of >8% $HgbA_{1c}$ is an indication that action needs to be taken, either by a change of medication or a reinforcement of education.

7. **(2)** Growth abnormalities are associated with anterior pituitary dysfunction and glucose intolerance with diabetes due to pancreas dysfunction. Coagulation abnormalities and fatigue would be associated with hematologic dysfunction. Hypoxia would be associated with oxygenation problems and jaundice with liver or biliary problems. Steatorrhea is associated with malabsorption syndrome and cystic fibrosis.

8. **(4)** Although the primary care provider may obtain TSH and antibody levels, the preferred diagnostic tool for the endocrinologist is the fine-needle aspiration biopsy. Scans, sonography, and x-ray tests can be used in initial screening; they do not assist in the determination of whether the nodule is malignant or not. The aspirate is sent for cytology and interpretation.

9. **(4)** The dexamethasone suppression test is the best screening test for Cushing's disease and a 24-hour urine free cortisol level is the best confirmatory testing for Cushing's. TSH

and T_4 levels may also be appropriate to rule out a thyroid condition, as some of the client's signs and symptoms are consistent with thyroid dysfunction. ANA and RF are ordered when rheumatoid arthritis or systemic lupus erythematosus is suspected; this client's clinical picture is not consistent with these conditions. A red blood cell count would be done to rule out anemia, a potential problem for this client based on the history of fatigue, but the rest of the clinical picture points to something more than anemia. There are no clinical findings to support blood for a calcium level being drawn.

10. **(2)** TSH levels should be decreased in a client with Graves' disease, because thyroid-stimulating immunoglobulins bind to TSH receptors, which increase T_4 synthesis and release, subsequently suppressing TSH levels.

11. **(3)** The correct procedure is to use a 10-gm (5.07 Semmes-Weinstein) filament and apply to ten sites on the foot (one on the top of the foot, nine on the heel, sole, and toes). The filament is to be applied perpendicular (90-degree angle) to the skin surface and have sufficient force applied for 1.5 seconds to cause the filament to bend. The filament should not be allowed to slide across the skin or make repetitive contact to each test site. Randomizing the selection of test sites (starting with big toe→heel→instep area→little toe→etc.) and the time between successive tests helps to reduce client guessing as does having the client close his/her eyes.

Disorders

12. **(2)** Type I diabetes is caused by destruction of the β cells mediated through the immune system. The other three choices refer to type II diabetes.

13. **(4)** An annual eye exam with the pupils dilated should be done by a specialist who can recognize subtle abnormalities. Although the other referrals can offer important contributions to diabetic care, it would be on an as-needed basis rather than annually.

14. **(3)** Because of the normal menstrual periods and androgen plasma level, this would be considered idiopathic. Diseases related to the ovaries would cause changes in the menstrual cycle, and with Cushing's syndrome they would have adrenal androgen overproduction.

15. **(4)** Testosterone production is regulated by the hypothalamic-pituitary-testicular (HPT) axis. Thus abnormalities in any one of these areas can affect the production of testosterone.

16. **(2)** It is important for diabetics to have their feet inspected daily either per self-exam or by a family member. Feet should be washed daily but never soaked. Corns and calluses should be cared for by a professional. Nails should be trimmed straight across to avoid injury to the nail beds.

17. **(1)** The normal serum glucose for adults ranges from 70–120 mg/dl. Diabetic acidosis is not of a concern until the glucose is >300 mg/dl. An $HgbA_{1c}$ of >8.0% indicates poor glucose control over the past few months.

18. **(1)** True hypoglycemia can be organized around whether it is fasting or postprandial. Postprandial hypoglycemia may be caused by early adult-onset diabetes or postgastrectomy syndrome. Fasting hypoglycemia is most commonly caused by excessive doses of insulin or sulfonylureas.

19. **(3)** The symptoms are suggestive of hypothyroidism and thyroid studies (TSH) would be the most useful.

20. **(2)** This middle-aged female client presents with many of the classic symptoms of early hyperthyroidism. A suppressed TSH level with an elevated free T_4 level establish the diagnosis of hyperthyroidism.

21. **(3)** The client's physical findings and habitus along with hypertension and hypokalemia are associated with Cushing's syndrome, which is a state of excessive cortisol production due to a pituitary tumor. A Cushing's-like syndrome is often associated with prolonged glucocorticoid administration. Obesity is the primary finding in Cushing's syndrome, along with the "moon face," "dowager" or "buffalo hump," truncal obesity, hirsutism in women, and impotence and loss of body hair in men. Addison's disease is characterized by hyperkalemia, hyponatremia, hypoglycemia, anemia, and hypercalcemia. Clients with hypoaldosteronism (impaired renin secretion) have hyperkalemia. Pheochromocytoma would be in the differential diagnosis of this client because of the hypertension; the other findings are not consistent with this diagnosis.

22. **(4)** Accumulation of hyaluronic acid in interstitial tissues increases capillary permeability to albumin and accounts for the interstitial edema that is noted in the face and eyelids of individuals with hypothyroidism.

23. **(2)** While alcohol abuse may be a cause for hypoglycemia, this client is presenting with classic symptoms of postprandial hypoglycemia. It would be a good idea to assess for alcohol abuse as the etiology of the diagnosis of hypoglycemia.

24. **(2)** Hyperparathyroidism accounts for hypercalcemia in more than 60% of clients and is likely to be the explanation for elevated serum calcium levels.

25. **(1)** While option #3 may explain the weight gain, Cushing's disease is correct for the constellation of symptoms of rapid weight gain, hypertension, and elevated blood sugar. These symptoms suggest adrenal dysfunction. Serum cortisol and adrenocorticotropic hormone levels should be checked.

26. **(1)** This woman is likely experiencing the life-threatening syndrome that can occur in decompensated hyperthyroidism. The clues were her symptom presentation and progression, the new "anti drug," and upcoming throat surgery.

27. **(3)** The symptoms describe the classic presentation of a client with hypothyroidism. A client with CHF would exhibit jugular venous distention, rales, and peripheral edema. The criteria for diagnosing DM are polydipsia, polyphagia, polyuria, and weight loss. Thyroid cancer commonly presents without physical symptoms, and often the only physical finding is a hard, fixed nodule on the thyroid gland.

28. **(2)** The client's blood sugars are low around lunch time, which is when the regular insulin is peaking (3–4 hours), so a reduction in the regular insulin would help this problem.

29. **(1)** The nurse practitioner's role in primary care for a client with a thyroid nodule involves initially the early identification of the thyroid nodule on physical examination, referring the client to an endocrinologist for further evaluation, and possibly obtaining some preliminary TSH and antibody testing. The endocrinologist performs the FNA. Levothyroxine may or may not be used to diminish the size of the nodule based on the findings from the FNA and the endocrinologist's chosen treatment plan.

30. **(4)** It is important for the diabetic client to understand that when they are sick their blood glucose level will probably increase, even when they are not eating. It is most important they monitor blood glucose levels every 2–4 hours and check urine for ketones, if the glucose level is above 240 mg/dl. In Option #3, these medications *should not* be given until the client's nausea and vomiting have subsided and they have resumed a normal diet (blood glucose monitoring is important during this period of time.)

31. **(2)** Graves' disease, an autoimmune condition also known as diffuse toxic goiter, is the most common cause of hyperthyroidism in this age group. Much less common causes include cancer of the thyroid, adenoma of the pituitary gland, and postpartum (or silent) thyroiditis.

32. **(1)** The TSH should be ordered to determine whether the client is euthyroid, hypothyroid, or hyperthyroid. The client should also be sent to an endocrinologist/

surgeon because all nodules of the thyroid should be biopsied to rule out malignancy. Watching and waiting is inappropriate without having a biopsy performed. Thyroid hormone replacement therapy would only be indicated in those clients found to be hypothyroid and in whom thyroid cancer has been ruled out. Thyroid ablation may be indicated in clients whose fine-needle biopsy results are positive for thyroid cancer, but this cannot be determined without a surgeon's intervention.

33. **(3)** Hypothyroidism often follows this treatment, with 50% of clients requiring replacement therapy in the first year, and nearly 100% within 10 years. For this reason, regular monitoring of TSH and T_4 levels should be performed. Clients emit a small amount of radioactivity after receiving the dose used to treat this condition, and do not require isolation for 7 days. Radioactive iodine is very safe, without an increased risk of gonad chromosomal abnormalities; therefore, there is no contraindication to becoming pregnant after therapy, although clients are counseled to avoid pregnancy while on treatment and to avoid children and pregnant women after receiving the oral ablation dose. This therapy is recommended for those clients who have cardiac disease associated with their thyroid condition.

Pharmacology

34. **(2)** The sulfonylureas reduce blood glucose by stimulating insulin release from the pancreas. Also, over a long period of time, they may actually increase insulin effects at the cellular level and decrease glucose production by the liver. This is the reason why sulfonylureas are used in type II diabetics who still have a functioning pancreas.

35. **(1)** Anorexia, nausea, and a metallic taste in the mouth are common side effects. Over time, the gastrointestinal (GI) symptoms subside and can be relieved by taking the medication with food or by starting at a lower dose.

36. **(4)** Antithyroid medications (propylthiouracil or methimazole) are relatively inexpensive and do cross the placenta. The client remains on the medication for 1–2 years with the hope of a permanent remission of symptoms when it is withdrawn.

37. **(2)** Both of these drug classifications tend to reduce insulin sensitivity and can cause hyperglycemia. ACE inhibitors, calcium channel blockers, and selective α-blockers are metabolically neutral or some may actually have a beneficial effect.

38. **(4)** The client's symptoms indicate hypothyroidism along with the elevated TSH; the normal range for TSH is 0.5–4.7 mU/L. Full replacement dose of levothyroxine (Synthroid) should be started based on the client's age, and the TSH level should be checked in 6 weeks, since it can take that long for a given dose to become effective. Loading doses should never be given except for coma, which is treated by IV medication in the hospital.

39. **(4)** Coronary clients found to be mildly to moderately hypothyroid can safely undergo urgent surgery (including bypass procedures) without prior replacement. The rate of complications is no greater than for nonhypothyroid clients and the cardiac risks are lessened compared to initiating replacement therapy preoperatively.

40. **(3)** Metformin is a better option in an obese client, as metformin is frequently associated with weight loss, while sulfonylureas may actually cause a weight gain. Insulin is also not a good choice, as it is an overly aggressive approach with mildly elevated glucose. Clients also tend to be less receptive to treatment requiring injections. Diet and exercise were unsuccessful, and the longer her blood sugar remains elevated, the greater the risk for end-organ damage.

41. **(2)** All but osteoporosis are related to acute overdosage of levothyroxine and can be relieved by omitting the dose for 3 days and then starting on a lower dose.

42. **(4)** In order to initiate treatment for elevated BP, it is recommended that three elevated readings be recorded on three separate occasions. There is no evidence to suggest that this client had an elevated BP on prior visits.

43. **(1)** This is the best answer, as the AM intermediate dose affects the glucose level before dinner. Altering the regular insulin will affect levels before lunch and before bedtime, and these levels are OK. In order to reduce the intermediate insulin while maintaining the level of regular insulin, the client will need to self-mix the intermediate and regular insulin using less of the intermediate.

44. **(4)** Pseudoephedrine (Sudafed) and other decongestant medications that contain sympathomimetics lead to adverse reactions of central nervous system (CNS) overstimulation, palpitations, headache, hypertension, nervousness, and the like. Robitussin in combination (i.e., Robitussin-CF [dextromethorphan, phenylpropanolamine, guaifenesin] or Robitussin-PE [pseudoephedrine, guaifenesin] can also cause palpitations and CNS overstimulation. Robitussin-DM (dextromethorphan, guaifenesin) usually has predominantly GI upset, drowsiness, headache, and rash as adverse effects.

45. **(2)** Infusion site problems and skin irritation are by far the most frequent complaints of a client who uses an insulin pump. Often, it is a major reason for the client's decision to discontinue using the pump. Clients also find it is more time consuming and costly. However, the Diabetes Control and Complications Trial (DCCT, 1993) reported a reduced risk of microvascular complications when insulin pumps and multiple daily injections were used.

46. **(3)** Prenatal clients are managed with insulin, not an insulin sensitizer. Troglitazone (Rezulin) acts by decreasing peripheral insulin resistance in skeletal muscle and adipose tissue without enhancing insulin secretion. It improves glucose tolerance and decreases insulin resistance in insulin-requiring type II

diabetics. Option #4 refers to the action of α-glucosidase inhibitors (e.g., acarbose [Precose] and miglitol [Glyset]).

47. **(3)** Older clients, especially with heart disease, need to be started on the smallest amount of thyroid medication replacement (0.025 mg, not 0.1 mg) and gradually increased until a therapeutic level is achieved. If replaced too quickly, the heart may decompensate. Two grains of thyroid extract is too much. Methimazole (Tapazole) is an antithyroid medication and is indicated for treatment of hyperthyroidism.

48. **(2)** The response to therapy is based on clinical symptomatology and a TSH assay approximately 4–6 weeks after initiation of therapy. This is continued until a stable dose is obtained. TSH and a free T_4 level are the two standard tests that can be used to monitor the status of the thyroid; a levothyroxine level cannot be drawn. Levothyroxine (Synthroid) is not a myelosuppressive agent.

49. **(3)** β-Blockers are initially prescribed to reduce the signs and symptoms of the condition and to reduce the peripheral conversion of T_4 to triiodothyronine (T_3); NSAIDs are indicated for reducing inflammation associated with thyroiditis; and antithyroid medications, such as propylthiouracil (PTU) or methimazole (Tapazole) are used to treat severe hyperthyroidism. Corticosteroids are sometimes used in the treatment of thyroiditis, but the remaining classes of medications are not routinely used in the management of hyperthyroidism (namely, antibiotics, ACE inhibitors, calcium channel blockers, and anxiolytics).

50. **(3)** Decreasing the dose of levothyroxine and evaluating the cardiac status of the patient are the appropriate interventions in this situation, in addition to involving the collaborating physician as to further work-up. Discontinuing the thyroid replacement would be inappropriate because the client remains hypothyroid and requires therapy to continue for life. An anxiolytic may be a helpful adjunct, but it is certainly not appropriate as the sole intervention, as it ignores the cardiac symptoms.

51. **(3)** Lactic acidosis is a potentially severe and fatal reaction to metformin. Metformin does not contribute to weight gain; it often helps with weight loss, and decreases LDL, triglycerides levels, and insulin requirements.

52. **(1)** Lispro (Humalog) is the first analog of human insulin that has several advantages over regular insulin, including a more rapid onset and shorter duration of action. It reaches peak activity in 1–2 hours and has a 4-hour duration, as compared to 6–8 hours of regular insulin. It is convenient for many clients, as it can be injected immediately before eating (10–15 minutes). Because it has been on the market only since June 1996, there is no long-term safety profile established and the teratogenicity is unknown. In addition, it is more expensive than insulin and some third-party payers may not reimburse clients.

10

Musculoskeletal

Physical Examination & Diagnostic Tests

1. A goniometer is used in a routine physical examination of geriatric clients. The nurse practitioner utilizes this tool to determine:

   1. The strength of the muscles in the extremities.
   2. The degree of joint flexion and extension.
   3. The range of motion of the extremities.
   4. The point of joint flexion that is painful.

2. The nurse practitioner places a client in the prone position with the knee flexed to 90 degrees. The tibia is firmly opposed to the femur by exerting downward pressure on the foot. The leg is rotated externally and internally. If locking of the knee occurs, this is accurately called a positive:

   1. Drawer sign.
   2. McMurray's test.
   3. Apley's sign.
   4. Bulge sign.

3. A client has numbness and tingling in the thumb and first two fingers when pressing the backs of the hands together (flexes wrists at 90 degrees) for 60 seconds. This is a positive:

   1. Tinel's sign.
   2. Drawer sign.
   3. McMurray's test.
   4. Phalen's maneuver.

4. What is the name of the sign that occurs when compressing the suprapatella pouch back against the femur and feeling for fluid entering the spaces?

   1. Drawer sign.
   2. Kernig's sign.
   3. Balloon sign.
   4. Bulge sign.

5. De Quervain's disease can be diagnosed in part by a positive:

   1. Finkelstein's sign.

   2. Tinel's sign.

   3. Phalen's maneuver.

   4. Lachman's sign.

6. The primary examination techniques to use for assessing the musculoskeletal system are:

   1. Inspection and percussion.

   2. Auscultation and palpation.

   3. Inspection and palpation.

   4. Palpation and percussion.

7. What can the nurse practitioner use to confirm a diagnosis of polymyalgia rheumatica?

   1. Chest radiograph.

   2. Serum protein electrophoresis.

   3. Corticosteroid challenge.

   4. Erythrocyte sedimentation rate (ESR).

8. When performing an assessment, the nurse practitioner understands that the metacarpophalangeal joints (MCP) are frequently involved with:

   1. Gout.

   2. Rheumatic fever.

   3. Rheumatoid arthritis.

   4. Osteoarthritis.

9. In the evaluation of polyneuropathy, which study would not be recommended?

   1. Sedimentation rate.

   2. Complete blood count (CBC).

   3. Glycosylated hemoglobin A_{1c} (HgbA$_{1c}$).

   4. Electromyography (EMG).

10. In accurately assessing a client who reports back injury, it is critical to question:

    1. Family history of back problems.

    2. Previous injury.

3. Personal history of chronic illness.

4. Mechanism of injury.

11. Tinel's sign and Phalen's maneuver are used in identifying a common workplace illness that the nurse practitioner recognizes as:

    1. Lateral epicondylitis.

    2. Carpel tunnel syndrome.

    3. Dupuytren's disease.

    4. Thoracic outlet syndrome.

12. An elderly client complains of fatigue, weakness, lightheadedness, and anorexia. He also complains of hot, swollen proximal interphalangeal (PIP) and metacarpophalangeal (MCP) joints. These symptoms occurred 5 months ago and have reoccurred a few days ago. Which lab findings would be most conclusive of these assessments?

    1. Mean corpuscular volume (MCV) 104, low serum ferritin.

    2. MCV 92, high serum ferritin.

    3. Elevation in the uric acid level.

    4. Elevation in the white blood cell (WBC) count.

13. In the talar tilt test:

    1. The examiner grasps the tibia with one hand and the heel with the other hand. The client's foot is held while backward pressure is applied to the tibia. Laxity of the ligament is graded.

    2. The ankle is gently inverted and laxity of the ligament is graded.

    3. The examiner passively inverts, everts, dorsiflexes, and plantar flexes the ankle.

    4. The client actively inverts, everts, dorsiflexes, and plantar flexes the ankle.

14. Varus pressure on a knee that is slightly flexed (30 degrees) tests:

    1. Medial collateral ligament stability.

    2. Lateral collateral ligament stability.

    3. Medial cruciate ligament stability.

    4. Lateral meniscus tear.

Disorders

15. A middle-aged male client presents with a complaint of waking up yesterday morning with his big toe swollen and painful. The client reports he has never had anything like this before and has not had any previous health problems. Physical exam finds his big toe to be red, hot, and tender in the joint with inflammation extending into the surrounding tissue. His temperature is 99.8°F and WBCs are mildly elevated. Needle aspiration of joint fluid reveals urate crystals. The best treatment choice the nurse practitioner could recommend for this client is:

    1. Bed rest, very-low-calorie diet, and increase fluid intake.

    2. Initiate pharmacologic therapy with allopurinal (Zyloprim) 200 mg PO qd and educate client on the need to remain on this medication for maintenance therapy once symptoms resolve.

    3. Start on naproxen (Naprosyn) 500 mg PO tid and instruct client to continue full-dose until symptoms resolve and then taper and discontinue over 72 hours.

    4. Administer an injection of intra-articular corticosteroid therapy to the affected joint.

16. The nurse practitioner realizes that the most common cause of shoulder pain is:

    1. Frozen shoulder.

    2. Thoracic outlet syndrome.

    3. Impingement syndrome.

    4. Osteoarthritis.

17. A 45-year-old female complains of knee pain when kneeling and a "clicking" noise when walking up steps. On exam, there is a slight knee effusion and tenderness when palpating the patella against the condyles. The diagnosis for this client is:

    1. Anterior cruciate tear.

    2. Dislocated patella.

    3. Chondromalacia patella.

    4. Tendinitis.

18. A client has been diagnosed with a complete rotator cuff tear of the left shoulder. The nurse practitioner would expect the client to have difficulty in:

    1. Abducting the left arm.

    2. Supinating the left forearm.

    3. Shrugging the shoulders.

    4. Touching the left hand to the right shoulder.

19. A client has been diagnosed with polymyalgia rheumatica. The nurse practitioner understands that this disorder is:

    1. An autoimmune, multisystem problem where the body makes antibodies to its own proteins.

    2. A degenerative disorder with no inflammatory changes, and where joint cartilage wears away with age and eventually causes bone spurs.

    3. An inflammatory disorder involving the axial skeleton and large peripheral joints.

    4. An inflammatory connective tissue disorder that primarily affects older women and is associated with giant cell (temporal) arteritis.

20. In teaching a client about fibromyalgia, the nurse practitioner includes what information?

    1. Diagnostic studies such as ESR and CBC are important tools to confirm the progress of the syndrome.

    2. Avoid stretching exercises and daily low-impact aerobics.

    3. Take ibuprofen (Motrin) 200 mg q4–6h prn for pain and amitriptyline (Elavil) 10 mg 1–2 hours before bedtime.

    4. Apply heat to or massage "trigger points" to reduce pain.

21. The nurse practitioner understands that chronic synovitis with pannus formation is the basic pathophysiologic finding in clients with:

    1. Systemic lupus erythematous (SLE).

    2. Ankylosing spondylitis (AS).

    3. Rheumatoid arthritis (RA).

    4. Osteoarthritis (OA).

22. The nurse practitioner is examining a client who is complaining of pain in her hips and knees. She has a history of osteoarthritis. On examination, the joints are painful to movement and are warm to touch. The best immediate therapy for this client is:

    1. Physical therapy for range of motion of affected areas.

    2. Decreased physical activity and immobilizing splints for affected joints.

    3. Moist heat and/or cold therapy on painful joints.

    4. ESR to determine level of activity.

23. The history of a client who may have contracted Lyme disease includes:

    1. Erythematous rash on bridge of nose and cheeks with discoid patches on the trunk.

    2. Immediate development of arthritis symptoms, especially in the knees.

    3. Expanding rash with central clearing occurring within a month of being bitten.

    4. Early symptoms of meningitis and myocarditis.

24. The nurse practitioner understands that finding Heberden's nodes on a physical exam of a client is a cardinal sign of:

    1. Septic arthritis.

    2. Rheumatoid arthritis.

    3. Gouty arthritis.

    4. Osteoarthritis.

25. Competing diagnoses for an adult male who presents with acute onset of unilateral inflammation, pain, and erythema of the first metatarsophalangeal joint could be:

    1. Gout, cellulitis, and osteoporosis.

    2. Cellulitis, rheumatoid arthritis, and gout.

    3. Osteoporosis, fibromyalgia, and cellulitis.

    4. Septic arthritis, rheumatoid arthritis, and osteoarthritis.

26. Diseases that often present as polyarthritic diseases include:

    1. Lyme arthritis, rheumatic heart disease, ankylosing spondylitis, and psoriatic arthritis.

    2. Rheumatoid arthritis, gout, Reiter's syndrome, and osteoarthritis.

    3. Gonococcal arthritis, systemic lupus erythematosus, and septic arthritis.

    4. Polymyalgia rheumatica, Lyme arthritis, pseudogout, and psoriatic arthritis.

27. The circumstances under which a common injury that can cause a meniscus tear to occur are:

    1. The knee is almost completely extended and the tibia is externally rotated.

    2. An external force that is strong enough to cause external rotation or hyperextension of the knee or a forceful direct blow to the knee.

    3. Valgus or varus pressure on the knee at full extension and at 30 degrees of flexion.

    4. An injury in which the knee is simultaneously twisted and flexed.

28. Pain in lumbosacral strain typically begins:

    1. Immediately with the injury.

    2. 1–2 hours after injury.

    3. 6–8 hours after injury.

    4. 12–36 hours after injury.

29. Acute onset of pain that shoots down to the lower leg and foot of an elderly obese adult is likely to be a symtom of:

    1. Lumbosacral strain.

    2. Herniated intervertebral disc injury.

    3. Osteomyelitis.

4. Osteoporosis.

30. Quadriceps setting is one exercise recommended for clients suffering patellofemoral syndrome. The nurse practitioner should teach the client to:

    1. Lie supine on the floor with legs extended. Dorsiflex the foot. Push the thigh into the floor.

    2. Sit on the floor leaning back on the elbows. Flex one knee to 90 degrees and extend one completely. Raise the straight leg until the thigh is parallel to the flexed knee. Hold for 5 seconds. Repeat for opposite leg.

    3. Lie on the floor and flex both knees to about 20 degrees with a rolled up towel underneath them. Extend one leg and hold for 5 seconds. Repeat for the opposite leg.

    4. Use resistance exercises with an elastic band.

31. Which risk factor is associated with gout?

    1. Female gender.

    2. Over age 20.

    3. Ingestion of salicylate medications.

    4. Overuse of the extremity.

32. In a third-degree ankle strain, there is:

    1. Moderate ecchymosis, moderate edema, and a stable joint.

    2. Moderate ecchymosis, moderate edema, and an unstable joint.

    3. Marked ecchymosis, marked edema, and a stable joint.

    4. Marked ecchymosis, marked edema, and an unstable joint.

33. A client with rheumatoid arthritis presents for follow-up. One of the best evaluative questions the nurse practitioner can ask that will help determine the severity of disease is:

    1. "Were you able to drive the car to your appointment today?"

    2. "Were you able to fix your dinner last night?"

    3. "How long does it take for your joints to loosen up after you get up in the morning?"

    4. "How many pounds can you carry?"

34. A 55-year-old female is seen with a complaint of diffuse musculoskeletal pain, stiffness, and fatigue for the past 3 months. The pain is worse in the morning and also with changes in the weather. She states she wakes up in the morning feeling tired and unrefreshed. Physical exam is normal except for pain on digital palpation in 12 tender points. Laboratory results are unremarkable. The most likely diagnosis is:

    1. Fibromyalgia.

    2. Myofascial syndrome.

    3. Rheumatoid arthritis.

    4. Depression.

35. When counseling a postmenopausal female client on prevention of osteoporosis, all of the following are therapeutic recommendations **except**:

    1. Cease smoking.

    2. Take 200 mg of calcium and 40 IU of vitamin D daily.

    3. Continue hormone therapy indefinitely.

    4. Monitor bone loss by dual-energy x-ray absorptiometry (DEXA) every 1–2 years for women who are not on hormone replacement therapy but are at increased risk.

36. A client presents with a complaint of sudden pain and swelling in the knee. He also is complaining of chills and fever. Upon exam the knee is warm, tender, and swollen with evidence of effusion. The family nurse practitioner would:

    1. Splint the affected joint.

    2. Obtain aspiration of synovial fluid from the affected joint.

    3. Initiate treatment with nonsteroidal anti-inflammatory drugs (NSAIDs).

    4. Recommend rest, ice, compresses, and elevation (RICE) of affected joint.

37. When determining the specific etiology of polyarticular complaints, the clinical clues most helpful for diagnosis are:

    1. Lab identification of antinuclear antibodies (ANA) and ESR.

    2. X-ray of affected joints.

    3. Affected joint pattern and presence of or lack of inflammation.

    4. Sexual history of client.

38. An older client with ankylosing spondylitis needs to be educated to manage his/her disease by all **except**:

    1. Regular exercise program.

    2. Maintenance therapy of systemic corticosteroids.

    3. Using indomethacin (Indocin) for discomfort.

    4. Watch for signs and symptoms of iritis.

39. Which of the diet selections indicate the older client understands the health education regarding the prevention of osteoporosis?

    1. Chicken and baked potato.

    2. A glass of skim milk and a toasted cheese sandwich.

    3. Hamburger and salad.

    4. Ice cream sundae with whipped cream.

40. During the history, which of the following questions would best assist the nurse practitioner in diagnosing osteoarthritis rheumatoid arthritis?

    1. "Is your joint pain symmetrical and localized?"

    2. "Does your morning stiffness usually last several hours?"

    3. "Have you experienced fatigue, weakness, and weight loss?"

    4. "Is your joint pain asymmetrical and worse with movement and relieved by rest?"

41. Primary treatment of joint injury involves:

    1. Rest, ice, compression, and elevation.

    2. Narcotic pain control and x-ray.

    3. Specialist referral and magnetic resonance imaging.

    4. Nonsteroidal anti-inflammatory agents and exercise.

42. The most common complaint in a client with back injury who had cauda equina syndrome, a surgical emergency, is:

    1. Urinary retention.

    2. Numbness below the level of injury.

    3. Weakness in the lower extremities.

    4. Pain.

43. Recognition of anular tears is important in the diagnosis of back pain because:

    1. They require immediate surgery.

    2. They are often misdiagnosed as strain or sprain and lead to herniation.

    3. They result in rapid paralysis.

    4. X-ray would reveal them, but x-rays are usually not ordered initially.

44. A chronic musculoskeletal problem that may occur after an injury and that is characterized by a 3-month history of pain on both sides of the body above and below the waist and tenderness in at least 11 of 18 specified points is:

    1. Chronic osteoarthritis.

    2. Reflex sympathetic dystrophy.

    3. Tendinitis.

    4. Fibromyalgia.

45. Which client is at highest risk for osteoporosis?

    1. A 55-year-old male smoker and retired athlete.

    2. A 60-year-old white postmenopausal female switchboard operator weighing 105 lb.

    3. A 42-year-old African-American female intensive care nurse who is lactose intolerant.

    4. A 50-year-old white obese female, wife of a dairy farmer, and mother of three.

46. A 53-year-old woman presents with complaints of morning stiffness in the neck and back. She has pelvic and shoulder pain and fatigue. Her laboratory studies reveal an elevated ESR, a normal rheumatoid factor, a normal creatine phosphokinase, and normochromic normocytic anemia. Physical examination reveals an elevated temperature, and bilateral pain and stiffness of the pectoral and pelvic muscles. Based on this information, the best diagnosis is:

    1. Polyarteritis nodosa.

    2. Wegener's granulomatosis.

    3. Polymyalgia rheumatica.

    4. Rheumatoid arthritis.

47. A 55-year-old woman with a prior diagnosis of polymyalgia rheumatica presents with headache, low-grade fever, aching, stiffness, fatigue, malaise, and anorexia. Based on this information, the nurse practitioner would make a preliminary diagnosis of:

    1. Influenza.

    2. Pneumonia.

    3. Temporal arteritis.

    4. Rheumatoid arthritis.

Pharmacology

48. The nurse practitioner is seeing a middle-aged, severely arthritic female who has been on maintenance therapy of prednisone 10 mg/day for the past 6 weeks. She now presents as acutely ill with signs and symptoms of acute pneumonia. She complains of feeling fatigued and weak, has a loss of appetite, and her blood pressure is lower than previous visit measurements. The nurse practitioner should:

    1. Immediately discontinue the prednisone.

    2. Increase dosage to 60 mg/day and then taper back to 10 mg/day.

    3. Gradually taper the prednisone from 10 mg/day to 1 mg/day.

    4. Maintain the dose of prednisone at 10 mg/day.

49. The primary drug of choice for a client with rheumatoid arthritis is:

    1. A nonsteroidal anti-inflammatory drug.

    2. Aspirin.

    3. Methotrexate.

    4. Hydrocortisone.

50. A client with rheumatoid arthritis is placed on prednisone 5 mg/day PO. In teaching the client about her medication, it would be important for the nurse practitioner to include what information?

    1. When the symptoms of arthritis subside, she will be able to quit taking her medication.

    2. It is important to take the medication as prescribed, even after the redness and swelling decrease.

    3. Increased fluid intake is important to prevent renal damage by the steroids.

    4. The medication should be taken about 30 minutes before eating.

51. A correct medication and dose for the treatment of an adult with an acute episode of gout is:

    1. Indomethacin (Indocin) 25 mg PO prn.

    2. Naproxen (Naprosyn) 100 mg PO bid.

    3. Colchicine 0.6 mg qid.

    4. Indomethacin (Indocin) 50 mg q8h for six to eight doses then decrease to 25 mg PM q8h until gout episode has resolved.

52. If a client's 24-hour urine indicates that the client is secreting too much uric acid (>900 mg/day), the nurse practitioner would prescribe:

    1. Aspirin 325 mg/day PO.

    2. Tylenol 325 mg q4–6h, PO prn.

    3. Indomethacin (Indocin) 25 mg PO q8h and then increase at weekly intervals by 25 mg daily.

    4. Allopurinol (Zyloprim) 100 mg PO × 1 week then increase the daily dose by 100 mg to a maximum of 300 mg/day.

53. Disease-modifying drugs for rheumatoid arthritis in adults include:

    1. Ibuprofen (Motrin, Advil), sulindac (Clinoril), salicylates (aspirin, Disalcid).

    2. Corticosteroids (prednisone, methylprednisolone).

    3. Misoprostol (Cytotec).

    4. Hydroxychloroquine (Plaquenil), sulfasalazine (Asulfidine), methotrexate, gold sodium thiomalate (Myochrysine).

54. Gold compounds are contraindicated in clients with all of the following **except**:

    1. Renal disease.

    2. Hepatic disease.

    3. Rheumatoid arthritis.

    4. Blood dyscrasia.

55. The most appropriate medication used to control pain for a client with osteoarthritis is:

    1. Acetaminophen.

    2. Systemic corticosteroids.

    3. Gold salts.

    4. Misoprostol.

56. What is a serious side effect of ibuprofen in the elderly client?

    1. Rebound headaches.

    2. Impairment of renal function.

    3. Neuropathy.

    4. Liver failure.

57. A client has been on methotrexate (Rheumatrex) for 6 weeks. This was the medication of choice for her severe refractory rheumatoid arthritis. What parameters should the nurse practitioner monitor?

    1. Monthly platelet count, CBC, and differential.

    2. Urinalysis, blood sugar, and electrocardiogram (ECG) every 2 weeks.

    3. Monthly CBC, urinalysis, and electrolytes.

    4. Coagulation studies, electrolytes, and CBC every week.

10 ▸ Answers & Rationales

Physical Examination & Diagnostic Tests

1. **(2)** The goniometer is used to determine the degree of joint flexion and extension. It provides a means of measuring degree of angle flexion and extension.

2. **(3)** Locking of the knee or the sound of clicks and pain may indicate a loose body, such as torn cartilage, and is performed to detect a torn meniscus and is called Apley's sign. The drawer sign tests the collateral ligaments with the client in a sitting and lying position, not prone. The McMurray's test is a test for medial meniscus injury. In this test, the knee is fully flexed and the tibia is externally rotated. Varus pressure is applied to the knee while it is extended. To test for medial meniscus tear, the test is performed while applying valgus pressure to the knee.

3. **(4)** This is called Phalen's maneuver and, when present, is suggestive of carpal tunnel syndrome. Tinel's sign is also a test for carpal tunnel syndrome, but is performed by lightly percussing over the median nerve on the palmar side of the wrist; an abnormal result would be tingling or shock-like sensations across the palm, thumb, and first two fingers. The drawer sign and McMurray's tests are used to assess the knee.

4. **(3)** The balloon sign occurs in instances when considerable fluid is in the suprapatellar pouch; ballottement of the patella may be possible. The bulge sign is for testing fluid in the knee joint and is ellicited with the knee extended by applying pressure to the medial aspect of the knee and watching for a bulge or fluid wave. A patellar tap suggests fluid in the knee as the patella clicks against the femur. The drawer sign tests the collateral ligaments with the client in a sitting and lying position. Kernig's sign is a sign of meningeal irritation and is the inability to extend the lower leg when that leg is flexed at the hip, or there may be resistance of pain during ellicitation of the sign.

5. **(1)** Pain with gentle deviation of a fist in which the thumb is tucked under the other four fingers to the ulnar side is a positive Finkelstein's sign and an indication of De Quervain's disease, which is swelling and tenderness over the volar portion of the "snuff box" resulting from chronic tenosynovitis. Treatment is usually a thumb splint, NSAIDs, and possible steroid injection into the area. A positive Tinel's sign (tapping gently over the carpal tunnel causing tingling in the thumb, index finger, and middle and lateral half of the ring finger) and a positive Phalen's sign (holding hands that are flexed at 90 degrees back to back with this same distribution of tingling) are indicative of carpel tunnel syndrome. A Lachman's sign is an indication of the stability of the cruciate ligament of the knee.

6. **(3)** The musculoskeletal system is examined by a visual inspection and palpation of bones, joints, and surrounding muscular tissue. Percussion is generally not done, and auscultation is not appropriate to the system being examined.

7. **(3)** Clients with polymyalgia rheumatica have a rapid, dramatic clinical response to corticosteroid therapy. The serum protein electophoresis is used to rule out myeloma. The ESR is elevated in a number of diseases and is not specific to polymyalgia rheumatica. The chest radiograph is used to diagnose diseases affecting the lungs and thorax.

8. **(3)** The wrist, MCP, and PIP joints along with other small joints of the hands and feet are involved with rheumatoid arthritis. The great toe is most often involved with gout. The large joints of the hip, knee, and shoulder along with the distal interphalangeal (DIP) joint and the base of the thumb are involved with degenerative joint disease (i.e., osteoarthritis).

9. **(2)** It would not be necessary to obtain a CBC. The HgbA$_{1c}$ would be ordered to evaluate the relative control of diabetes. The EMG is most often performed to evaluate both nerve conduction and needle electrode examination. Many toxins and inflammatory processes are involved with polyneuropathy, hence the sedimentation rate would be a helpful diagnostic tool.

10. **(4)** A thorough history is very important in assessing any client with injury, but in the event of a back injury, the mechanism of injury will provide the greatest clue as to the extent of injury and the proper path to take in diagnosis and treatment.

11. **(2)** Carpel tunnel syndrome, a compression of the median nerve at the wrist, is commonly caused by repetitive finger motion and results in a positive Tinel's sign and Phalen's maneuver. Tinel's sign is considered positive when tapping over the nerve with a reflex hammer causes tingling in the distribution of the nerve. Phalen's maneuver is performed by fully flexing the wrist passively and noting tingling in the thumb or fingers.

12. **(2)** The clinical assessments point to a chronic inflammatory process such as rheumatoid arthritis. The dizziness, fatigue, lightheadedness, and weakness may be a problem with anemia. The anemia of chronic disease is either a microcytic or normocytic anemia. The value that differentiates the anemia of chronic disease from other anemias is the serum ferritin (iron stores). The value will be either normal or high. The MCV of 104 indicates a macrocytic anemia, which would not include the anemia of chronic disease. The low serum ferritin would not be considered a possibility with this disorder. The uric acid level would be elevated in gout. The WBC count does not address the signs of anemia.

13. **(2)** Gentle inversion of the affected ankle in an ankle injury is compared with the unaffected ankle in the talar tilt test. Anterior ankle stability is tested in the anterior drawer test, in which the tibia is grasped by the examiner's one hand while the heel is firmly grasped and backward pressure is applied to the tibia with the examiner's other hand. In passive range of motion, the examiner inverts, everts, dorsiflexes, and plantar flexes the foot and ankle. The client puts the foot and ankle through complete range of motion in active range of motion.

14. **(2)** Varus pressure on a slightly flexed knee tests for lateral collateral ligament stability. Valbus pressure tests for medical collateral ligament stability. Cruciate ligaments are tested with the anterior drawer test. The McMurray's test is a test for medial meniscus injury. In this test, the knee is fully flexed and the tibia is externally rotated. Varus pressure is applied to the knee while it is extended. To test for medial meniscus tear, the test is performed while applying valgus pressure to the knee.

Disorders

15. **(3)** Nonsteroidal anti-inflammatory agents are recommended treatment for an acute gout attack in clients able to take NSAID therapy. Allopurinal (Zyloprim) is contraindicated in an acute attack and can even precipitate an attack in the early stages of treatment. Low-calorie diets increase risks of gouty attacks. Joint injection would not be first-line choice of treatment. However, in refractory cases in clients unable to take oral medication, it may be an option.

16. **(3)** Impingement syndrome is usually caused by rotator cuff tendinitis, which is when internal/external rotation is impaired.

Frozen shoulder can occur after a rotator cuff injury, especially if a sling is used for a prolonged period of time. Thoracic outlet syndrome would be indicated by a decrease of loss of radial pulse when the client abducts arm, holds a deep breath, while simultaneously hyperextending the neck and turning the chin toward the raised arm.

17. **(3)** These are common symptoms of chondromalacia patella. With anterior cruciate tears, the client generally cannot bear weight on the extremity without it buckling or giving way. With a dislocated patella, there would be considerable effusion (loss of normal knee hollow on sides of patella) and possible patellofemoral compartment.

18. **(1)** With a complete rotator cuff tear (rupture of the supraspinatus tendon), the client would have difficulty abducting the arm and impaired internal/external rotation. Touching the hand to the opposite shoulder is adduction.

19. **(4)** Also, anemia is common in polymyalgia rheumatica, along with an elevated ESR. Common complaint of morning stiffness; rheumatoid factor is negative. Option #1 is characteristic of systemic lupus erythematosus. Option #2 is characteristic of osteoarthritis. Option #3 is characteristic of ankylosing spondylitis.

20. **(3)** Diagnostic studies are of little value and benefit, except to rule out other causes, such as polymyalgia rheumatica, hypothyroidism, and so forth. Treatment is symptomatic, usual drugs are amitriptyline (Elavil), NSAIDs, cyclobenzaprine (Flexeril), temazepam (Restoril), and triazolam (Halcion). Daily, slow, low-impact aerobics, preferably in the late afternoon or early evening, is encouraged. Heat and massage are helpful, but not on the "trigger points."

21. **(3)** The chronic inflammatory disorder of RA has synovial hypertrophy from chronic synovitis and pannus formation that results in progressive destruction of the cartilage, ligament, tendons, and bone. Ankylosing spondylitis usually involves the large peripheral joints (i.e., sacroiliac), and is characterized by extreme kyphosis. There is no inflammation with osteoarthritis. SLE has a distribution of symptoms similar to that of RA, but no pannus formation.

22. **(3)** Moist heat or cold is appropriate to use on acutely affected joints, whichever relieves the pain more effectively. Physical therapy is recommended after the acute involvement of the joint, and care must be taken to decrease repetitive movements. Immobilization is avoided, as it tends to increase the stiffness of the joint. The ESR is not an appropriate indicator of activity of osteoarthritis.

23. **(3)** Option #1 describes the malar or "butterfly" rash of systemic lupus erythematosus. The arthritis symptoms and other complications (meningitis and myocarditis) occur later in the disease process, especially if the client is not treated with antibiotics (usually tetracycline, doxycycline, or amoxicillin).

24. **(4)** Finding deformities (bony protuberances) of the distal DIP joints (called Heberden's nodes) is a cardinal signs of osteoarthritis. The DIP joints are seldom involved with rheumatoid arthritis. Gouty arthritis most often affects the great toe. Joints are warm, red, tender, and swollen with septic arthritis.

25. **(2)** Cellulitis usually presents with warm, erythematous, painful areas of the skin. Symptoms of erythema, edema, and pain of the first metatarsophalangeal joint are a common presentation for gout. Symptoms that can be present in rheumatoid arthritis are similar: red, swollen, painful joint(s). The inflammation of rheumatoid arthritis is usually symmetrical but can present as erythematous, swollen joints. Systemic symptoms may also be present. Osteoporosis most often occurs in postmenopausal women due to bone loss that occurs with the decline of the estrogen in the blood. Bone thinning leads to fractures, not inflammation of joints or skin. Osteoarthritis presents as pain and stiffness with decreased range of motion, and stiffness in the morning for a few minutes. Joint effusions occur occasionally. Point tenderness in 11 of 18 sites with digital palpation is present in fibromyalgia. Joint swelling and erythema are not present. In septic arthritis, joint pain, inflammation, and erythema would be accompanied by systemic symptoms of fever and chills. It would be considered in the differential for this client.

26. **(1)** Lyme arthritis, rheumatic heart disease, ankylosing spondylitis, psoriatic arthritis, rheumatoid arthritis, Reiter's syndrome, osteoarthritis, gonnococcal arthritis, systemic lupus erythematosus, and polymyalgia rheumatica commonly occur as polyarthritic diseases. Most often gout, septic arthritis, and pseudogout occur as monoarthritis.

27. **(4)** A client that sustained a meniscal tear can usually recall a twisting injury of the knee followed by pain and effusion over the joint line. A strong force or injury that causes external rotation or hyperextension of the knee is a common mechanism of injury for collateral or cruciate ligament injuries. A test for stability of the knee joint involves applying medial and lateral pressure to the knee during full extension and flexion of 30 degrees.

28. **(4)** As the soft tissue swells, pain onset is usually about 12–36 hours after injury.

29. **(2)** Herniated intervertebral disc pain typically shoots to the lower leg and foot. Lumbosacral strain causes pain in the back, buttock, and sometimes thigh. Osteomyelitis must be preceded by an event that permits an infectious agent to enter the bone. Osteoporosis occurs most commonly in postmenopausal women.

30. **(1)** In quadriceps setting, with the foot dorsiflexed the thigh is pressed down against the floor and held for 5 seconds. The straight leg raise involves lifting an extended leg while sitting on the floor and leaning back on the elbows with the opposite leg flexed to 90 degrees. A terminal arc extension requires that the client lie on the floor supine with extended legs flexed to 20 degrees over a rolled-up towel. The client then extends one leg and holds for 5 seconds. The exercise is repeated for the opposite leg. All of the above exercises can be used to stretch and strengthen the quadriceps muscles in those suffering from patellofemoral stress syndrome. Resistive exercises with an elastic band are general exercises that can be done with the extremities.

31. **(3)** Gout generally affects men over 30 and is associated with obesity, lead intoxication, starvation, and use of some medications, including salicylates, diuretics, pyrazinamide, and alcohol.

32. **(4)** A third-degree strain is a complete tear of the ligament resulting in marked edema, ecchymosis, pain, and an unstable joint.

33. **(3)** Morning stiffness or activity and the length of time it takes for maximal improvement is one of the American Rheumatism Association Classification criteria for RA and is a useful, measurable tool for effects of treatment. The other questions are good indicators of quality of activities of daily living but do not give a full overall, measurable picture of the client's joint discomfort.

34. **(1)** This client meets classification criteria for fibromyalgia based on history of widespread pain and pain in 11 of 18 tender points. Myofascial syndrome symptoms are more focal and there is no associated fatigue or sleep disorder. Rheumatoid disease would have abnormal serologic studies. Depression may cause musculoskeletal pain and fatigue but would not have reproducible tender points.

35. **2)** This is a subtherapeutic amount of calcium and vitamin D. The other choices are recommendations for prevention of osteoporosis.

36. **(2)** Symptoms are indicative of septic arthritis, which is a medical emergency; if it is not treated promptly, the joint may be destroyed. Examination of the joint fluid is the single most important diagnostic test. Other choices may provide some symptomatic relief, but the first goal of treatment is to determine if the joint is septic.

37. **(3)** When developing the differential diagnosis, the history and physical exam will help narrow the differentiation. Other procedures are important in completing the evaluation, but the most important information is the pattern of joints affected and whether it is inflammatory versus noninflammatory disease.

38. **(2)** Corticosteroids have limited value in treating AS, and long-term effects are associated with many serious side effects. Important treatment includes regular

exercise to strengthen supporting muscles and use of NSAIDs for pain. Approximately one third of clients have recurrent attacks of acute iritis.

39. **(2)** The calcium intake is important in minimizing the development of osteoporosis. Both of these contain calcium. The other distractors are not focused on the calcium intake.

40. **(4)** Signs and symptoms of osteoarthritis include asymmetrical joint pain worse with movement and relieved by rest; stiffness of short duration (<15 minutes) after inactivity, or in the morning; and pain that may be described as aching and poorly localized. Options #1, #2, and #3 are indicative of rheumatoid arthritis.

41. **(1)** The RICE principle is used for initial treatment: rest, ice, compression, and elevation. All other treatments mentioned may be appropriate but not in the primary treatment.

42. **(1)** Although all of the above symptoms may be associated with cauda equina syndrome, urinary retention is the most important clue to the immediate need for surgery.

43. **(2)** Anular tears are the first step toward herniation, and early recognition can help to avoid the need for surgical repair of a subsequent herniation.

44. **(4)** Fibromyalgia is correct. This is a poorly understood condition that can prolong the normal treatment course of an injury considerably and is very difficult to treat. Osteoarthritis may follow an injury, as can reflex sympathetic dystrophy or tendinitis, but they do not have specified tender points.

45. **(2)** This example demonstrates five of the risk factors for osteoporosis, which include female gender, Caucasian or Asian, over age 45, low body weight, postmenopausal, sedentary lifestyle, low calcium intake, and smoker.

46. **(3)** Polymyalgia rheumatica (PMR) is an inflammatory disorder of the proximal muscles presenting as described. Polyarteritis nodosa is an inflammatory disorder affecting the small arteries. It

presents with muscle weakness, myalgias, headache, and subcutaneous nodules along the arteries in the extremities. Wegener's disease presents with mild anemia, dyspnea, cough, chest pain, hemoptysis, and abnormal urinalysis.

47. **(3)** Up to 40% of clients with temporal arteritis have a previous history of PMR. Presenting complaints include headache, low-grade fever, aching and stiffness of PMR, fatigue, malaise, and anorexia.

Pharmacology

48. **(2)** Clients on chronic steroid therapy should be evaluated for adrenal insufficiency during an acute illness, which increases stress. Signs and symptoms indicate subtle clinical manifestations of adrenal insufficiency. Recommended treatment is to empirically treat with stress-dose corticosteroid during acute illness. Stopping the medication or maintaining at the same dose may precipitate acute adrenal insufficiency.

49. **(2)** Aspirin is the first choice. NSAIDs can be used, but the anti-inflammatory and antipyretic effects of aspirin, plus low cost, make it the drug of choice. Methotrexate is used for severe cases that do not respond to either aspirin or NSAIDs. Steroids may be given, but are not drugs of choice.

50. **(2)** The client needs to understand the importance of maintaining her dose of the steroids. When symptoms decrease, the medication is effective. It is not influenced by fluids and it should be taken with food.

51. **(3)** This is the only effective dose listed for the treatment of an acute episode of gout. The other doses are incorrect or insufficient as dosed.

52. **(4)** Allopurinol works to keep the serum uric acid level lower. The goal of therapy is a serum uric acid level of <6.5 mg/dl. The other medications listed do not help to lower serum uric acid levels and aspirin can precipitate a gout attack.

53. **(4)** These drugs modify the disease when nonsteroidal anti-inflammatory agents (ibuprofen, sulindac, salicylates) have not worked. Corticosteroids can be used until the disease-modifying agents begin to work. Misoprostol (Cytotec) is used to prevent ulcer development related to long-term medication use.

54. **(3)** Gold is indicated for treatment of rheumatoid arthritis and is contraindicated in the presence of these other diseases.

55. **(1)** Acetaminophen or NSAIDs are generally used for pain relief for clients with osteoarthritis. Systemic corticosteroids are not indicated in osteoarthritis. Gold salts may be one of several pharmacologic approaches to the treatment of rheumatoid arthritis. Misoprostol is used to minimize the development of NSAID-induced gastric ulcers.

56. **(2)** Renal function may be already reduced in the elderly and ibuprofen can further impair renal function, which in turn can result in nephrosis, cirrhosis, and congestive heart failure.

57. **(1)** The client should be monitored for blood dyscrasias on a monthly basis.

11

Neurology

Physical Examination & Diagnostic Tests

1. To evaluate the neurologic system for appropriate sensory system functioning in the geriatric client, stereognosis is determined. This is done by having the client:

    1. Rapidly touch the index finger and then the nose.

    2. Distinguish between a coin and key by touch.

    3. Stand with heels together and eyes closed.

    4. Close eyes and identify familiar odors.

2. To determine cerebellar functioning in the geriatric client, the nurse practitioner evaluates:

    1. Ability of the client to balance on one foot then the other.

    2. Ability to discriminate between two familiar objects.

    3. Ability to recall names of three U.S. presidents.

    4. Range of motion and ability to move extremities.

3. What is considered a "soft" neurologic (or equivocal) sign?

    1. Positive Babinski's reflex in an adult.

    2. Mirroring hand movements of the extremities.

    3. Brudzinski's sign.

    4. Kernig's sign.

4. A client is having problems controlling her seizures and is referred to have an electroencephalogram (EEG) performed. Prior to the test, the nurse practitioner explains to the client that:

    1. This test will cause some discomfort and she will be given a sedative before the test.

    2. It will be important for her to take her regular dose of fluoxetine (Prozac) and phenytoin (Dilantin) prior to the test.

    3. The procedure is painless and she will not be in any discomfort or experience electrical shock during the procedure.

    4. After the test, she will be on bed rest for 8 hours and will be given full liquids for 12 hours.

5. Which cranial nerve is being tested when the nurse practitioner asks the client to raise his eyebrows, smile, frown, or puff out his cheeks?

   1. Hypoglossal nerve.

   2. Acoustic nerve.

   3. Glossopharyngeal nerve.

   4. Facial nerve.

6. The nurse practitioner notes in a healthy individual an absent knee jerk reflex. What might the nurse practitioner ask the client to do?

   1. Lift both arms above the head and count to 5 slowly as the reflex is tested.

   2. Raise both legs slowly and then lower and immediately test for the reflex.

   3. Clench both hands together and pull while the reflex is tested.

   4. Close eyes and hold breath while examiner tests for the reflex.

7. The nurse practitioner gently flexes a client's neck in the direction of the chin touching the chest. If there is pain and resistance to the flexion and the hips and knees flex at the same time, the nurse practitioner accurately describe this finding as:

   1. Phalen's sign.

   2. Romberg's sign.

   3. Kernig's sign.

   4. Brudzinski's sign.

8. The nurse practitioner understands that dysdiadochokinesia refers to:

   1. Trouble with speech.

   2. Memory.

   3. Trouble with attempts at rapidly alternating movements.

   4. A neurologic triad of symptoms with gait, memory, and speech.

Disorders

9. The nurse practitioner understands that the most common form of facial paralysis in the adult client is:

   1. Facial nerve fasciitis.

   2. Trigeminal neuralgia.

   3. Bell's palsy.

   4. Herpes zoster.

10. A client has a history of injury at thoracic level 5 (T5) and his condition has stabilized. The nurse practitioner understands that with this level of injury the client is most likely not going to be able to:

   1. Perform coordinated movements with his hands, such as writing.

   2. Achieve lower body strength and coordination for walking.

   3. Have upper body strength adequate to drive a car.

   4. Maintain upper body coordination required to feed himself.

11. An older client, who as a young child recovered very quickly after extensive initial impairment due to poliomyelitis, is diagnosed with postpolio syndrome. The most common symptoms are:

   1. Gastrointestinal upset, headache, and malaise.

   2. New onset of weakness, fatigue, and pain.

   3. Sudden onset of lower limb paralysis following an acute infection.

   4. Headache, fever, and elevated blood pressure and pulse.

12. A client has Parkinson's disease. The nurse practitioner is discussing safety measures for the home environment. It would be important for the nurse practitioner to include what information?

   1. Sleep on a firm mattress that is high off the floor to facilitate getting into and out of bed.

2. Pour hot liquids with the cup or container placed on the table to avoid spilling.

3. Place a sheepskin pad on the bed to decrease the development of decubiti.

4. Perform passive and active range of motion twice daily to prevent contracture.

13. A client is admitted after a diving accident to a rural clinic. The nurse practitioner suspects a spinal cord injury at cervical level 5 (C5). While awaiting emergency transport services, the nurse practitioner assesses for the development of complications by:

1. Checking for voluntary movement of extremities and sensation below level of injury.

2. Assessing breath sounds and evaluating movement of diaphragm with respirations.

3. Maintaining cervical flexion to facilitate airway until cervical traction is initiated.

4. Beginning neurologic checks with careful documentation of location of pain sensations.

14. Many clients who suffer from recurrent headaches have similar symptoms with each episode. Which is a sign that a headache may be from a more serious cause?

1. It occurs on the right side.

2. Rhinorrhea occurs with the headache.

3. The headache continuously becomes more and more painful.

4. A client is able to sleep through the pain of the headache.

15. Epidemic meningococcal meningitis occurs rarely. This control is due to:

1. Use of active immunization.

2. Lower community carrier rates.

3. Improved socioeconomic conditions.

4. Earlier detection and recognition of outbreaks.

16. The nurse practitioner understands that benign paroxysmal positional vertigo:

1. Is described as vertigo and nystagmus with positional change and occurs most commonly in the elderly.

2. Is more common in the young and occurs suddenly and in episodes that include vertigo, tinnitus, hearing loss, feeling of fullness in the ears, and nausea and vomiting.

3. Follows a viral syndrome (upper respiratory or gastrointestinal) with exacerbation of the vertigo with position change without hearing loss or tinnitus.

4. Involves gradual hearing loss and tinnitus along with vertigo. Eventually facial numbness and weakness develop.

17. All of the following are included in the differential diagnosis of a client with facial paralysis **except**:

1. Herpes zoster.

2. Bell's palsy.

3. Trigeminal neuralgia.

4. Otitis media.

18. What would be appropriate to include in the treatment plan for health promotion in a client with a diagnosis of multiple sclerosis?

1. Avoid aerobic exercise due to muscle weakness.

2. Keep warm (especially extremities) to improve neurologic function.

3. Avoid antioxidants (vitamins C and E, beta-carotene), as they contribute to loss of myelin sheath.

4. Consume a low-fat, high-fiber diet, with daily cranberry juice, and calcium supplement.

19. A cerebrovascular accident (CVA) client is incontinent of urine. The family should be taught to:

1. Restrict fluid intake.

2. Insert a Foley catheter.

3. Establish a scheduled voiding pattern.

4. Reposition the client often to reduce the discomfort of urgency.

20. The best way to test the hearing of a client with Bell's palsy would be:

    1. Stand out of sight of the client and ask the client to move or do something.

    2. Use a tuning fork to test for lateralization of sound.

    3. Stand in front of the client and whisper, "Raise your hand."

    4. Snap your fingers next to the client's ear and ask if the sound was heard.

21. The physical examination findings on a 50-year-old female client who wears a left lower leg brace are: weight 100 lb, height 65 inches, vital signs within normal limits. In assisting this client who has developed postpolio syndrome, the nurse practitioner suggests that the client:

    1. Gain weight to prevent further disability.

    2. Exercise all muscle groups vigorously to prevent disuse syndrome.

    3. Avoid exposure to cold or chilling, as it may cause a loss of strength in the affected muscle.

    4. Reduce the amount of time using the brace for joint support to prevent further loss of strength.

22. Inflammation and swelling of the seventh cranial nerve with resultant unilateral facial muscle paralysis is called:

    1. Bell's palsy.

    2. Transient ischemic attack.

    3. Facial droop.

    4. Trigeminal neuralgia.

23. A skin change associated with carpal tunnel syndrome is:

    1. Rapidly appearing and disappearing wheals.

    2. Lichenification of skin of the flexor surface of the elbow.

    3. Vesicular lesion of the hand.

    4. Dry skin on the thumb, index, and middle finger.

24. Which is a pathophysiologic reason for a headache?

    1. Vascular constriction of the middle meningeal artery.

    2. Muscle strain.

    3. Dysregulation of the ascending brainstem serotonergic system.

    4. Inflammation of the scalp.

25. A symptom that can occur in an older client who has experienced a transient ischemic attack in the anterior cerebral circulation is:

    1. Bilateral vision disturbance and/or diplopia.

    2. Dysarthria (speech disturbance).

    3. Disorders of behavior and cognition.

    4. Motor and sensory problems on both sides of the body at once.

26. Many visits to emergency departments by older adults are prompted by headaches. One symptom that may help the nurse practitioner differentiate a headache that is life threatening is:

    1. It is preceded by an "aura."

    2. It occurs mainly behind one eye and tends to be grouped.

    3. The onset is sudden and is accompanied by nuchal rigidity.

    4. The headache occurs mainly on awakening.

27. An adult older client presents with a complaint of facial paralysis that started suddenly. In making a diagnosis, the nurse practitioner considers the following symptoms of Bell's palsy:

    1. Concurrent paralysis of the opposite arm and leg.

    2. Pain in the ear that accompanies or precedes the paralysis.

    3. Loss of bowel control.

    4. Loss of hearing on the opposite side.

28. The nurse practitioner is evaluating an elderly client's tremor. Which assessment

would assist in differentiating an essential tremor from a parkinsonian tremor?

1. The handwriting is not affected.

2. The tremor occurs with purposeful movements.

3. The tremor occurs at rest.

4. The tremor gets worse with β-blockers or alcohol.

29. Which assessment may be evaluated in a client with Parkinson's disease?

1. Macrographia.

2. Micrographia.

3. Exaggeration of rapid successive movements.

4. Increased swinging of arms while walking.

30. A 50-year-old female client has had several episodes of incontinence, weakness, visual loss, and some ataxia. Physical exam reveals slight swelling of the optic disc on funduscopic exam, difficulty in walking heel-to-toe, lower extremity weakness, 2+ deep tendon reflexes. The nurse practitioner suspects:

1. Multiple sclerosis.

2. Parkinson's disease.

3. Amyotrophic lateral sclerosis.

4. Postpolio syndrome.

31. A client has a history of recurrent headache for the past 3 years, occurring one or two times per month and lasting 12–18 hours for which she takes acetaminophen. The client has been using acetaminophen 6 gm in the past 12-hour period and has had no relief and presents to the clinic. The nurse practitioner would:

1. Refer client to a neurologist for headache work-up.

2. Consider analgesic rebound relative to dose of acetaminophen taken.

3. Order naproxen (Anaprox) for prophylactic treatment of the headaches.

4. Order an EEG and magnetic resonance image (MRI) to rule out pathology.

32. A client presents to the emergency room with the "worst headache of my life"; the most common diagnosis and most important to rule out is:

1. Brain tumor.

2. Migraine.

3. Onset of newly diagnosed seizure disorder.

4. Subarachnoid hemorrhage.

33. An elderly client with a recent history of a left hemisphere stroke returns to the clinic for a checkup. What symptoms would the nurse practitioner anticipate the client to exhibit?

1. Left-sided weakness.

2. Bilateral weakness of lower extremities.

3. Difficulty with speech.

4. Left visual field deficit.

34. The nurse practitioner is evaluating a group of geriatric clients for risk factors of an embolic stroke. Which condition would be least likely to precipitate this type of stroke?

1. Mitral valve disease.

2. Atrial fibrillation.

3. Endocarditis.

4. Diabetes mellitus.

35. An elderly lady comes to the clinic complaining of having difficulty when she tries to do her needlework. She walks straight, although somewhat slowly, and no rigidity is noted on movement. She states the shaking in her hands stops when she holds her hands in her lap. The nurse practitioner makes a tentative diagnosis of:

1. Parkinson's disease.

2. Transient ischemic attack.

3. Benign essential tremor.

4. Simple partial seizure activity.

36. A client with a history of myasthenia gravis presents with ptosis, facial weakness, dysphagia, and generalized weakness. What is important for the nurse practitioner to establish initially?

    1. When did the symptoms first begin, and have they increased in severity?

    2. What medications is the client on and when did he last take them?

    3. What activity was the client participating in when the symptoms began?

    4. Has the client experienced any seizure activity with the increase in symptoms?

37. The nurse practitioner is reviewing the records of an older client who is recovering from a stroke (brain accident). The records indicate the client is experiencing homonymous hemianopia. This is interpreted as:

    1. Partial loss of visual acuity in the peripheral area of the visual field.

    2. Diplopia in the eye contralateral to the cerebral lesion.

    3. Nystagmus in both eyes but movements are dissimilar.

    4. Loss of vision in both eyes in either the right or left halves of the visual field.

Pharmacology

38. An elderly client is diagnosed with herpes zoster. To reduce the occurrence of postherpetic neuralgia, the nurse practitioner orders which medication?

    1. Prednisone (Deltasone).

    2. Acyclovir (Zovirax).

    3. Ketorolac (Toradol).

    4. Carbamazepine (Tegretol).

39. A client is on antiepileptic medication. The nurse practitioner understands that antiepileptic medication:

    1. Must be taken indefinitely.

    2. Is usually discontinued after 4 years of no seizure activity, following an EEG test to confirm lack of seizure activity.

    3. Is usually given in combination with other antiepileptics or sedatives to reduce the seizure threshold.

    4. Must be given to all clients who experience a seizure.

40. A medication and dose that can be used for abortive therapy for an adult client with symptoms of a migraine headache are:

    1. Sumatriptan (Imitrex) 6 mg IM.

    2. Ergotamine (Ergostat) 2 mg SL.

    3. Ketorolac (Toradol) 100 mg IM.

    4. Amitriptyline (Elavil) 100 mg PO.

41. The family of a Parkinson's client brings him to the clinic because his tremors and difficulty walking have increased. The nurse practitioner increases the client's trihexyphenidyl (Artane) from 3 mg/day to 5 mg/day in divided doses. What is important for the nurse practitioner to teach the family regarding the increase in the dose of this medication?

    1. There may be an increase in the fluctuations of his symptoms.

    2. There will be increased tendency for urinary retention.

    3. Initially an increase in confusion is not uncommon.

    4. Closely observe the client for dizziness when he stands up.

Answers & Rationales

Physical Examination & Diagnostic Tests

1. **(2)** Sterognosis is the ability to determine familiar objects by shape rather than visual identification. Option #1 determines fine motor and coordination; Option #3 determines proprioception (balance, posture); and Option #4 determines the functioning of the first cranial nerve (i.e., olfactory).

2. **(1)** The cerebellar area controls gross motor movements and balance, as well as fine motor movements of the upper and lower extremities. Discriminatory sensations are controlled by the sensory system, and remote memory is mental status examination involving the cerebral cortex.

3. **(2)** Soft neurologic signs involve slight deviations of the central nervous system (CNS) that are present occasionally or inconsistently. Examples are short attention span, clumsiness, frequent falling (disturbances of gait), hyperkinesis, left handed but right footed, language disturbances, anisocoria, and mirroring movements of the extremities (when one hand performs; the other is in motion). The other three options indicate CNS problems that occur consistently (i.e., Brudzinski's and Kernig's sign indicate meningeal irritation; positive Babinski's sign in an adult may indicate an upper motor lesion of the corticospinal tract).

4. **(3)** The procedure is painless, and there is no danger of electrical shock. Anticonvulsants, antidepressants,

stimulants (caffeine, tobacco), and alcohol should not be taken. There is no restriction on movement or diet after the procedure.

5. **(4)** The facial nerve is tested by facial movement, taste, sensation, and corneal reflex. The hypoglossal nerve is tested by the client sticking out his tongue. The acoustic nerve is tested by a hearing test. The glossopharyngeal nerve is tested by taste, gag reflex, and giving the client a drink and asking him to swallow.

6. **(3)** Augmentation of the knee jerk reflex can be obtained by having the client isometrically tense muscles not directly involved with the reflex arc being tested. This is called Jendrassik's maneuver.

7. **(4)** This describes Brudzinski's sign. Phalen's sign is elicited in carpal tunnel syndrome. Romberg's test is done to assess gross swaying by asking the client to stand with feet together and eyes closed for 5 seconds. Kernig's sign (inability to extend the lower leg when the leg is flexed at the hip or when there is resistance or pain during the process) along with Brudzinski's sign indicate meningeal irritation and should be further evaluated.

8. **(3)** Dysdiadochokinesia is trouble with attempts at rapidly alternating movements (i.e., finger to nose).

Disorders

9. **(3)** The most common form of facial paralysis is Bell's palsy, which is a disorder affecting the facial nerve and characterized by muscle flaccidity of the affected side of the face. Trigeminal neuralgia is a disorder of cranial nerve V characterized by an abrupt onset of pain in the lower and upper jaw, cheek, and lips. Herpes zoster affects the dermatomes and does not cause a paralysis, but pain and possible postherpetic neuralgia occur.

10. **(2)** T5 injuries do not affect the coordination or capacity of the upper body, arms, and hands; the lower body is paralyzed. The client should be able to do all of the activities listed except walk.

11. **(2)** The cardinal signs of postpolio syndrome include onset of new weakness, fatigue, and pain along with hot or cold intolerance, and swallowing, speech, breathing, and/or sleep disturbances.

12. **(2)** Pouring liquids is frequently a complicated task for this client due to his tremors. If the cup or container in which the client is pouring the liquid is placed on the table, there is less chance of spilling the contents.

13. **(2)** At this level of injury (C5), the intercostal muscles and diaphragm can be affected and the client will have respiratory compromise. Airway maintenance and avoiding flexion of the neck are critical.

14. **(3)** If a headache becomes more and more severe, if there is new onset of severe headache in a client over 35 years old, if the headache's character or progression is different from other headaches, of if there is vomiting but no nausea, there could be a new and serious cause for the headache. The side on which the headache occurs, accompanying rhinorrhea, and sleeping through a headache may or may not be significant, depending on other symptoms.

15. **(3)** Undoubtedly, improved sanitary and socioeconomic conditions have led to the marked reduction in the number of cases of epidemic meningitis. There is no research to support increased cases in communities with higher carrier numbers.

16. **(1)** Benign paroxysmal positional vertigo usually occurs in older clients. In younger persons, symptoms such as sudden episode of vertigo, tinnitus, hearing loss, sensation of fullness, and nausea and vomiting are typical of Meniere's disease. Peripheral vestibulopathy usually follows upper respiratory or gastrointestinal viral illness and involves nearly incapacitating vertigo that increases with positional changes but not hearing loss or tinnitus. Suspect an acoustic neuroma if gradual hearing loss, tinnitus, and vertigo develop before the facial numbness and weakness develop.

17. **(3)** The differential diagnosis for facial paralysis includes numerous problems: bacterial infections of the ears, Lyme disease, herpes zoster, mumps, temporal bone fracture, acoustic neuroma, other types of tumors, and demyelinating diseases. Trigeminal neuralgia is associated with intense facial pain, not paralysis.

18. **(4)** In addition to the factors listed, keeping cool, not warm, is associated with improvement of neurologic function. A regular exercise program is encouraged along important aspects of promoting health: daily intake of a multiple vitamins, antioxidants, and low-dose aspirin (81 mg); maintaining ideal body weight, having rest periods or naps daily; and becoming informed about the disease process.

19. **(3)** Re-establishing regularity will assist in maintaining bladder control. A catheter exposes the client to infection. Fluids should not be restricted.

20. **(1)** Bell's palsy involves a sensorineural hearing loss. In contrast to the client being able to read lips, he must be able to hear the direction of sound without any visual prompting. The tuning fork assists in differentiating between air or bone conduction of sound.

21. **(3)** In addition to encouraging the client to have regular health maintenance visits, the client should be advised to avoid gaining weight and exercising to the point of muscle pain. Cold temperatures can cause a loss of muscle strength in the affected muscle

groups and should be avoided. Assistive or orthotic devices (canes, walkers, braces, etc.) should be used along with periodic evaluation of muscle strength and function.

22. **(1)** The symptoms describe Bell's palsy, which is believed to be caused by a virus. This sudden onset of unilateral facial paralysis usually resolves within a couple of weeks but can endure for months. A few clients can have residual problems. Transient ischemic attacks last <24 hours. Facial droop occurs with Bell's palsy due to paralysis of the muscles innervated by the facial nerve (seventh cranial nerve). Trigeminal neuralgia is sudden pain along the fifth cranial nerve.

23. **(4)** These changes are typical of carpal tunnel syndrome. Rapidly appearing and disappearing wheals are known as urticaria and could have one of many causes including allergic response to a substance that was ingested. A vesicular lesion of the hand could be caused by one of many etiologies, including a burn, local allergic reaction, and friction.

24. **(3)** Stimulation of pain-sensitive structures, vessel and meningeal inflammation, vasodilation, severe muscle contraction in the head and neck area, and dysregulation of the ascending brainstem serotonergic system are causes for headaches.

25. **(3)** A wide variety of changes can occur in behavior and cognition after a transient ischemic attack. Bilateral vision disturbance, diplopia, dysarthria (speech disturbance), and motor/sensory problems on both sides of the body are problems associated with a transient ischemic attack in the posterior cerebral circulation.

26. **(3)** Classic migraine headaches are accompanied by auras. Cluster headaches occur behind one eye and are grouped. Headaches associated with hypertension occur mainly on awakening. A sudden onset and nuchal rigidity may indicate a subarachnoid hemorrhage.

27. **(2)** Bell's palsy is typically preceded or accompanied by pain in the ear on the paralyzed side. The paralysis is confined to the fact and there is no bowel involvement.

28. **(2)** The differentiating feature between the two tremors is that the essential tremor occurs with purposeful movements. Handwriting may be affected with both tremors. The tremor with Parkinson's disease occurs at rest. Essential tremors improve with β-blockers as well as with alcohol.

29. **(2)** Micrographia is a classic manifestation of Parkinson's disease. There is an impairment of rapid successive movements and a loss in automatic movements such as swinging the arms while walking.

30. **(1)** Involvement of more than one area of the CNS, age 15–60 years, two or more separate episodes of symptoms involving different sites, or a gradual progression over at least 6 months meets the criteria for multiple sclerosis.

31. **(2)** The recommended dose for acetaminophen is no more than 4 gm/day. This client may be experiencing analgesic rebound headache. Appropriate prophylactic medications for migraine include β-blockers (propanolol), tricyclic antidepressants (amitriptyline), selective serotonin reuptake inhibitors (fluoxetine), monoamine oxidase inhibitors (phenelzine), and calcium channel blockers (verapamil). It is not necessary to order expensive tests for clients with migraine or tension headache. Usually, a careful, thorough history is sufficient.

32. **(4)** This is a common complaint of the client with subarachnoid hemorrhage headache. This client should be immediately referred to a neurologic surgeon.

33. **(3)** The speech center (Broca's area) is most often located in the left hemisphere. The client would experience weakness of the right side of the body and a right-sided visual deficit as well.

34. **(4)** Options #1, #2, and #3 precipitate the development of an embolus that can result in an embolic stroke (brain accident). Diabetes will precipitate occlusive disease of the cerebral arteries and the possible development of a thrombotic stroke, not an embolic stroke.

35. **(3)** The characteristics of a benign tremor are a fine to course rhythmic tremor of the hands and feet that increases with activity, and that may be absent at rest. Frequently, the voice is also involved. Ingestion of a small amount of alcohol may decrease symptoms.

36. **(2)** It is important to determine if the client has stayed on his medication schedule. The symptoms may be the result of missed medication, or may also occur due to too much medication. This is especially true with pyridostigmine bromide (Mestinon). This should be addressed first. The symptoms may also be exacerbated by exercise and heat.

37. **(4)** Homonymous hemianopia is the loss of vision in one half of the visual field. Either the right or left field of vision may be affected. It is most often caused by a lesion or pathology to the optic tract or the occipital lobe.

Pharmacology

38. **(1)** Elderly clients are particularly susceptible to postherpetic neuralgia, which is pain at the site that may last for months or years. Management of discomfort is alleviated by pain medication. Systemic corticosteroids may reduce the occurrence of postherpetic neuralgia. Usually, 60 mg prednisone qd for 2 weeks with a rapid taper is prescribed. Acyclovir is used for immunocompromised clients.

39. **(2)** Although most medication is discontinued after 4 years of no seizure activity, this should be confirmed by an EEG. Not all seizure clients require medication; referral and monitoring by a neurologist are appropriate.

40. **(2)** The correct dose is ergotamine (Ergostate) 2 mg SL. Sumatriptan (Imitrex) is given SC or 100 mg PO. Ketorolac (Toradol) is dosed 30–60 mg IM. Amitriptyline (Elavil) is not used for abortive therapy.

41. **(2)** Trihexyphenidyl (Artane) is an anticholinergic medication. Geriatric men frequently have problems with benign prostatic hypertrophy and are more likely to develop a problem with urinary retention when on Artane.

12

Gastrointestinal & Liver

Physical Examination & Diagnostic Tests

1. The nurse practitioner is preparing to examine the abdomen of a client. What is the correct sequence in which to conduct the examination?

   1. Inspection, palpation, percussion, auscultation.

   2. Palpation, percussion, auscultation, inspection.

   3. Percussion, palpation, auscultation, inspection.

   4. Inspection, auscultation, percussion, palpation.

2. When obtaining a history from a client with abdominal pain, the following areas are to be examined:

   1. The quality, quantity, and location of the pain.

   2. The location, the way in which the pain developed (gradually over hours or suddenly), if the pain has changed since onset, and associated symptoms.

   3. If the pain is referred to other sites, what aggravates or alleviates the pain and the client's past medical history and medication history.

   4. All of the above.

3. To test for a positive obturator sign in a client with abdominal pain, the nurse practitioner:

   1. Passively rotates the right hip from the 90-degree hip/knee flexion position.

   2. Asks the client to take a deep breath while applying pressure in the area of the gallbladder.

   3. Percusses over the costovertebral angles.

   4. Positions the client supine with hips flexed and auscultates for bowel sounds then palpates the abdomen, beginning with superficial palpation of nontender areas.

4. Serologic features* of acute hepatitis B are:

   1. HBsAg, HBeAg, and a high titer of immunogloblin M (IgM) anti-HBc.

   2. HBeAg- and HBsAg-positive.

   3. HBeAg- and HBsAg-negative.

   4. IgM anti-HBc- (high titer) HBsAg-negative.

5. The nurse practitioner is performing a physical examination on a middle-aged man. The history reveals the client's father died of colon cancer. What diagnostics are used to screen this client?

   1. Barium enema (BE) and upper gastrointestinal (GI) series.

   2. Carcinoembryonic antigen titer (CEA).

   3. Proctoscopy and biopsy.

   4. Colonoscopy and Hemoccult.

6. The Anti-HCV test indicates the client has:

   1. Acute hepatitis C.

   2. Chronic hepatitis C.

   3. Resolved hepatitis C.

   4. Acute, chronic, or resolved hepatitis C.

7. The diagnosis of early acute pancreatitis will be considered by the nurse practitioner based on physical findings and the following laboratory result:

   1. A white blood cell (WBC) count of 10,300/mm^3.

   2. A serum amylase of 75 U/L.

   3. A serum amylase of 300 U/L.

   4. A serum lipase of 75 U/L.

8. An elderly woman who is overweight has right upper quadrant pain that radiates to her right subscapular area, is severe, and is persistent. She is also experiencing anorexia, nausea, and has a fever. For her last meal, she ate a double quarter-pound hamburger with cheese, French fries, and a vanilla shake. Based on this information,

the nurse practitioner examines the abdomen for costovertebral angle tenderness. The abdomen is tender in the right upper quadrant, and if there is a positive:

   1. Obturator sign, the client has appendicitis.

   2. Costovertebral angle tenderness, the client has a urinary tract infection.

   3. Murphy's sign, the client has cholecystitis.

   4. McBurney's sign, the client has a strangulated hernia.

9. A client complains of extreme pain in his abdomen and points to the right lower quadrant. In examining the acute abdomen, the nurse practitioner would:

   1. Immediately order a WBC, abdominal x-ray.

   2. Percuss the abdomen in all quadrants followed by auscultation and gentle palpation.

   3. Palpate the right side of the abdomen first, paying close attention for guarding in the area of pain.

   4. Palpate the left side of the abdomen then gently palpate the right side noting guarding and tenderness.

Disorders

10. Diarrhea is often associated with:

    1. Infectious gastroenteritis, inflammatory bowel disease and diverticulitis.

    2. Diseases of the colon or rectum.

    3. Fever and abdominal pain in sexually transmitted diseases.

    4. Dysuria and flank pain in urinary tract infections.

11. Esophageal pain may radiate to the:

    1. Infrascapular area.

    2. Right shoulder.

*HBeAg, hepatitis B e antigen; anti-HBc, antibody to hepatitis B core antigen; HBsAg, hepatitis B surface antigen; anti-HBs, antibody to hepatitis B surface antigen.

3. Neck and left arm.

4. Periumbilical area.

12. The most important goal of assessing a client with abdominal pain is to:

1. Palpate the area of pain right away.

2. Rule out emergent conditions.

3. Determine the exact etiology of the pain on the first visit for every client.

4. Determine what tests to order.

13. When the nurse practitioner suspects peritonitis in a client, the best action is to:

1. Percuss over the costovertebral angle and watch for signs of pain.

2. Perform a rectal exam and test the stool for blood.

3. Auscultate the abdomen for decreased bowel sounds.

4. Palpate for a tense, hard abdomen and check for a positive obturator sign.

14. Under what circumstances should peptic ulcer disease **not** be treated empirically before diagnostic studies are done? When the client's ulcer pain:

1. Awakens him/her from sleep early in the morning.

2. Can be relieved by food, antacids, or vomiting.

3. Is worsened by food ingestion.

4. Is atypical or occurring with anemia, blood in the stool, or weight loss.

15. A careful history of a client with a chief complaint of diarrhea reveals that this adult has recurrent abdominal pain and diarrhea that alternates with constipation. The most likely diagnosis is:

1. Drug-induced diarrhea.

2. Inflammatory bowel disease.

3. Giardiasis.

4. Irritable bowel syndrome (IBS).

16. Clients with dysphagia due to motility disorders usually complain of:

1. More difficulty swallowing solids than liquids.

2. Can have a stricture due to esophagitis following a long history of reflux disorder.

3. Cold liquids causing pain.

4. Marked weight loss.

17. The pathogenesis of gastroesophageal reflux disease (GERD) is:

1. Frequent and excessive retograde movement of stomach contents into the esophagus due to an abnormal lower esophageal sphincter (LES) function.

2. Due to a hiatal hernia that leads to the esophageal irritation and inflammation.

3. Due to reflux of the gastric contents after meals when a client is in the upright position often after a period of vigorous exercise.

4. Initiated by erosion of the gastrointestinal mucosa into the LES causing weakening of LES pressure and a burning sensation in the stomach.

18. A client comes to emergent care concerned about pain and swelling in his groin. He tells the nurse practitioner that his doctor told him that he has an incarcerated hernia. The examination of the client reveals a hernia that:

1. Easily moves back and forth across the abdominal wall.

2. Protudes from the groin area and cannot be reduced into the abdomen.

3. Is very painful to palpation with significant abdominal swelling.

4. Decreases in size when the client increases intra-abdominal pressure.

19. Which of the following findings would indicate a need for endoscopy in clients with peptic ulcer disease (PUD)?

    1. All new cases of dyspepsia.

    2. Symptoms persisting after 6–8 weeks of therapy.

    3. All clients with dyspepsia who smoke and use alcohol.

    4. Good response to empiric treatment after 7–10 days.

20. The nurse practitioner's understanding of which principle will be helpful in educating clients with GERD?

    1. A hiatal hernia is always a coexisting and major contributing factor.

    2. The LES has become a poor antireflux barrier.

    3. The amount of acid reflux is dependent on a familial tendency for GERD.

    4. Overeating and use of caffeine and alcohol cause GERD.

21. Inflammatory toxigenic gastrointestinal illness is characterized by:

    1. Fecal leukocytes, dysentery, site: proximal small bowel.

    2. No fecal leukocytes, watery diarrhea, site: distal small bowel.

    3. Fecal leukocytes, secretory diarrhea, site: colon.

    4. Fecal leukocytes, watery diarrhea, site: colon.

22. The nurse practitioner understands that hepatitis B can be transmitted in blood and blood products. Another common mode of transmission of hepatitis B is:

    1. Respiratory contact.

    2. Contaminated fluid.

    3. Fecal–oral route.

    4. Perinatal exposure.

23. An older adult client presents to the nurse practitioner's office with a chief complaint of intermittent heartburn, which became worse 2 months ago from job stress. The discomfort is worse after eating and at night and is relieved temporarily by antacids. The client also states that several times in the last 14 days he has regurgitated very bitter tasting material into the mouth. The physical exam by the nurse practitioner is unremarkable. The nurse practitioner's most likely diagnosis is:

    1. Viral esophagitis.

    2. Irritable bowel syndrome.

    3. Gastroesophageal reflux disease.

    4. Carcinoma of the esophagus.

24. All of the following should be referred to an internist for management due to the high rate of chronic hepatitis **except**:

    1. Hepatitis A.

    2. Hepatitis B.

    3. Hepatitis C.

    4. Hepatitis D.

25. An indirect inguinal hernia:

    1. Is a portion of the bowel or omentum that protrudes directly through the floor of the inguinal canal and exits through the external inguinal ring.

    2. Occurs mainly in middle and later years.

    3. Is due to a weakness in the abdominal structure.

    4. Passes through the internal abdominal ring, traverses the spermatic cord through the inguinal canal, and exits at the external inguinal ring.

26. Which is true about enterobiasis?

    1. The parasite is in the soil and enters the body through the feet. It can cause anemia.

    2. The parasite causes pruritus around the anus because the gravid females exit through the anus at night and lay eggs on the skin. The human is the only host of this parasite.

    3. The eggs of this parasite enter the body by ingestion of dirt (pica) or dirt on unwashed vegetables that contain the eggs or through water containing eggs.

4. This parasite is a protozoan. The source is usually contaminated water but it is spread from person to person by oral–fecal contamination.

27. The therapeutic energy diet modification in GERD consists of which type of diet?

   1. Low energy.
   2. Energy controlled.
   3. High energy.
   4. Small feedings.

28. Nonpharmacologic management of GERD includes the following:

   1. Weight reduction, sleep with head of bed elevated 4–6 inches with blocks.
   2. Lying down and resting after meals, weight reduction.
   3. Drinking large amounts of fluids with meals, avoiding alcohol.
   4. Avoiding mint, orange juice, and high-energy diet.

29. An organism associated with etiology of peptic ulcer disease is:

   1. *Streptococcus pneumoniae.*
   2. *Helicobacter pylori.*
   3. *Moraxella catarrhalis.*
   4. *Staphylococcus aureus.*

30. The most common cause of cirrhosis is:

   1. Hepatitis A.
   2. Hepatitis B.
   3. Hepatitis D.
   4. Alcoholic hepatitis.

31. Prolapse of a vascular anal cushion through the anal canal with resultant entrapment by the internal anal sphincter describes a:

   1. Prolapse of the rectal mucosa.
   2. Hemorrhoid.
   3. Tumor.
   4. Hernia.

32. An acute febrile illness with jaundice, anorexia, and malaise; an incubation period of 45–160 days having a chronic and an acute form; and transmitted by parenteral, sexual, and perinatal routes describes:

   1. Hepatitis A.
   2. Hepatitis B.
   3. Hepatitis C.
   4. Hepatitis D.

33. A client presents to the nurse practitioner's office with a history of cholelithiasis. Which client complaining of increased pain would require immediate admission to the hospital for possible prompt intervention?

   1. A client who is human immunodeficiency virus (HIV)-positive.
   2. A 75-year-old diabetic.
   3. A client with a history of diverticulosis.
   4. A client who is vomiting and has a slight fever.

34. An older adult male presents to the nurse practitioner for evaluation of "heartburn." The client states that he has been taking antacids and an oral histamine, (H₂)-blocker. The client states that after eating he feels like there is a knot in his stomach. He also gives a history of being a cigar smoker. What differential diagnosis must the nurse practitioner consider first?

   1. Gastric ulcer.
   2. Acid reflux.
   3. Esophageal tumor.
   4. Lung tumor.

35. An older adult male presents to the nurse practitioner complaining of weakness and vomiting. The client gives a history of "several" drinks per day for the past 12 years. The nurse practitioner observes that the client's lips appear to have dark blood on them. What emergent condition does the nurse practitioner suspect?

   1. Seizure disorder.
   2. Cerebral hemorrhage.
   3. Pancreatitis.
   4. Esophageal varices.

36. A usually benign diagnosis that can result in small bowel obstruction and infarction and which requires immediate referral to a surgeon is:

    1. Gastric ulcer.

    2. Endometriosis.

    3. Hernia.

    4. Ectopic pregnancy.

37. A previously benign condition that can cause a client severe rectal pain and can be the cause of an emergency visit to the nurse practitioner is:

    1. Hookworms.

    2. Pinworms.

    3. Thrombosed hemorrhoid.

    4. Cystitis.

38. An elderly client presents with fever, leukocytosis, left lower quadrant pain, and diarrhea alternating with constipation. The nurse practitioner would make the diagnosis of:

    1. Appendicitis.

    2. Diverticulitis

    3. Irritable bowel syndrome.

    4. Pancreatitis.

39. Which clients would be the lowest risk for developing diverticular disease?

    1. Vegetarians.

    2. Type A personality.

    3. The elderly.

    4. Fad dieters.

40. The nurse practitioner knows that the following symptom is characteristic of left-sided colon cancer:

    1. Anemia.

    2. Tenesmus.

    3. Bright red rectal bleeding.

    4. Change in bowel habits.

41. The nurse practitioner knows that a history of pancolonic ulcerative colitis requires careful surveillance because of an increased risk of:

    1. Colon cancer.

    2. Anemia.

    3. Depression.

    4. Perforation.

42. Which is true of peptic ulcer disease in the elderly?

    1. Smoking does not increase the risk of peptic ulcer disease.

    2. Duodenal ulcers are more common in the elderly.

    3. Perforation is a rare complication.

    4. Weight loss and anorexia are often the only symptoms.

43. Which is true of early cancer of the esophagus in the elderly client?

    1. Alcoholism and smoking increase the risk for cancer of the esophagus.

    2. It is usually an adenocarcinoma.

    3. Dysphagia for liquids, cough, and hoarseness are early symptoms.

    4. A boring-type midchest pain indicates mediastinal involvement and requires immediate surgery.

44. A client has a history of colon polyps. The nurse practitioner knows:

    1. Polyps of the cecum are most likely to be malignant.

    2. Polyps <1 cm are suspicious for malignancy.

    3. Villous polyps are rarely malignant.

    4. Sessile polyps are more likely to be malignant than pedunculated.

45. The nurse practitioner identifies which of these conditions as most conducive to the development of the metabolic alkalosis in an older adult?

    1. Severe anxiety resulting in hyperventilation.

2. Excessive vomiting related to gastroenteritis.

3. Depressed respirations from excessive narcotics ingestion.

4. Decreased renal function with glomeruli damage.

46. What is the most consistent finding in clients with acute appendicitis?

1. An elevated WBC count.

2. High fever.

3. Periumbilical dull pain.

4. Nausea and vomiting.

Pharmacology

47. An adult client has been treated on and off for PUD for the past 12 years. He has always responded quickly to cimetidine (Tagamet) and antacids. He continues to smoke. He presents to the nurse practitioner's office with severe epigastric pain, weakness, and lightheaded feelings. The stool guaiac is positive and his hemoglobin is 11.2 gm/dl. His weight has decreased slowly over the past 6 months for unknown reasons. Based on this information, what should the nurse practitioner do next?

1. Refill his medications.

2. Give medications and refer to smoking cessation clinic.

3. Discontinue cimetidine and start omeprazole (Prilosec).

4. Consult with a physician.

48. The nurse practitioner is examining an elderly obese man who is complaining of indigestion and heartburn with a strong acid taste in the mouth about an hour after meals. The history is negative for chronic illnesses. A diagnosis of GERD is made. The best way to treat this client is:

1. Lie down after meals, eat five smaller meals per day.

2. Pro-Banthine 15 mg tid 30 minutes prior to eating.

3. Decrease weight, ranitidine (Zantac) 150 mg bid.

4. Omeprazole (Prilosec) 40 mg once a day, antacids.

49. Which of the following would be prescribed as initial treatment for uncomplicated PUD?

1. Cimetidine (Tagamet) 400 mg bid.

2. Doxepin (Sinequan) 25 mg qhs.

3. Omeprazole (Prilosec) 20 mg qd.

4. Pirenzepine 50 mg tid.

50. Which drug would be most useful for the nurse practitioner to prescribe for a client to prevent ulcers due to nonsteroidal anti-inflammatory drugs (NSAIDs)?

1. Misoprostol (Cytotec).

2. Cimetidine (Tagamet).

3. Doxepin (Sinequan).

4. Pirenzepine.

51. After percutaneous or permucosal exposure to an HBsAg-positive source:

1. In an unvaccinated person, begin with the hepatitis B series.

2. In a known hepatitis B responder with an adequate response, no treatment is necessary.

3. In a known hepatitis B responder with inadequate HBsAg, give hepatitis B immunoglobulin and initiate a new hepatitis B vaccine series.

4. In an unknown hepatitis B responder who completed the entire hepatitis B vaccine series, give a hepatitis B booster.

52. *Helicobacter pylori* has been found to be a causative factor in many cases of PUD. Successful treatment requires therapy with which regimen?

1. Combination of H_2 blockers, antacids, and omeprazole (Prilosec).

2. Combination of Pepto-Bismol, amoxicillin (Amoxil), and metronidazole (Flagyl).

3. Combination of lifestyle changes, Pepto-Bismol, and cimetidine (Tagamet).

4. Combination of H_2 blocker, amoxicillin (Amoxil), and antacid.

53. A primary therapy for clients with mild ulcerative colitis is:

    1. Metronidazole (Flagyl).

    2. Sulfasalazine (Azulfidine).

    3. Amoxicillin (Amoxil).

    4. Cephalexin (Keflex).

54. The stepwise approach to management of GERD is:

    1. Lifestyle changes and antacids as needed and cimetidine (Tagamet) 800 mg qd at bedtime.

    2. Lifestyle changes and antacids as needed followed by lifestyle changes plus ranitidine (Zantac) 150 mg bid.

    3. Lifestyle changes and antacids as needed followed by lifestyle changes plus omeprazole (Prilosec) 20 mg qd.

    4. Cisapride (Propulsid) 10 mg taken 15 minutes before meals and at bedtime. Lifestyle changes can be added if this therapy is not effective.

55. After exposure to household or sexual contacts with hepatitis A, the nurse practitioner would:

    1. Give immunoglobulin 0.02 ml/kg as soon as possible but no later than 2 weeks after exposure.

    2. Give hepatitis B immune globulin (HBIG) × 1 and immunoglobulin 0.02 ml/kg as soon as possible.

    3. Give immunoglobulin 0.02 ml/kg and HBIG × 2.

    4. Understand that no injections are needed.

56. Shigellosis is treated by:

    1. No medication intervention, careful toileting and bathroom sanitation, and keeping the perineal area clean.

    2. Symptomatic treatment and antidiarrheal agents.

    3. Symptomatic treatment and trimethoprim-sulfamethoxazole (TMP-SMX; Septra) dosed for age and weight bid × 5 days.

    4. Boiling water and quinacrine HCl (Atabrine) 100 mg PO tid × 5 days.

57. Pharmacologic management of nausea and vomiting includes:

    1. Emetrol 15–30 ml PO in adults.

    2. Promethazine (Phenergan) 25 mg for children over 6 years old and adults.

    3. Hydroxyzine hydrochloride (Vistaril) 1 mg IM for adults.

    4. Trimethobenzamide (Tigan) 10 mg PO prn for adults.

58. The two major factors that lead to disruption of the gastrointestinal mucosa with subsequent development of an ulceration are:

    1. Alcohol consumption and NSAIDs.

    2. NSAIDs and smoking.

    3. NSAIDs and *Helicobacter pylori*.

    4. *Helicobacter pylori* and smoking.

59. A 55-year-old presents with a history of recent unprotected sexual activity with a partner now diagnosed with hepatitis B. She is currently asymptomatic and she does not recall having a vaccine in the past. The best action for the nurse practitioner is:

    1. Draw a hepatitis B e antibody test (anti-HBe).

    2. Administer one dose of HBIG.

    3. Administer two doses of HBIG and initiate vaccination.

    4. Administer one dose of HBIG and initiate vaccination.

60. What condition is a contraindication for the administration of the hepatitis B vaccine?

    1. Pregnancy.

    2. Lactating mothers.

    3. Severe hypersensitivity.

    4. Age >60 years.

61. A 78-year-old client is diagnosed with enterocolitis and the physician prescribes vancomycin (Vancocin) 125 mg PO qid. The nurse practitioner will follow the progress of the client. What areas will be monitored with regard to the medication tolerance?

1. Complete blood count (CBC), platelet count, clotting studies.

2. Serum creatinine, blood urea nitrogen (BUN), hearing changes.

3. Serum electrolytes, urinalysis, ataxia.

4. Changes in bowel habits, diarrhea, electrocardiographic changes.

62. A client with PUD is treated with a regimen that includes bismuth subsalicylate (Pepto-Bismol), tetracycline, and metronidazole (Flaygl). The client calls the nurse practitioner to report that his stools are unusually dark. He is not experiencing any gastric discomfort, orthostatic hypotension, or increased lethargy. The nurse practitioner's interpretation of this information is:

1. He is probably bleeding and should come in immediately.

2. He ate something to affect the color of his stool.

3. His stools are dark secondary to the Pepto-Bismol.

4. The stool discoloration is due to the metronidazole (Flagyl).

Answers & Rationales

Physical Examination & Diagnostic Tests

1. **(4)** Inspection and auscultation should be conducted first in order to prevent undue guarding. If the examination is painful initially, the client is going to be very uncomfortable with allowing the examiner to continue.

2. **(4)** All of the information is important in sorting out the cause of abdominal pain. The location and character may help identify the origin of the pain. Abrupt onset of pain usually has a different etiology than pain that develops over hours. Whether or not the pain has changed since onset can help in determining if a larger area of the abdomen is becoming involved or if the pain is subsiding. Both visceral and parietal pain can be referred to remote sites along shared nerve pathways. Aggravating and alleviating factors can provide clues as to the origin of the pain. Fever, chills, vomiting, diarrhea, constipation, and urogenital associated symptoms are important in determining the cause of the abdominal pain. Past medical history and medication history can give clues to known conditions and to medications that may be causing the symptoms or are being used for conditions that can cause abdominal pain. For example, a client taking ranitidine (Zantac) may fail to mention a history of GERD.

3. **(1)** If abdominal pain results from passive internal rotation of the right hip from the 90-degree hip/knee flexion position, the client has a positive obturator sign, which is suggestive of appendicitis. In a positive Murphy's sign (Option #2), pain and a brief inspiratory arrest results when a client takes a deep breath while the examiner applies pressure over the gallbladder. This is suggestive of cholecystitis. Percussion over the costovertebral angles that elicits pain is a positive costovertebral angle tenderness suggestive of pyrelonephritis. Positioning of the client in a supine position with hips flexed and then auscultating and palpating the abdomen, beginning with light palpation in nontender areas, is the sequence for examining the abdomen.

4. **(1)** HBsAg is found in active or chronic hepatitis B disease. HBeAg indicates active replication of the virus. IgM anti-HBsAg indicates chronic disease. Positive HBsAg indicates chronic disease, and negative HBsAg indicates prior exposure.

5. **(4)** These are standard diagnostics used for screening a client with a high risk for colon cancer. CEA is used more to determine recurrence of cancer; BE, upper GI, and proctoscopy do not provide as reliable information for detecting the malignancy.

6. **(4)** This is the surface marker for hepatitis C; at present there is no way to differentiate the diffuse forms of hepatitis C, as the viremia level is well below the threshold of most assays.

7. **(3)** Options #2 and #3 are almost identical. (*Note: use the testing strategy; both are wrong or one is the correct answer.*) In acute pancreatitis the serum amylase increases within 3–6 hours of onset. The serum lipase elevates after the increase in amylase. (Normal levels of serum amylase in adults are 50–180 U/L; levels of serum lipase are 55–417 U/L).

8. **(3)** The history, right upper quadrant pain that radiates to the right subscapular area, and a positive Murphy's sign are all commonly associated with cholecystitis. A positive obturator sign at McBurney's point is a sign associated with appendicitis. Clients with strangulated hernias have colicky abdominal pain, nausea, vomiting, abdominal distention, and hyperperistalsis. Those with reducible hernias are asymptomatic or have only mild pain.

9. **(4)** Always palpate the nontender areas first, before going to the area of pain and tenderness. Option #2 is not described in the correct order of assessing an abdomen, which is inspection, auscultation, percussion, and palpation. Although Option #1 may be done, it does not answer what the question is asking.

Disorders

10. **(1)** Diarrhea is a common symptom in infectious gastroenteritis, inflammatory bowel disease, diverticulitis, and early intestinal obstruction. Diseases of the colon or rectum are often associated with constipation that clearly precedes the onset of abdominal pain. With sexually transmitted disease, abdominal pain can often occur with vaginal discharge or bleeding and sometimes irregular menses. Dysuria, flank pain, hematuria, and urinary frequency are common signs and symptoms of upper or lower urinary tract infections or ureteral calculi.

11. **(3)** Esophageal pain may radiate to the neck and left arm. Gallbladder pain can radiate to the infrascapular area, diaphragm pain to the right shoulder, and the pain of appendicitis to the periumbilical area.

12. **(2)** The most important goal in evaluating a client who presents with abdominal pain is to rule out emergent conditions. Palpation is done after auscultation. Begin in an area away from the site of the pain. It is important to rule out emergent causes and ideal to make an exact diagnosis every time. However, due to the sometimes complicated nature of abdominal pain, it is not always possible to do this. Ordering appropriate laboratory tests is important but is not the most important goal.

13. **(4)** A tense, hard abdomen, verbal refusal or severe pain when asked to jump, or a positive obturator sign are positive peritoneal signs. Costovertebral angle tenderness is a sign of a renal disorder. Stool for occult blood is not a test for peritonitis. Decreased bowel sounds could be present in appendicitis or bowel obstruction but is not a peritoneal sign.

14. **(4)** Atypical pain or pain that occurs with hematochezia, anemia, or weight loss could be caused by a disorder other than peptic ulcer, such as gastric cancer, or the client's ulcer could be bleeding. Pain that awakens a client early in the morning from sleep or is relieved or worsened by food ingestion is typical of peptic ulcer pain.

15. **(4)** Irritable bowel syndrome presents with abdominal pain and/or altered bowel habits. These symptoms can be aggravated by psychological stresses. Symptoms disappear while sleeping. Bacterial or viral gastroenteritis presents as abdominal pain with diarrhea and vomiting of abrupt onset. Drug-induced diarrhea follows initiation of drug therapy and in this situation, there is no mention of previous drug therapy. In inflammatory bowel disease, nocturnal diarrhea and abdominal pain are often accompanied by rectal fistula, fever, and/or skin lesions. Diarrhea occurring with giardiasis is malodorous. Weight loss occurs over a period of weeks.

16. **(3)** Cold liquids causing pain, dysphagia for both liquids and solids, and repeated swallowing or performance of a rapid Valsalva maneuver that helps food or liquid pass into the stomach are experiences reported by clients with dysphagia caused by a motility disorder. Those with dysphagia due to obstruction have more difficulty swallowing solids than liquids, can have a stricture due to esophagitis resulting from longstanding esophageal reflux, and may report marked weight loss if a tumor is present.

17. **(1)** Esophageal inflammation caused by excessive reflux that overpowers the normal mucosal defense mechanism leads to symptoms of reflux. People with and without a hiatal hernia can experience gastroesophageal reflux. Physiologic or normal reflux occurs in most people after eating when they are in an upright position, especially during vigorous exercise, but its low frequency and small volume do not lead to symptoms. Symptoms of peptic ulcer disease are initiated by erosion of the gastrointestinal mucosa.

18. **(2)** The most common hernia is an inguinal hernia protruding at the inguinal canal. Incarcerated means the hernia cannot be reduced or returned to the abdominal cavity. Reducible hernia easily moves across the abdominal wall. There should be no abdominal swelling and if the hernia is particularly painful and associated with nausea and vomiting, then incarceration should be considered.

19. **(2)** All cases of recurrent, not new, dyspepsia indicate a need for endoscopy. Endoscopy is reserved for those clients with no response to empiric therapy after 7–10 days and symptoms persisting after 8 weeks of therapy. Dyspepsia can be characterized by fullness, belching, and regurgitation and can include PUD and gastroesophageal reflux. Smoking should be discontinued and alcohol intake should be decreased to a moderate level in PUD and GERD, but endoscopy is not indicated for these clients.

20. **(2)** The factor contributing most to reflux is an abnormal antireflux barrier, the LES. Hiatal hernia is not believed to play an important role in the etiology of reflux. Reflux occurs postprandially in the upright position and may be exacerbated by meals, but overeating is not a direct cause. Alcohol and use of caffeine excessively may affect the lower esophageal sphincter pressure.

21. **(3)** The etiologic agents that produce inflammation and cause diarrhea are characterized by positive fecal leukocytes. Viral diarrhea is free of pus, thus no fecal leukocytes would be found on the smear. Noninflammatory diarrhea is usually caused by a rotavirus. Toxigenic bacteria cause diarrhea by elaborating toxins that have been released after bacterial growth in the intestines. These poisonous substances result in secretory diarrhea.

22. **(4)** A common means of hepatitis B transmission is from mother to baby, perinatally. Other mechanisms of transmission are by infected body fluids, sexual contact, and parenterally. Hepatitis E virus is spread in contaminated water. Hepatitis A's mode of transmission is fecal–oral and person-to-person.

23. **(3)** The client is presenting with the most reliable symptoms of GERD. GERD is most often related to inappropriate relaxation of the lower esophageal sphincter, which allows reflux of gastric acid and pepsin into the distal esophagus. Common presentations of IBS are differentiated by cramping, abdominal pain, or altered bowel habits predominating. Clients with esophagitis complain of the acute onset of chest pain, dysphagia, and odynophagia. Bleeding is associated with carcinoma.

24. **(1)** Hepatitis A and E do not have a chronic stage, and generally resolve without any long-term effects.

25. **(4)** Because indirect hernias are due to a congenital defect in which the processus vaginalis remains patent, they occur more often in younger persons. A portion of the bowel and/or the omentum comes through the internal abdominal ring, traverses the spermatic cord through the inguinal canal, and exits at the external inguinal ring. In a direct hernia, the omentum or bowel protrudes directly through the floor of the inguinal canal and exits through the external inguinal ring. Because it is due to a weakness in the abdominal structures, it

occurs more often in the middle and later years of life.

26. **(2)** These parasites reside in the intestine. Females lay eggs on the skin outside the anus, resulting in extreme pruritus. The only host is humans. Hookworm larvae reside in the soil, enter the body through the feet, and can cause anemia. When dirt containing roundworm eggs is ingested due to pica, or unwashed vegetables or contaminated water is consumed, an intestinal infestation occurs. Giardiasis results from ingestion of the protozoan *Giardia lamblia* through contaminated water or via oral–fecal transmission.

27. **(4)** The small-feedings diet used for GERD results in decreased gastric volume and decreased likelihood of continued reflux. Low-energy diets are used in obesity for weight loss. Energy-controlled diets are used for clients with diabetes mellitus for increased glucose tolerance. High-energy diets are used for clients with anorexia for increased weight and fat.

28. **(1)** A high-energy diet is used for clients with anorexia. Management of GERD includes weight reduction, avoid lying down after meals, avoid large meals, avoid exercise after meals, and elevate the head of the bed. Certain foods and drinks, such as alcohol, mint, and orange juice, should be avoided as they may cause symptoms of heartburn.

29. **(2)** *Helicobacter pylori* has been implicated in the etiology of ulcer disease. The other organisms listed are implicated in other types of infections, such as acute otitis media and skin infections.

30. **(4)** Alcohol is the most important cause of cirrhosis in the United States. Especially in men, one six-pack of beer or four glasses per day of wine significantly increases the risk for long-term hepatic injury leading to cirrhosis. The corresponding amount is about half that for women. Hepatitis A is a self-limited infection without a known chronic state. Hepatitis B and D acute infections do not directly result in a high incidence of cirrhosis.

31. **(2)** A hemorrhoid results when a vascular anal cushion prolapses through the anal canal and is entrapped by the internal anal sphincter. In a rectal mucosa prolapse, the wall of the rectum prolapses. A tumor is not a vascular anal cushion.

32. **(2)** These characteristics describe hepatitis B. Hepatitis A has similar symptoms but can be transmitted by the oral–fecal or oral–genital route and has an incubation period of 15–50 days and no chronic form. Hepatitis C infection rarely causes jaundice. It is transmitted parenterally and has an incubation period of 14–140 days and a chronic form. Hepatitis D coexists with hepatitis B, is transmitted parenterally, and can also become chronic. Hepatitis E is characterized by oral–fecal transmission associated with contaminated food and water, an incubation period of 14–60 days, and no chronic disease state.

33. **(2)** While most clients need eventual intervention, those who are elderly and diabetic are at increased risk and should be hospitalized for prompt diagnosis, intravenous fluids, pain control, and surgical consultation.

34. **(3)** A typical description of a "knot" is described by clients who have esophageal tumors. The symptom of heartburn caused by either gastric ulcer or acid reflux should be controlled by the H_2-blocker.

35. **(4)** Clients with a history of heavy alcohol intake are at increased risk for cirrhosis and portal hypertension, which may result in variceal bleeding. These clients often present clinically with bleeding, hypotension, and eventual shock.

36. **(3)** A strangulated hernia is irreducible and the blood supply to the trapped bowel is compromised, resulting in bowel infarction. Ulcers, endometriosis, and ectopic pregnancy can cause abdominal pain and can be surgical emergencies but they do not cause bowel obstruction.

37. **(3)** Thrombosed hemorrhoids can cause severe pain for clients and should be quickly decompressed. While irritating and causing itching, pinworms do not cause rectal pain. Hookworms penetrate the soles of the feet and cystitis usually causes lower abdominal, not rectal, pain.

38. **(2)** Diverticular disease presents with change in bowel habits (diarrhea alternating with constipation or both), blood in stool, and if diverticulitis develops, flatus, low-grade fever, and leukocytosis may be present. The majority of clients with diverticulosis may have no symptoms; some may have abdominal pain in the left lower quadrant. Appendicitis may present with pain in the right lower quadrant and may not be severe until perforation occurs. Other signs may include nausea and vomiting, and leukocytosis; fever may or may not be present. Irritable bowel syndrome may present with aching or cramping periumbilical or lower abdominal pain often precipitated by meals and relieved by defecation. Pain may radiate to left chest or arm, and there are alternating episodes of diarrhea and constipation. Pancreatitis may present with epigastric pain or tenderness that lasts for hours and may radiate to the back, fever, nausea and vomiting, mental confusion, and jaundice.

39. **(1)** High-fiber diet is the treatment for this disease, and vegetarians eat increased amounts of fruits, vegetables, grains, and cereals. Options #2, #3, and #4 are at higher risk because they do not address the concept of fiber.

40. **(4)** Colorectal cancer occurs most commonly in individuals over age 50. A change in bowel habit with reduced caliber of stool and blood mixed with the stool are characteristic of left-sided colon cancer, which is the most common site. Anemia is found with right-sided lesions. Bright red rectal bleeding and tenesmus are characteristic of rectal cancer.

41. **(1)** Colon cancer risk in pancolonic ulcerative colitis increases by 2% per year after the tenth year of diagnosis.

42. **(4)** Peptic ulcer disease in the elderly often does not cause the usual pain and indigestion associated with the disease in younger individuals. Smoking does increase the risk, and without the pain perforation is common. Gastric ulcers are more commonly seen.

43. **(1)** Cancer of the esophagus is found mostly in elderly men. Alcoholism and smoking are the primary risk factors of cancer of the esophagus. The cell type is usually squamous cell. Symptoms include dysphagia for liquids, cough and hoarseness, as well as boring midchest pain, and indicate late disease, which does not usually respond to any treatment, including surgery.

44. **(4)** Flexible sigmoidoscopy and colonoscopy are screening tools for colorectal cancer recommended after age 50. It is useful for identifying adenomatous polyps, which are considered premalignant. Sessile or flat polyps are more suspicious for malignancy. The polyps of the cecum and polyps <1 cm are less likely to be malignant and villous polyps are often malignant.

45. **(2)** Excessive vomiting with loss of acid is a common problem with metabolic alkalosis. Respiratory problems do not precipitate primary metabolic acid-base imbalance and renal disease most often causes metabolic acidosis.

46. **(3)** Appendicitis usually begins as dull periumbilical pain accompanied by anorexia and nausea, but not necessarily vomiting. Within a few hours there may be low-grade fever. Most laboratory tests are normal. A WBC count of >15,000/mm^3 is often noted but neither confirms nor excludes the diagnosis of appendicitis.

Pharmacology

47. **(4)** For clients with reoccurring symptoms after a course of treatment for PUD, consult a physician. The client is having symptoms of active bleeding and endoscopy may be indicated at this point. The physician should be consulted regarding the next step. Omeprazole (Prilosec), a proton pump inhibitor, inhibits acid secretion, is useful for hypergastrinemia, and may be useful in PUD clients not controlled by H$_2$ antagonists in the absence of active bleeding.

48. **(3)** H$_2$ blockers, changes in diet, and weight reduction are the first line of treatment for GERD. The client should be advised to sit up after meals, and sleep with his head elevated. Anticholinergics (Pro-Banthine) may increase the problem by lowering the

LES pressure. Omeprazole is not recommended for the first phase of treatment.

49. **(1)** Goals of PUD treatment include relief of pain, healing of ulcer, and cost-effectiveness. The H$_2$ receptor antagonists heal 90% of duodenal ulcers and 70% of gastric ulcers. The proton pump inhibitors such as omeprazole are recommended for ulcers unresponsive to the receptor antagonists after 8–12 weeks with full dosing and GERD. The anticholinergic drugs doxepin (Sinequan) and pirenzepine are useful when used with the H$_2$ receptors but are limited by side effects, and used only in Canada and Europe at this time.

50. **(1)** The prostaglandins, such as misoprostol (Cytotec), are used to decrease recurrent ulcerations in clients who require NSAIDs. They have not, however, been shown to increase ulcer healing. Cimetidine (Tagamet) has been shown to increase healing. Doxepin (Sinequan) and pirenzepine are not prescribed in the United States as of this date.

51. **(2)** If a person exposed to a client known to be positive for hepatitis B has sufficient immunity to hepatitis B, no treatment is necessary. If this same person had not been vaccinated, in addition to initiation of the hepatitis B vaccine series, HBIG 0.06 ml/kg IM is also administered. If an exposed person has had an inadequate immune response to the hepatitis B vaccine series, a hepatitis B booster is to be given. There is no need to repeat the series. If the response to the hepatitis B vaccine series is unknown, test the exposed person's hepatitis D surface antigen level and decide what intervention, if any, is needed.

52. **(2)** Therapy for clients with refractory ulcers due to *H. pylori* are most successfully treated with the triple-drug therapy of Pepto-Bismol, amoxicillin or tetracycline, and metronidazole (Flagyl). Less effective but well-tolerated regimens consist of omeprazole (Prilosec) and amoxicillin.

53. **(2)** Sulfasalazine (Azulfidine) therapy for clients with mild ulcerative colitis results in symptomatic improvement in 50–75% of cases. If no response is seen after 2–4 weeks, the addition of prednisone is recommended. This drug prevents relapse of ulcerative colitis once remission is induced. The other drugs listed are not recommended as first-line treatment.

54. **(2)** Since 25% of clients are effectively treated with lifestyle changes, therapy should begin with use of these measures. If these are not completely effective, an H$_2$ receptor antagonist can be added. Twice-daily dosing is recommended. Omeprazole (Prilosec) is recommended only for refractory cases. Cisapride (Propulsid) can be effective, but lifestyle changes and antacid tablets as needed is the recommended starting point for therapy.

55. **(1)** To minimize the risk of a contact developing hepatitis A, immunoglobulin 0.02 ml/kg should be given as soon as possible after exposure. It has not been shown to be effective if administered more than 2 weeks after exposure.

56. **(3)** Treatment with trimethoprim-sulfamethoxazole shortens the course and prevents further spread of the organism. Prevention of dehydration that can result from the diarrhea is accomplished through symptomatic treatment (clear liquids for 24–48 hours, no dairy products, electrolyte-rich sports drinks, advance diet as tolerated). Antidiarrheal medications are not recommended because intestinal motility is important in recovery. Option #4 would be appropriate treatment for nonpregnant adults who have giardiasis.

57. **(1)** The Emetrol dose for adults is 15–30 ml. Phenergan 25 mg can be given to children over 12 years old (not 6 years old) and adults. The older child and adult dose for hydroxyzine hydrochloride (Vistaril) is 25–100 mg. Trimethobenzamide (Tigan) is dosed at 200 mg, not 10 mg.

58. **(3)** Nonsteroidal anti-inflammatory agents are more often associated with mucosal disruptions causing gastric ulcers. *Helicobacter pylori* is associated with mucosal disruption that leads to peptic ulcer disease. Alcohol and smoking are not causes of gastrointestinal mucosal disruption.

59. **(4)** For clients with exposure to hepatitis B and who are unvaccinated, administer one dose of HBIG and initiate the vaccine. For clients who thinks they may have been vaccinated but do not know if they responded, the nurse practitioner may have a prevaccination antibody testing done. The HBe antibody is drawn to determine the potential for transmission; it generally appears about 3 months after the onset of the infection.

60. **(3)** The only contraindication to the hepatitis B vaccine is a prior anaphylaxis or severe hypersensitivity to the vaccine or components of the vaccine.

61. **(2)** This medication causes problems with nephro- and ototoxicity (eighth cranial nerve). Laboratory tests to monitor renal function should be determined on a regular basis. The client should be frequently evaluated for any hearing loss. The geriatric client is particularly susceptible to the complications and toxicity.

62. **(3)** This is a common observation for a client on Pepto-Bismol. He may also experience a problem with discoloration of his tongue.

13

Hematology

Physical Examination & Diagnostic Tests

1. On physical examination, a palpable, firm, nontender, supraclavicular lymph node is noted on the left side of the body. This information is consistent with a diagnosis of:

   1. Bacterial infection draining from the internal jugular chain.

   2. Thoracic or abdominal malignancy.

   3. Inflammation of the tonsils and adenoids.

   4. Non-Hodgkin's lymphoma.

2. The nurse practitioner describes a "shotty" lymph node as:

   1. Tender, mobile, and >5 mm.

   2. Small and pellet-like.

   3. Discrete and cystic.

   4. Irregular, soft, and fixed to surrounding tissue.

3. A macrocytic, normochromic anemia is diagnosed in an elderly man. The next test(s) that should be ordered is (are):

   1. Serum iron and total iron-binding capacity (TIBC) levels.

   2. Bone marrow biopsy.

   3. Colonoscopy.

   4. Vitamin B_{12} and red blood cell (RBC)-folate levels.

4. After confirming the diagnosis of iron deficiency anemia in an adult client based on standard laboratory values (complete blood count [CBC], peripheral smear, serum iron, TIBC, serum ferritin), what would be the next essential test for the nurse practitioner to order?

   1. Stool guaiac $\times$ 3.

   2. Prothrombin time and partial thromboplastin time.

   3. Liver function tests.

   4. Endoscopy.

5. Evaluation of an elderly male client reveals a macrocytic, normochromic anemia. Subsequent testing shows a folate level that is normal, and a decreased vitamin B_{12} level. Further evaluation should include:

   1. Referral to a hematologist for a bone marrow biopsy.

   2. Schilling's test.

   3. Upper gastrointestinal (GI) series.

   4. No tests are indicated at this time.

6. The most sensitive test for the diagnosis of sickle cell anemia is:

   1. CBC with a peripheral smear.

   2. Bone marrow biopsy and aspiration.

   3. Hemoglobin electrophoresis.

   4. Hemoglobin and hematocrit.

7. An elderly male presents to the nurse practitioner's office with complaints of fatigue, dizziness, decreased activity tolerance, and occasional bounding heart rate. Physical examination reveals pallor (including mucous membranes), tachycardia, and general appearance of lethargy. The following tests are ordered: CBC with differential, peripheral smear, serum iron, TIBCs, serum ferritin. These tests are ordered because there is a high index of suspicion of:

   1. Sideroblastic anemia.

   2. Pernicious anemia.

   3. Folic acid deficiency anemia.

   4. Iron deficiency anemia.

8. Anemia of chronic disease would reveal which lab findings?

   1. Decreased iron, decreased TIBC, and decreased serum ferritin.

   2. Decreased iron, decreased TIBC, and increased serum ferritin.

   3. Decreased iron, increased TIBC, and decreased serum ferritin.

   4. Decreased iron, increased TIBC, and increased serum ferritin.

Disorders

9. Sickle cell anemia is caused by:

   1. Exposure to ionizing radiation.

   2. A genetically induced production of abnormal hemoglobin S.

   3. A deficiency of dietary folic acid.

   4. Long-term use of thiazide diuretics.

10. An adult client presents to the nurse practitioner with a history of erythrocytosis. One common complaint that could cause a serious complication for this client is:

    1. A laceration.

    2. Vomiting and diarrhea.

    3. Coughing.

    4. Dizziness.

11. A client has a folic acid deficiency anemia. The nurse practitioner teaches the client to eat foods rich in folic acid such as:

    1. Green leafy vegetables, nuts, and liver.

    2. Carrots, salmon, and avacados.

    3. Cottage cheese, yogurt, and skim milk.

    4. Lima beans, brussel sprouts, and potatoes.

12. Which of the changes occur in the RBC indices for pernicious anemia?

    1. Microcytic, normochromic.

    2. Microcytic, hypochromic.

    3. Normocytic, normochromic.

    4. Macrocytic, normochromic.

13. Iron deficiency anemia is an example of:

    1. Macrocytic, normochromic anemia.

    2. Macrocytic, hypochromic anemia.

    3. Microcytic, hypochromic anemia.

    4. Normocytic, normochromic anemia.

14. A client with pernicious anemia may present with which signs and symptoms?

1. Paresthesias, unsteady gait, lethargy, and fatigue.

2. Hepatomegaly, jaundice, and right upper quadrant pain.

3. Hypertension, angina, and peripheral edema.

4. Blurred vision, diplopia, and decreased visual acuity.

15. Anemia of chronic disease is a:

   1. Normochromic, normocytic anemia.

   2. Normochromic, microcytic anemia.

   3. Hypochromic, microcytic anemia.

   4. Hypochromic, macrocytic anemia.

16. An adult presents to the clinic for a routine checkup. History is unremarkable, and on physical exam, an enlarged (2-cm) mobile, nontender and rubbery lymph node is palpated on the left posterior cervical chain. The nurse practitioner's next step is:

   1. Order a throat culture and monospot test.

   2. Referral to a surgeon for a lymph node biopsy.

   3. Order a stat chest x-ray.

   4. No intervention is necessary at this time.

17. The nurse practitioner understands that "B" symptoms associated with non-Hodgkin's lymphoma (NHL) include:

   1. Bruising and bleeding.

   2. Peripheral edema, shortness of breath, and ascites.

   3. Fever, night sweats, and unexplained weight loss (>10% of body weight).

   4. Headache, fatigue, and weakness.

18. In teaching a client with anemia to include foods rich in iron in their diet, the nurse practitioner encourages the client to eat:

   1. Cheese, milk, and yogurt.

   2. Red beans, whole-grain bread, and bran cereal.

   3. Tomatoes, cabbage, and citrus fruits.

   4. Beef, spinach, and peanut butter.

19. Anemia of chronic disease is associated with:

   1. Malnutrition and B_{12} deficiency.

   2. Infections, inflammation, and neoplasms.

   3. Traumatic injuries and folate deficiency.

   4. Excessive menstrual flow, trauma, and heredity.

20. The nurse practitioner understands that most adult clients with Hodgkin's disease present with:

   1. Nausea, vomiting, and diarrhea.

   2. Night sweats, weight loss, and fever.

   3. Painless, movable mass in the neck, axilla, or groin.

   4. Hepatosplenomegaly with a painful mass in the mediastinum.

21. What is the most common leukemia found in the older adult and is typically asymptomatic and characterized by a median survival rate of approximately 10 years?

   1. Acute myelogenous.

   2. Chronic myelogenous.

   3. Acute lymphocytic.

   4. Chronic lymphocytic.

Pharmacology

22. The nurse practitioner determines that an adult male client has an iron deficiency anemia, and has ruled out GI bleeding as the cause. The nurse practitioner:

   1. Refers the client to a hematologist.

   2. Refers the client to a GI specialist.

   3. Prescribes ferrous sulfate 300 mg PO tid, and has the client return in 1 month for a repeat CBC, serum iron, and TIBC.

   4. Has the client return in 6 months for additional stool guaiac testing.

23. Teaching clients regarding the treatment of vitamin B_{12} deficiency includes:

    1. The client will receive vitamin B_{12} tablets given twice daily for 1 year.

    2. Oral folic acid supplements will be given daily for the client's lifetime.

    3. Monthly cyanocobalamin (vitamin B_{12}) injections will be given for the client's lifetime (after being given weekly for the first month).

    4. Iron supplementation and monthly blood transfusions will be required until the deficiency is corrected.

24. Treatment of anemia of chronic disease should include:

    1. A folic acid supplement, 1 mg PO qd.

    2. Iron sulfate ($FeSO_4$) supplement, 300 mg PO tid.

    3. Treatment of the underlying condition.

    4. Weekly epoetin alfa (Epogen) injections.

13   Answers & Rationales

Physical Examination & Diagnostic Tests

1. **(2)** A Virchow's node in the left supraclavicular region is of concern due to the high correlation with abdominal or thoracic malignancy. Infections and inflammatory conditions produce tender inflamed lymph nodes.

2. **(2)** Shotty, or small and pellet-like, lymph nodes that are movable, cool, nontender, discrete, and up to 3 mm in diameter are usually considered normal.

3. **(4)** It is important to determine which type of macrocytic anemia a client has, so that the appropriate therapy can be ordered. Therefore, the vitamin B_{12} and RBC-folate levels would be ordered. These tests would determine if the client has a pernicious anemia (the most common type), or a folate deficiency (also common in the elderly). Serum iron and TIBC would be ordered if an iron deficiency anemia was suspected (it is not in this case because it is a microcytic anemia). There is no indication for a colonoscopy. It would be premature to order a bone marrow biopsy at this point, without performing initial testing and potentially overlooking an easily treated condition (i.e., pernicious anemia, folate deficiency anemia).

4. **(1)** Stool guaiac would identify blood loss from the GI tract, the most common cause of iron deficiency anemia. The other tests should be done if the stool guaiacs are positive. Finding the cause of the iron deficiency is paramount, and the stool guaiac is an easy, noninvasive method of ruling out bleeding as the cause.

5. **(2)** A Schilling's test will determine the cause of the vitamin B_{12} deficiency. It will distinguish between inadequate intake, an intrinsic factor deficiency, or a malabsorption problem. This will allow the practitioner to prescribe the most appropriate therapy for the client. A bone marrow biopsy and an upper GI series are not indicated at this time.

6. **(3)** Normal and abnormal hemoglobins can be detected by electrophoresis, which matches hemolyzed red cell material against standard bands for the various known hemoglobins, including hemoglobin S (the abnormal hemoglobin that is associated with sickle cell anemia). CBC with peripheral smear, and hemoglobin/hematocrit would not yield enough information to diagnose sickle cell anemia. Bone marrow biopsy would not be necessary and would not indicate the presence of hemoglobin S.

7. **(4)** This client's clinical picture is a classic presentation for anemia. Further testing would be needed to determine the type of anemia involved. The most common cause in elderly males is GI bleeding, which would cause an iron deficiency anemia. The tests that were ordered would confirm or rule out this diagnosis; the peripheral smear is especially important in diagnosing the specific type of anemia. If the smear ruled out the diagnosis of iron deficiency anemia, it would lead the practitioner to other diagnoses (including the remaining choices) and appropriate laboratory tests required for confirmation.

8. **(2)** Normal to increased iron stores (serum ferritin) with concurrent low serum iron is the hallmark finding of anemia of chronic disease. The serum iron is decreased along with the total iron-binding capacity. Options #1 and #4 contain incorrect information for the anemias. Option #3 contains the findings for iron deficiency anemia.

Disorders

9. **(2)** Sickle cell anemia is a genetic disorder characterized by the production of hemoglobin S, an anemia secondary to shortened erythrocyte survival, microvascular occlusion by sickle-shaped erythrocytes, and an increased susceptibility to certain infections. Exposure to ionizing radiation has been associated with the development of certain malignancies, especially leukemia. A deficiency of dietary folic acid does not cause sickle cell anemia, although folic acid is used in the treatment of these clients to help increase hematopoiesis and aid in recovery from aplastic events. Long-term use of thiazide diuretics has been implicated in the development of hemolytic or aplastic anemias, in very rare cases.

10. **(2)** Erythrocytosis (or polycythemia) can be worsened by dehydration from any cause. Coughing and dizziness will have no effect on the condition and a laceration may actually improve the symptoms due to the blood loss.

11. **(1)** Green leafy vegetables, nuts, and liver are excellent sources of folic acid. Also, cereals and breads are now fortified with folic acid. The other foods are not significant sources of folic acid.

12. **(4)** A macrocytic (MCV >100), normochromic anemia resulting from atrophic gastric mucosa not secreting intrinsic factor is the definition for pernicious anemia. These indices could also include folic acid deficiency anemia. Options #1 and #2 could include iron deficiency anemia or anemia of chronic disease. Option #3 could also include anemia of chronic disease.

13. **(3)** Iron deficiency anemia is a microcytic, hypochromic anemia. The red blood cells are smaller (microcytic) due to the decrease in hemoglobin production caused by inadequate amounts of iron. This also makes the cell appear pale (hypochromic). The other selections describe other types of anemia, and would be determined by the peripheral smear.

14. **(1)** A deficiency in vitamin B_{12} can cause neurologic signs and symptoms including paresthesias, an unsteady gait, lethargy, and fatigue. These findings are specific to pernicious anemia, and so must always be assessed for in any client who presents with an anemia. The other signs and symptoms are not characteristic of pernicious anemia.

15. **(1)** Anemia of chronic disease is a chronic normochromic, normocytic anemia. There is normal production of hemoglobin, along with normal maturation of red blood cells.

16. **(2)** Lymphadenopathy as described, without evidence of infection, should always be referred to a surgeon for biopsy, because biopsy is the only definitive test to rule out a malignancy (a frequent cause of lymphadenopathy not caused by infectious processes). There are no signs or symptoms to suggest the need for a throat culture, monospot, or chest x-ray. Not intervening is not appropriate because the cause of lymphadenopathy needs to be determined.

17. **(3)** This constellation of symptoms (fever, night sweats, weight loss) is used in the staging of non-Hodgkin's lymphoma, the presence of which is considered to be a poor prognostic indicator. The other symptoms may occur depending on the amount of disease involvement, but are not considered

"B" symptoms, also known as constitutional symptoms.

18. **(4)** Beef, spinach, and peanut butter are iron-rich foods. The remaining selections are examples of foods rich in calcium, fiber, and vitamin C, respectively.

19. **(2)** Anemia of chronic disease is associated with infections (i.e., tuberculosis), chronic inflammatory conditions (i.e., systemic lupus erythematosus, rheumatoid arthritis), and malignancies. Excessive blood loss from menstrual flow or traumatic injuries would more likely cause an iron deficiency anemia. Malnutrition can contribute to iron, vitamin B_{12}, and folate deficiencies.

20. **(3)** Most clients present with a painless, movable mass in the neck, axilla, or groin. Older clients may present with fatigue, weight loss, or persistent fever, and night sweats. Often, there is pain in diseased areas after consuming alcohol (an unexplained finding). Hepatosplenomegaly presents with advanced disease.

21. **(4)** Chronic lymphocytic leukemia (CLL) is found primarily in the middle and older adult; fewer than 10% of all clients are under the age of 50. Acute myelogenous leukemia (AML) incidence increases with age, and approximately 50% are younger than 50 years of age. Chronic myelogenous leukemia (CML) occurs most often at a median age of 45. Acute lymphocytic leukemia (ALL) is most common in children and gradually increases in frequency in later life.

Pharmacology

22. **(3)** Treatment with iron orally for at least 6 months is necessary to correct both the anemia and the depleted body stores. The client should have the hemoglobin, hematocrit, iron, and TIBC rechecked after 1 month on iron supplementation. If there is not improvement in all parameters, most notably a rise in the hemoglobin by 1 gm/dl, the client should be referred to a hematologist. There is no need to refer to a GI specialist or repeat the guaiac, because there is no indication that this client's condition is caused by bleeding.

23. **(3)** If the deficiency is not due to inadequate intake, the client will require lifetime supplementation of vitamin B_{12}. It must be given in the form of an intramuscular or subcutaneous injection to ensure absorption. Oral folic acid, iron, and blood transfusions would not treat the cause of the deficiency, and therefore the resulting anemia would not be corrected.

24. **(3)** Treatment of the underlying condition leads to resolution of the anemia of chronic disease. Folic acid and iron supplements are indicated for folate and iron deficiency anemias, respectively. Epoetin alfa (Epogen) injections are indicated for those conditions that affect erythropoiesis, (i.e., chronic renal failure, chemotherapy-induced anemia, and acquired immunodeficiency syndrome).

Urinary

14

Physical Examination & Diagnostic Tests

1. When taking a history on voiding patterns in adults, the nurse practitioner knows:

   1. Adults normally void q2–3h in a 24-hour period (8–12 times a day).

   2. The first sensation to void occurs when the bladder fills to 200–300 ml.

   3. Normally, 15–20 minutes pass between when the first urge to void occurs and the functional capacity is reached.

   4. Adults typically reach functional (comfortable) capacity at 200–300 ml and may experience some leakage if voiding is delayed.

2. A urinalysis that suggests a urinary tract infection shows:

   1. Protein only.

   2. Alkaline pH and positive nitrite and leukocyte esterase.

   3. Hematuria and pyuria only.

   4. Red color without the presence of red blood cells.

3. An intravenous urography and voiding cystourethrography assists in diagnosing:

   1. Congenital anomalies, stone formation, or foreign bodies.

   2. Renal size and the presence of stone.

   3. A problem in the urethra, prostate, or bladder.

   4. Visualization of the ureter and renal pelvis.

165

4. According to the Agency for Health Care Policy and Research (AHCPR) Guideline Panel, the basic continence evaluation for the primary care provider includes:

   1. History, physical examination, measurement of postvoid residual volume, and urinalysis.

   2. Measurement of postvoid residual volume, blood urea nitrogen (BUN) serum creatinine, and urinalysis.

   3. History, physical examination, serum glucose, BUN, serum creatinine, and urinalysis.

   4. Urodynamic, endoscopic, and imaging tests; urinalysis and serum creatinine.

5. The nurse practitioner expects which findings on examination of an older client with dehydration?

   1. Tongue furrows and skin tenting on the forehead.

   2. Specific gravity of urine 1.004.

   3. Pulse rate 58 strong and regular; blood pressure (BP) 100/62.

   4. Geographic tongue and reduced saliva pool.

Disorders

6. An older adult female client explains to the nurse practitioner that she has been having frequent and painful urination. The nurse practitioner orders a clean-catch urine for routine urinalysis and culture and sensitivity. The laboratory culture and sensitivity report is as follows: 10^5 *Escherichia coli* and 10^4 *Staphylococcus epidermidis* per ml. The nurse practitioner would:

   1. Treat the *E. coli*.

   2. Order penicillin.

   3. Treat the *S. epidermidis*.

   4. Encourage citric fruit juices.

7. An elderly female client is incontinent of urine. What should the nurse practitioner advise the family caretaker to avoid using on the skin in the perineal area?

   1. Petrolatum.

   2. Moisture-barrier films.

   3. Mild soap and water.

   4. Zinc oxide ointment.

8. Which plan would be most appropriate for an older client with functional incontinence:

   1. Evaluate need for pads.

   2. Limit fluid intake in the evenings.

   3. Perform Credé's maneuver.

   4. Provide a bedside commode.

9. A male client presents with recurrent urinary tract infections. What is the most likely cause?

   1. Balanitis.

   2. Epididymitis.

   3. Chronic bacterial prostatitis.

   4. Benign prostatic hypertrophy.

10. A possible cause of transient urinary incontinence, which can be reversed, is:

    1. Poor pelvic support causing hypermobility of the base of the bladder in females.

    2. Lower urinary tract problems, such as carcinoma.

    3. Cystocele or uterine prolapse in women.

    4. Ingestion of certain medications, such as sedatives, diuretics, anticholinergic agents, α-adrenergic agents.

11. Functional incontinence is:

    1. Leakage of urine during activities that increase abdominal pressure, such as coughing, sneezing, laughing, or other physical activities.

    2. Mainly caused by factors outside the urinary tract, such as dementia or immobility, that prohibit proper toileting habits.

3. Characterized by the inability to delay urination, with an abrupt and strong desire to void.

4. The occurrence of incontinence with overdistention of the bladder.

12. The two most common pathogens in community-acquired urinary tract infections are:

1. *Klebsiella pneumoniae* and *Proteus mirabilis.*

2. *Staphylococcus saprophyticus* and *Escherichia coli.*

3. *Proteus mirabilis* and *Staphylococcus saprophyticus.*

4. *Escherichia coli* and *Proteus mirabilis.*

13. Recurrent urinary tract infections in older adult females are due to relapse or reinfection. The nurse practitioner understands that relapse:

1. Is less common than reinfection and occurs within 2 weeks of the completion of drug therapy for the infection.

2. Is responsible for most recurrent urinary tract infections in females.

3. May occur due to residual urine after voiding due to a prolapsed uterus or bladder or to lack of estrogen.

4. Can be treated with the same medication regimen as the original infection.

14. A client has a renal stone that consists of uric acid. What is the best diet to order for this client to decrease the incidence of the stone formation?

1. Alkaline ash diet and low purine.

2. High purine and an acid ash diet.

3. Increased fluid intake and high doses of vitamin C.

4. High complex carbohydrates and decreased protein.

15. The nurse practitioner understands that the treatment of pyelonephritis:

1. In females is suggestive of a structural problem.

2. Requires hospitalization, parenteral antibiotic therapy, and an intravenous voiding pyelogram in males.

3. In females requires hospitalization, parenteral antibiotic therapy, and an intravenous voiding pyelogram.

4. Requires no follow-up.

16. A client is diagnosed with renal failure and the origin of the problem is thought to be postrenal. What would the nurse practitioner identify as a possible precipitating cause of this client's renal failure?

1. History of myocardial infarction with severe hypotensive episode.

2. Advanced prostate hypertrophy with hematuria.

3. Renal vascular changes secondary to long history of diabetes.

4. Exposure to carbon tetrachloride on his job site.

17. Urinary incontinence associated with conditions such as Parkinson's disease, Alzheimer's disease, and stroke is termed:

1. Stress incontinence.

2. Urge incontinence.

3. Frequency incontinence.

4. Overflow incontinence.

18. A male client presents with complaints of blood in his urine; it is painless and he has no difficulty with voiding. The nurse practitioner obtains a urinalysis to confirm the presence of blood and there is no bacteria present. What is the priority diagnosis that must be ruled out on this client?

1. Cancer of the prostate.

2. Prerenal failure.

3. Renal calculi.

4. Cancer of the bladder.

19. The nurse practitioner is taking a history on a client who has been diagnosed with renal calculi. What information in the history would the practitioner identify as a precipitating factor in the development of renal calculi?

    1. Increased incidence of urinary tract infections over the past 3 years.

    2. Drinking 6–8 oz of milk daily.

    3. History of fractured femur and prolonged bed rest.

    4. High intake of citrus fruit and high-fiber carbohydrates.

20. A nurse practitioner recognizes what factors as contributing to the development of prerenal failure?

    1. History of an anaphylactic reaction that rendered the client unconscious.

    2. Extended treatment of an infection with gentamicin (Garamycin).

    3. Acute pyelonephritis and consequently glomerulonephritis.

    4. Renal vascular changes that occur secondary to atherosclerotic disease.

21. The nurse practitioner is teaching a female client some guidelines regarding bladder health, which include all **except**:

    1. Drink at least six to eight glasses of water per day.

    2. Avoid doing Kegel's exercises.

    3. Avoid constipation.

    4. Consider estrogen replacement after menopause.

Pharmacology

22. The nurse practitioner has selected nitrofurantoin (Macrodantin) for treatment of a chronic urinary tract infection in a female geriatric client. What parameter should be evaluated prior to the administration of this medication?

    1. Determine creatinine clearance to be >50 ml/min.

    2. Evaluate levels of serum alanine aminotransferase (ALT).

    3. Any current medications that include anticoagulant agents.

    4. History of allergic reactions to sulfa-based medications.

23. A client is diagnosed with benign prostatic hypertrophy. Which medication should be recognized by the nurse practitioner as likely to aggravate this condition?

    1. Glyburide (DiaBeta).

    2. Oral buspirone (Buspar).

    3. Inhaled ipratropium (Atrovent).

    4. Ophthalmic timolol (Timoptic).

24. Which of the following agents can be useful for stress incontinence?

    1. Propantheline (Bro-Banthine) 7.5–30 mg, three to five times a day.

    2. Oxybutynin (Ditropan) 2.5–5 mg tid to qid.

    3. Doxepin (Sinequan) 10–25 mg pd/bid/tid initially to a maximum total daily dose of 25–100 mg.

    4. Conjugated estrogen (Premarin) 0.3–1.25 mg/day orally or vaginally, medroxyprogesterone (Progestin) 2.5–10 mg/day either continuously or intermittently.

25. In order to decrease the production of uric acid stones, the nurse practitioner orders what medication?

    1. Allopurinol (Zyloprim).

    2. Potassium citrate (Urocit-K).

    3. Bethanechol (Urecholine).

    4. Phenazopyridine (Pyridium).

26. A 70-year-old woman is treated with oxybutynin (Ditropan) for her urinary frequency and urgency. The nurse practitioner would explain to the client she will probably experience:

    1. Increased sensitivity to sunlight.

    2. Dizziness when she stands up.

3. A dry mouth and increased thirst.

4. Increased bruising.

27. All of the following medications can cause urinary incontinence in the older adult **except**:

    1. Hypnotics.

    2. Antibiotics.

    3. Sedatives.

    4. Antidepressants.

28. A 46-year-old man with a history of renal calculi presents with complaints of severe flank pain radiating to his groin area; he is also experiencing nausea and vomiting. His temperature is 99°F. What is the best initial order for the nurse practitioner to give at this time?

    1. Morphine sulfate 10 mg SC now.

    2. Ibuprofen (Advil) 600 mg PO now and q6h.

    3. Increase fluid intake and strain all urine.

    4. Trimethobenzamide (Tigan) 250 mg PO now.

29. The nurse practitioner is prescribing nitrofurantoin (Macrodantin) for a woman who is experiencing problems with urinary tract infections. What specific directions are given to this client regarding the administration of this medication?

    1. Medication should be taken with food and anticipate the urine to have brown discoloration.

    2. Do not take medication with milk products, take on empty stomach for better absorption.

    3. Take the medication four times a day until the symptoms have subsided for at least 24 hours.

    4. Acetaminophen (Tylenol) and/or ibuprofen (Advil) should not be taken with this medication.

30. A young woman presents with complaints of burning on urination, frequency, and urgency. Phenazopyridine (Pyridium) is prescribed by the nurse practitioner. What specific directions are given to the client regarding this medication?

    1. May discolor contact lens; if sclera begin to turn yellow, return to the office.

    2. Always take the medication on an empty stomach to increase absorption.

    3. Do not take any medication containing aspirin or salicylate.

    4. May interfere with effectiveness of minipill for birth control.

14 Answers & Rationales

Physical Examination & Diagnostic Tests

1. **(2)** Adults normally void four to six times in a 24-hour period (q4–6h). Most usually do not get up in the middle of the night, unless they have a medical problem (e.g., benign prostatic hypertrophy, urge incontinence). The feeling of the bladder filling occurs around 90–150 ml, with first urge occurring at 200–300 ml. Normally, 1–2 hours pass between when the first urge to void occurs and the functional capacity is reached. Adults typically reach functional (comfortable) capacity at 300–600 ml and should *never* experience leakage if voiding is delayed.

2. **(2)** These are results indicating the presence of a urinary tract infection. Proteinuria alone suggests glomerulonephritis. Hematuria and pyuria without bacteria may indicate chlamydia, gonorrhea, viral infection or, less commonly, tuberculosis. If a dipstick test is negative for red blood cells but the urine color is red, a substance that can change the color of the urine is likely the cause.

3. **(1)** In an intravenous urography and voiding cystourethrography, congenital anomalies, stone formation, or foreign bodies can be identified. Renal size and the presence of stones can be seen in flat plate and upright films of the abdomen. In a cystoscopy, the urethra, prostate, and bladder can be visualized. A urethroscopy can visualize the ureter and renal pelvis.

4. **(1)** The 1996 AHCPR Guideline Panel encourages primary health care providers to initiate the basic evaluation of urinary incontinence by performing a history and physical examination, measurement of postvoid residual volume, and urinalysis. The other tests may be performed based on the findings from the initial evaluation.

5. **(1)** The classic sign of dehydration in the older adult is lack of skin turgor along with skin tenting on the forehead, concentrated urine (specific gravity >1.025), oliguria, sunken eyes, lack of axillary moisture, orthostatic blood pressure changes, tachycardia, dry mucous membranes of the mouth and nose, and absent or small saliva pool. It is important to examine the mouth, as it reveals reliable assessment data in the older adult suspected of having dehydration. A geographic tongue (patchy papillary loss giving rise to a map-like appearance) should not be confused with tongue furrows and tongue coating.

Disorders

6. **(1)** *E. coli* is the most common organism causing urinary tract infections in the young adult female, and counts of 10^5 are diagnostic and should be treated with trimethoprim-sulfamethoxazole (Bactrim DS) or any suitable, sensitive antiinfective agent. *S. epidermidis* is more often a contaminant due to inappropriate clean-catch specimen collection technique.

7. **(2)** Although moisture-barrier films may protect the skin from urine, they often contain alcohol and can further burn and irritate denuded skin. Cleansing with a mild soap and water helps prevent infections. Petrolatum and zinc oxide, which are types of moisture-barrier ointments, are used to prevent or treat irritant dermatitis.

8. **(4)** Functional incontinence is an inability to toilet appropriately due to impaired mobility. Providing physical assistance and guidance such as with wheelchairs, bedside commodes, appropriate clothing that can be removed easily, and accessible facilities are effective with this type of incontinence. Evaluating the need for pads is effective with stress incontinence. Limiting fluid intake in the evenings to reduce nocturnal incontinence is appropriate for urge incontinence. Performing the Credé's maneuver is appropriate for overflow incontinence.

9. **(3)** Chronic bacterial prostatitis is the most likely cause, as it is difficult to treat due to the bacteria being harbored in the prostatic calculi and in corpora amylacea. A 3- to 4-month treatment with trimethoprim-sulfamethoxazole or a quinolone may be necessary to prevent urinary symptoms.

10. **(4)** Sedative-hypnotics, diuretics, anticholinergic agents, α-adrenergic agents, and calcium channel blockers can cause transient reversible urinary incontinence. Poor pelvic support is a possible cause of stress incontinence. Urge incontinence, or the inability to delay urination with a sudden and powerful urge to void, is a possible result of lower tract problems. A prolapsed uterus or bladder can cause overflow incontinence with overdistention of the bladder.

11. **(2)** Functional incontinence results from a client's inability to toilet appropriately. Stress incontinence is leakage from the bladder during activities that increase intra-abdominal pressure and, therefore, increase the pressure on the bladder, forcing some urine out. An inability to delay urination with a strong, abrupt urge to void is urge incontinence and is due to bladder hyperactivity or a hypersensitive bladder. The client often has little warning before urine passes out of the bladder.

Incontinence with overdistention of the bladder is called overflow incontinence and is due to an underactive detrusor or one that will not contract or to bladder outlet or urethral obstruction. It is characterized by frequent urination in small amounts.

12. **(2)** *Escherichia coli* is the pathogen in 80–90% of community-acquired infections. Gram-positive *Staphylococcus saprophyticus* is the second most common pathogen. *Klebsiella pneumoniae* and *Proteus mirabilis* are also possible common pathogens. In hospital settings, *Escherichia coli* is less prevalent.

13. **(1)** Relapse is an uncommon cause of recurrent urinary tract infections in women, and occurs within 2 weeks of completion of antibiotic therapy. It may need to be treated for 2–12 weeks. Reinfection is the cause of most urinary tract infections in women and may be due to residual urine resulting from a prolapsed uterus or bladder or to lack of estrogen in perimenopausal women. If the client has two or fewer urinary tract infections in a year, the single-dose or 3-day regimen of antibiotic therapy may be used.

14. **(1)** With an acid stone, the rule of thumb is to promote a diet that will render the urine more alkaline, which is an alkaline ash diet. A high-purine diet contributes to the development of the renal stones, so the client needs decreased purine. Foods that are high in purines include liver, spinach, chicken, and dried peas. Milk is allowed on an alkaline ash diet. An increased fluid intake is recommended in all stones, but does not particularly correlate with vitamin C intake. High-carbohydrate diets do not contribute to the stone formation.

15. **(2)** Pyelonephritis in men is suggestive of a structural abnormality and is usually an indication for hospitalization, parenteral antibiotics, and an intraveneous voiding pyelogram. Pyelonephritis in women is usually a result of invasion of the urinary tract by bacteria that have ascended the urethra from the introitus of the urethra. If bacteremia is suspected, women need to be hospitalized, also. Suggested follow-up is by telephone contact within 12–24 hours of initiation of antibiotic therapy and at 2 weeks and 3 months for posttreatment urine cultures.

16. **(2)** Postrenal failure is the development of a complication that presents an obstructive problem distal to the kidney. The hypotensive episode is prerenal, and the vascular changes due to diabetes and the exposure to nephrotoxic chemicals are all intrarenal.

17. **(2)** Urge incontinence is associated with conditions that involve the central nervous system causing detrusor motor and/or sensory instability.

18. **(4)** Painless hematuria is the most common symptom in the client with bladder cancer. This often occurs early; it may be the only symptom the client will exhibit. There is no evidence of renal failure, renal calculi are characterized by flank pain, and cancer of the prostate will often present with the other symptoms of benign prostatic hypertrophy.

19. **(3)** Sedentary lifestyle or episodes of immobilization can predispose a client to the development of stones. Urinary tract infections usually do not precipitate problems with stones; however, the presence of stones will predispose the client to urinary tract infections. Six to 8 oz of milk daily is not excessive, and the increased intake of citrus and high-fiber carbohydrates is good.

20. **(1)** The precipitating factor in prerenal failure is most often an incident that precipitated renal ischemia, most often a shock situation. Nephrotoxic medications, pyelonephritis, and renal vascular changes are all causes of intrarenal failure.

21. **(2)** Kegel's (pelvic floor) exercises keep the bladder support strong. Weak pelvic floor muscles contribute to urinary incontinence, especially with activity. In addition, the teaching should include avoiding bladder irritants such as caffeine, alcohol, and spicy foods.

Pharmacology

22. **(1)** If there is any impairment of renal function, the antibacterial concentration in the urine is inadequate and there is increased risk of toxicity. With normal doses there should be no serum or tissue accumulation of the medication. Liver function studies may be indicated if the client experiences adverse reactions to the medication. Anticoagulants and sulfa-based medications have not been reported as producing any significant drug interactions.

23. **(3)** Benign prostatic hypertrophy is a common cause of urinary retention in older men. Atrovent is an atropine-like bronchodilator used to treat chronic bronchitis, and its anticholinergic agent may aggravate urinary retention. Neither glyburide nor buspirone have an effect on the urinary system, and timolol does not have a systemic effect.

24. **(4)** Combination hormone replacement therapy can be useful for management of stress incontinence. Propantheline and oxybutynin may be useful in urge incontinence; research is limited on the use of these drugs for urge incontinence.

25. **(1)** To decrease the formation of uric acid stones, a urinary alkylating agent such as allopurinol (Zyloprim) is frequently used.

26. **(3)** The medication produces anticholinergic side effects. Dry mouth is very common. Other reactions are not consistent with oxbutynin.

27. **(2)** Sedatives and hypnotics lead to sedation and muscle relaxation. Antidepressants have anticholinergic effects and lead to sedation. Antibiotics have not been implicated in the development of incontinence in the older adult.

28. **(1)** The severe pain of renal calculi should be addressed prior to other treatments or diagnostics. Ibuprofen may be used for beginning pain, but severe pain needs to be treated with morphine or meperidine (Demerol). Tigan can be used, but only after the pain relief has been initiated.

29. **(1)** The most common side effect is gastrointestinal upset. This can be decreased if the medication is taken with food or milk. The discoloration of the urine is a very common occurrence. The medication should be taken for at least 3 days after sterile urine is obtained.

30. **(1)** Yellow discoloration of the sclera may indicate poor renal excretion. Pyridium should be administered with food, and there is no drug interaction with aspirin or with birth control pills.

Male Reproductive

Physical Examination & Diagnostic Tests

1. Which organ is **not** palpable on physical examination of a male client?

   1. Vas deferens.

   2. Testes.

   3. Epididymis.

   4. Cowper's glands.

2. A review of a lab report with an elevated serum gonadotropin would raise suspicion of which disorder?

   1. Seminal vesiculitis.

   2. Vas deferens disease.

   3. Testicular disease.

   4. Benign prostatic hypertrophy (BPH).

3. Which of the following structures can be palpated during an external examination of a male client?

   1. Epididymis.

   2. Cowper's ducts.

   3. Seminal vesicles.

   4. Ejaculatory ducts.

4. What would be most helpful in diagnosing gynecomastia?

   1. History and physical examination.

   2. Liver function test.

   3. Thyroid function test.

   4. Mammogram.

5. The correct position to place a healthy, adult male client to examine the rectum and prostate is:

   1. Left lateral Sims' position with right knee flexed and left leg extended.

   2. Supine position with hips and legs flexed and feet positioned on the examining table.

   3. Modified knee-chest position with client prone and knees flexed under hips.

   4. Leaning over the examination table with chest and shoulders resting on the table.

6. Which test is a tumor marker used to diagnose advanced prostatic cancer?

   1. α-Fetoprotein (AFP).

   2. Prostate-specific antigen (PSA).

   3. Prostatic acid phosphatase (PAP).

   4. Human chorionic gonadotropin (hCG).

7. Which statement is correct about the PSA test?

   1. It can be elevated in clients with BPH.

   2. It is not elevated in clients with prostatitis.

   3. Prostatic massage will not elevate levels.

   4. It does not increase in reoccurrence of prostate cancer.

8. Which procedure is used in screening males (age 40) for prostate cancer, but is not diagnostic?

   1. Prostate-specific antigen test.

   2. Digital-rectal exam (DRE).

   3. Urinalysis and complete blood count (CBC).

   4. Prostate-specific antigen test and digital-rectal exam.

9. When examining the scrotum of an adult Hispanic male, a normal finding is:

   1. Symmetrical scrotal sac with two movable testes.

   2. Smooth, rubbery sac-like surface that is sensitive to gentle compression.

   3. Asymmetrical sac with the left side lower than the right side.

   4. A reddened color that is darker than body skin with sebaceous cysts.

10. Which test is a useful tumor marker for testicular cancer?

    1. α-fetoprotein.

    2. Prostate-specific antigen.

    3. Prostatic acid phosphatase.

    4. Alkaline phosphatase.

Disorders

11. Which statement is correct concerning circumcision?

    1. Circumcision is helpful in preventing phimosis.

    2. Circumcision is a cause of paraphimosis.

    3. Balanoposthitis is the direct result of circumcision in older men.

    4. Circumcision increases the incidence of cancer of the penis.

12. Which of the following are true statements about impotence?

    1. Impotence can be caused by antihypertensives.

    2. Impotence is caused by infections only.

    3. Impotence is not the result of multicausal factors.

    4. Impotence is not the result of vascular problems.

13. Which statement is true about the prostate?

    1. It secretes fluid that is acid.

    2. It secretes fluid that is alkaline.

    3. It secretes androgens.

    4. It produces sperm.

14. An elderly man presents to the clinic with complaints of difficulty voiding and hematuria. The rectal examination reveals a very firm prostate about 5 cm in diameter, asymmetrical, with firm nodules. The PSA level is 14. The next action is to:

    1. Medicate with finasteride (Proscar), 5 mg PO daily, and re-evaluate in 3 months.

    2. Advise the client to avoid caffeine, alcohol, and over-the-counter decongestants.

    3. Obtain a urinalysis to determine the presence of infection and amount of hematuria.

    4. Refer to urologist for biopsy and diagnostic evaluation for prostatic cancer.

15. An older adult male presents with a history of burning on urination and difficulty urinating that has been increasing over the past few days. A stat urinalysis reveals the presence of leukocytes and bacteria. The primary diagnosis considered by the nurse practitioner is:

    1. Bladder cancer.

    2. Testicular torsion.

    3. Benign prostatic hyperplasia.

    4. Renal failure.

16. The client with localized prostate cancer will exhibit which symptoms?

    1. Hesitancy, frequency, and dysuria.

    2. Fatigue, severe constipation, and dysuria.

    3. Hematuria, nocturia, and weight loss.

    4. Myalgia, confusion, and lethargy.

17. An uncircumcised male client presents with a complaint of not being able to retract the foreskin over the glans penis. The most likely diagnosis is:

    1. Lateral phimosis.

    2. Phimosis.

    3. Peyronie's disease.

    4. Paraphimosis.

18. A middle-aged uncircumcised client presents with red pinpoint pustules and papules on the prepuce and glans. The most likely diagnosis is:

    1. Peyronie's disease.

    2. Balanitis.

    3. Phimosis.

    4. Paraphimosis.

19. A male client is diagnosed with balanitis; the mostly likely cause is:

    1. Candidiasis.

    2. Herpes genitalis.

    3. Lichen planus.

    4. Psoriasis.

20. A male client presents with a complaint of sexual dysfunction. The nurse practitioner understands that sexual dysfunction is impairment of:

    1. Erection only.

    2. Emission only.

    3. Ejaculation only.

    4. Erection or emission or ejaculation.

21. A client presents with a complaint of dysuria, enlarged scrotal tenderness over the epididymis, and abdominal pain. The most likely diagnosis is:

    1. Testicular torsion.

    2. Vas deferens inflammation.

    3. Epididymitis.

    4. Balanitis.

22. In response to a male client's question concerning a possible cause of prostate cancer, which is correct?

    1. Syphilis.

    2. Gonorrhea.

    3. Cryptorchidism.

    4. Balanitis.

23. A male client complains of impotence. Which one may be a contributing factor?

    1. Antihypertensives.

    2. Intercourse.

    3. Smoking.

    4. Masturbation.

24. An older male presents with gynecomastia. The most likely cause is:

    1. Cirrhosis.

    2. Diabetes mellitus.

    3. Hypergonadism.

    4. Peptic ulcer disease.

25. Concerning the male breast, which is a correct statement?

    1. Gynecomastia is the result of low estrogen and normal levels of testosterone.

    2. Most breast cancers in men are estrogen-receptor positive.

    3. Breast cancer in males is very common.

    4. Gynecomastia is a nonhormonal or tissue alteration.

26. Which is true of prostate cancer?

    1. Rarely diagnosed in men over 50 years of age.

    2. Soft, indiscrete, symmetrical nodules of the prostate.

    3. Rarely have obstructive symptoms.

    4. Asymmetrical, discrete, hard nodules of the prostate.

27. The nurse practitioner knows that erectile dysfunction is:

    1. Primarily psychological in origin.

    2. Primarily associated with the 70+ older male.

    3. Is the persistent inability to achieve and maintain an erection adequate for sexual intercourse.

    4. Is the physiological dysfunction when smooth muscle contracts causing a lack of adequate amount of blood in the penis to render a rigid, larger penis.

28. Which statement is correct concerning testicular cancer?

    1. This is a very common problem in men over 50 years.

    2. This problem is directly related to testicular trauma.

    3. Testicular cancer presents suddenly with pain.

    4. Testicular cancer is primarily found in young men.

29. Which statement is correct about acute bacterial prostatitis?

    1. It is characterized by recurrent urinary tract infections.

    2. It is an ascending infection of urinary tract.

    3. It always occurs in men under 30.

    4. The usual treatment is a 12-week course of antibiotics.

30. What are common symptoms of BPH?

    1. Dribbling, hesitancy, and loss of stream volume and force, and recurrent urinary tract infections.

    2. Dysuria, urgency, frequency, nocturia, and suprapubic heaviness or discomfort.

    3. Obstructive symptoms, such as a weak urinary stream, abdominal straining to void, hesitancy, incomplete bladder emptying, and terminal dribbling.

    4. Acute onset of fever, chills, flank pain, headache, malaise, costovertebral angle tenderness, and possibly hematuria.

Pharmacology

31. A client has been on doxazosin (Cardura) 2 mg PO daily for 3 weeks for treatment of his BPH. He returns to the clinic and is complaining of feeling dizzy when he stands up. The nurse practitioner:

    1. Determines his blood pressure with him lying down, standing, and sitting.

    2. Orders a urinalysis to determine hematuria and presence of bacteria.

    3. Reviews with the client his symptoms over the past 3 weeks.

    4. Performs a DRE to determine if the prostate is smaller than previously noted.

32. In planning the treatment for a client with balanitis, the nurse practitioner orders:

    1. Rest, ice, and elevation.

    2. Massage.

3. Antifungals.

4. Emergency circumcision.

33. An adult male presents with complaints of fever, low back pain, perineal pain, and intense pain on voiding. Rectal exam reveals a tender, swollen, firm, warm prostate. Based on the client's symptoms, the treatment of choice is:

   1. Trimethoprim-sulfamethoxazole (TMP-SMX; Septra DS) 1 tablet bid × 30 days.

   2. Tetracycline (Achromycin) 250 mg qid × 10 days.

   3. Amoxicillin (Amoxil) 500 mg tid × 14 days.

   4. Erythromycin Ilosone 250 mg q6h × 24 days.

34. A 70-year-old man complains of scrotal pain with dysuria and frequency that has been increasing over the past 2 weeks. Physical examination reveals extreme tenderness and swelling of the scrotum, there is a urethral discharge, and the testes are normal in size and position. A urinalysis reveals pyuria. Based on the client's symptoms, the treatment of choice for this client is:

   1. Nitrofurantoin (Macrodantin) 100 mg PO qid × 14 days.

   2. TMP-SMX (Septra DS) 1 tablet PO bid × 10 days.

3. Doxazosin (Cardura) 1 mg PO qd × 10 days.

4. Oxbutynin (Ditropan) 5 mg PO tid × 10 days.

35. Finasteride (Proscar) is prescribed for a 50-year-old man who is experiencing a problem with urination secondary to an enlarged prostate. The nurse practitioner would teach this client that while on this medication it is important for him to:

   1. Increase his fluid intake.

   2. Restrain from sexual activity.

   3. Use contraceptives.

   4. Increase intake of folic acid.

36. A 75-year-old client is diagnosed with chronic bacterial prostatitis and the nurse practitioner selects TMP-SMX (Septra DS) as the treatment. How should the TMP-SMX (Septra DS) be prescribed for this client?

   1. 2 tablets bid × 10 weeks.

   2. 1 tablet tid × 3 days then 2 tablets × 10 days.

   3. 2 tablets qid × 2 days, then 1 tablet bid × 14 days.

   4. 1 tablet bid × 30 days.

15   Answers & Rationales

Physical Examination & Diagnostic Tests

1. **(1)** Cowper's glands (bulbourethral glands) are located near the prostate and beside the urethra near the base of the penis. These glands are part of the internal and nonpalpable genitalia that consists of glands and ducts. The testes, vas deferens, and epididymis are part of the external genitalia.

2. **(3)** Elevated gonadotropin is elevated in testicular disease, whereas PSA is elevated in disease of the prostate such as BPH.

3. **(1)** The epididymis is part of the external genitalia, whereas the ducts and glands are part of the internal genitalia. The epididymis is palpated on the posterolateral surface of each testis and is a comma-shaped structure. The seminal vesicles (pair of glands) lie behind the urinary bladder in front of the rectum. These vesicles join the ampulla of the vas deferens to form the ejaculatory duct.

4. **(1)** A complete history and physical will usually provide the cause of gynecomastia without further testing, since it can be caused by medication, starving and refeeding, or lack of androgen (atrophying testes), which change the estrogen/androgen ratio.

5. **(4)** For client comfort and ease of examination, the healthy, ambulatory adult client is asked to lean over the examination table with his chest and upper body resting on the table. Although Option #1 is correct,

it is the position used for examining a client who is confined to the bed.

6. **(3)** Prostatic acid phosphatase is an enzyme marker. An increased value is the result of increased metabolism and catabolism of cancer cells of the prostate; in three fourths of clients the cancer arises in the posterior lobe of the prostate. This marker is also used to monitor therapy with antineoplastic drugs and cancer metastatic to bone (osteoblastic lesions). AFP (oncofetal antigen) is produced by fetal liver, yolk sac, and intestinal epithelium, and disappears from blood soon after birth and is not present in healthy individuals. It is increased in primary hepatocellular cancer, embryonal cell (nonseminomatous germ cell) cancer, testicular tumors, and others. PSA (protein marker), which is more sensitive than PAP, increases in prostate cancer and in BPH. hCG (hormone marker) is produced by placental syncytiotrophoblasts and is not usually found in sera of healthy, nonpregnant women, but increases in seminomatous and nonseminomatous testicular cancer.

7. **(1)** The PSA level can be elevated in clients with BPH as well as those with prostatitis, and following prostate gland massage; it does increase with the increasing burden of the tumor such as in the reoccurrence of prostate cancer.

8. **(2)** Recommended screening for prostate cancer should begin at age 40 with DRE

with PSA testing to begin at age 50, if there are no risk factors or symptoms. Urinalysis and CBC are used in an annual physical as screening procedures, but are not indicated in screening for prostate cancer. *PSA testing and DRE are indicated for men over 50 years.*

9. **(3)** The scrotal sac is asymmetrical, darker than body skin and often appears reddened in red-haired men (abnormal finding if found in clients without red hair), and has a surface that may be coarse with small lumps on the skin which are sebaceous or epidermoid cysts that may have an oily discharge.

10. **(1)** AFP (oncofetal antigen) is produced by fetal liver, yolk sac, and intestinal epithelium and disappears from blood soon after birth and is not present in healthy individuals but increases in primary hepatocellular cancer, embryonal cell (nonseminomatous germ cell) cancer, testicular tumors, and others. PAP is an enzyme marker, the increased values of which are the result of increased metabolism and catabolism of cancer cells of the prostate; in three fourths of clients the cancer arises in the posterior lobe of the prostate. This marker is also used to monitor therapy with antineoplastic drugs and cancer metastatic to bone (osteoblastic lesions). PSA (protein marker), which is more sensitive than PAP, increases in prostate cancer and in BPH. ALP increases in osteosarcoma, hepatocellular carcinoma, cancer metastatic to liver, and primary or secondary bone tumors.

Disorders

11. **(1)** Circumcision is helpful in preventing phimosis and paraphimosis, as both are retraction dysfunctions of the prepuce. In phimosis, the foreskin is too tight to be retracted backward over the glans penis. In paraphimosis, once the foreskin has been retracted behind the glans penis, it is too constricted to return to a position of covering the glans penis.

12. **(1)** Impotence can be caused by antihypertensives such as propranolol

(Inderal, Inderal LA). The nonselective β-blockers are believed to decrease vascular resistance and central effect. Erectile dysfunction is reported to begin at doses of 120 mg/day. Other causes include infections or multicausal factors such as vascular, psychological, and trauma.

13. **(2)** The prostate secretes fluid that is alkaline and helps sperm survive in the acidic environment of the female reproductive tract. Androgens are produced by the Leydig's cells of the testes. Sperm are produced in the seminiferous tubules of the testes.

14. **(4)** The DRE and levels of PSA are the primary indicators of prostatic cancer. These should be thoroughly evaluated. Other options are directed toward treatment of BPH. Only after prostatic cancer has been ruled out should these be utilized.

15. **(3)** Benign prostatic hyperplasia is commonly seen in men over 50 years old. Bladder cancer should be ruled out as a diagnosis.

16. **(1)** All of the symptoms listed can be found in the client with prostate cancer, but only the symptoms listed in Option #1 are localized. Many times the client will be asymptomatic.

17. **(2)** Phimosis is a retraction disorder of the penile foreskin or prepuce and can occur at any age and is usually the result of poor hygiene and chronic infection (the foreskin cannot be retracted back over the glans penis). Peyronie's disease is a fibrotic condition that causes lateral curvature of the penis during erection. Paraphimosis is the inability to retract the foreskin from behind the glans penis.

18. **(2)** Inflammation of the glans penis and prepuce is usually associated with poor hygiene and usually found in men with poorly controlled diabetes and candidiasis. Peyronie's disease is a fibrotic condition that causes lateral curvature of the penis during erection. Phimosis and paraphimosis are retraction disorders of the penis. Phimosis is the inability to retract the prepuce over the glans penis, whereas paraphimosis is the inability to retract the prepuce from behind the glans penis.

19. **(1)** Candidiasis is the usual cause for balanitis, which is inflammation of the glans penis and prepuce that is usually associated with poor hygiene and usually found in men with poorly controlled diabetes and candidiasis.

20. **(4)** In sexual dysfunction, erection, emission, or ejaculation may not be functioning due to multifactorial causes, such as vascular, neuropathy, or trauma. Peyronie's disease and priapism are examples of erection dysfunction.

21. **(3)** Epididymitis presents as above, and on palpation the epididymis will often feel like a bag of worms in the scrotal sac rather than a fairly smooth cord.

22. **(3)** Males with undescended testicles are more prone to developing prostate cancer. The other conditions are not causes of prostate cancer.

23. **(1)** Antihypertensive drugs such as propranolol (Inderal, Inderal LA) and other antihypertensives as well as infections can cause impotence. Multicausal factors such as vascular, psychological, and trauma also play a role in impotence. The nonselective β-blockers are believed to decrease vascular resistance and central effect. Erectile dysfunction is reported to begin at doses of 120 mg/day.

24. **(1)** Cirrhosis and diseases of the hepatic system are often a cause of gynecomastia. It is thought that cirrhosis and other hepatic disease alter the estrogen/androgen ratio. None of the other diseases have been implicated in gynecomastia.

25. **(2)** Gynecomastia is the result of an increased estrogen/androgen ratio in men; as a result, their breast cancers are estrogen-receptor positive.

26. **(4)** Prostate cancer in men is usually found in those over the age of 50 years, which causes rapid onset of urinary obstructive symptoms. On palpation, asymmetrical, discrete, hard nodules are located.

27. **(3)** This is the correct definition of erectile dysfunction which statistics reveal that 40% of 40-year-old males and 70% of 70+ year-old males may experience. It involves a hemodynamic mechanism of smooth muscle relaxation which increases the amount of blood flow in the penis and ultimately causes venous trapping (compression of the subtunical venules) causing rigidity.

28. **(4)** Testicular cancer is primarily found in young men and presents as nonpainful nodules of the involved testicle. Trauma is not a causal factor.

29. **(2)** Acute bacterial prostatitis is caused by an infection in the urinary tract moving up the urethra into the prostate. The most common organisms are *Escherichia coli*, *Pseudomonas*, and *Streptococcus faecalis*. The condition tends to occur in men between 30 and 50 years old, but can be associated with BPH in older men. Chronic bacterial prostatitis is characterized by recurrent urinary tract infections, with the usual course of antibiotic treatment lasting for 12 weeks (due to blockage by fibrosis in the prostatic tissue to the antibiotics).

30. **(3)** Obstructive symptoms are common in BPH. Dribbling, hesitancy, loss of normal urine stream, and recurrent urinary tract infections are present in chronic bacterial prostatitis. Dysuria, urgency, frequency, nocturia, and suprapubic heaviness are common symptoms of cystitis. Fever, chills, flank pain, headache, malaise, and costovertebral angle tenderness of acute onset with or without hematuria are indications of pyelonephritis.

Pharmacology

31. **(1)** Doxazosin (Cardura) is also used an an antihypertensive agent; the client may be experiencing orthostatic hypotension. Other answers are directed toward evaluating his BPH, which has already been diagnosed and has not had sufficient time to respond to the medication.

32. **(3)** Antifungals are the treatment of choice (e.g., topical nystatin [Mycostatin] or Ciclopirox [Loprox]). If recalcitrant, oral fluconazole (Diflucan) 150 mg/day or itraconazole (Sporanox) 100 mg/day should be given. All the other treatments are inappropriate.

33. **(1)** The client is presenting with classic symptoms of acute bacterial prostatitis. The treatment of choice is TMP-SMX. It is important to treat the client for at least 30 days to prevent relapse. Treatment is started pending the results of the culture and sensitivity.

34. **(2)** The client is presenting with classic symptoms of epididymitis. The treatment of choice is TMP-SMX. Nitrofurantoin is a urinary antiseptic, doxazosin is given for BPH, and oxbutynin is indicated for incontinence or enuresis. On differential diagnosis the gradual onset of pain, voiding problems, urethral discharge, and swelling are more indicative of epididymitis than testicular torsion.

35. **(3)** It is important that women of child-bearing age are not exposed to the sperm of a client on finasteride. Pregnant women and those of child-bearing age should avoid handling crushed tablets.

36. **(4)** The recommended treatment is for at least 30 days to prevent reoccurrence. Clients may require continued suppression therapy for an extended period of time.

16

Women's Health

Physical Examination & Diagnostic Tests

1. When obtaining a cervical specimen for a Pap smear, the nurse practitioner:

   1. Lubricates the speculum with a water-soluble lubricant to assist in the insertion of the instrument.

   2. Utilizes the cervical brush when obtaining the cervical cells on a prenatal client due to the presence of the cervical mucous plug.

   3. Uses warm water to lubricate the speculum to assist in the insertion of the instrument.

   4. Completes the bimanual portion of the examination first in order to determine the relative position of the cervix to assist in a comfortable insertion of the speculum.

2. To promote client comfort prior to performing a pelvic exam, the nurse practitioner:

   1. Asks the client to bear down slightly as the speculum is inserted.

   2. Has the client empty her bladder.

3. Explains each step of the procedure in a calm manner.

4. Carefully reassures the client that the exam will only take a few minutes.

3. What finding is considered a normal surface characteristic of the cervix?

   1. Small, yellow, raised round area on cervix.

   2. Red patchy areas with occasional white spots.

   3. Friable, bleeding tissue at opening of cervical os.

   4. Irregular, granular surface with red patches.

4. The primary role of a breast ultrasound is:

   1. As a screening test for breast cancer.

   2. For definitive diagnosis of breast cancer.

   3. To determine if a breast lesion is cystic or solid.

   4. To locate small lesions prior to surgery.

185

5. Potassium hydroxide (KOH) use when doing a wet mount assists in the diagnosis of:

   1. Bacterial vaginosis and candida vaginitis.

   2. Trichomonas and chlamydia.

   3. Syphilis and gonorrhea.

   4. Herpes and condyloma.

6. The nurse practitioner is reviewing the lab results of an older client seen recently for a Pap smear. The results are as follows: Classification—high-grade squamous intraepithelial lesion; endocervical cells seen; adequate smear. The nurse practitioner phones the client and tells her which of the following?

   1. "Your Pap smear was normal. Follow-up in 1 year, sooner if problems arise."

   2. "Your Pap smear shows invasive cancer. I would like you to see a gynecologic oncologist for treatment."

   3. "Your Pap smear shows abnormal tissue that needs to be evaluated. Please schedule an appointment for a colposcopy."

   4. "Your Pap smear shows a minor abnormality. Sometimes this can signify a disease process just beginning. Please schedule another Pap smear in 4 months for follow-up."

7. When describing the findings from a normal breast examination, the nurse practitioner documents on the client record:

   1. Left nipple everted, several coarse black hairs arising from the areola, enlarged axillary lymph nodes palpated bilaterally, and tender nodes in supraclavicular area.

   2. No dimpling or retraction; 1-cm hard, fixed, stellate mass noted next to nipple with scant nipple discharge; no pain or tenderness on palpation.

   3. Right breast slightly larger and denser than left with no nipple discharge, right areola dark pink in color and inverted, left areola dark brown in color and everted, breasts tender to palpation with no axillary nodes noted.

   4. Pendulous breasts with no dimpling, retraction, nipple discharge or areas of discoloration; numerous small nevi near areola with Montgomery's tubercles noted; no supraclavicular or axillary lymph nodes palpated.

8. The nurse practitioner is reviewing the lab work of a 61-year-old adult client seen recently for a Pap smear. She has been treated for breast cancer with mastectomy and tamoxifen (Nolvadex). She is not and has never been on hormone replacement therapy. The results to her Pap smear are as follows: Atrophic changes—scant endocervical cells; adequate smear. What is appropriate for the nurse practitioner to tell the client when she phones her with her result?

   1. "Your Pap smear is slightly abnormal. I would recommend the use of some estrogen vaginal cream nightly for 3 weeks, then return to the office to have the Pap smear repeated."

   2. "Your Pap smear is normal but shows a mild thinning of the tissue. This is to be expected in someone who is not on hormones and it does not pose a threat to your health. Please return to the office in 1 year for your annual exam, sooner if needed."

   3. "Your Pap smear shows that you do not have enough endocervical cells. Please make an appointment for endocervical curettage."

   4. "Your Pap smear is abnormal. This could signify a disease state of the cervix. Please schedule a colposcopy at your earliest convenience."

9. Which test is the "gold standard" for the diagnosis of chlamydia?

   1. Use of KOH wet mount "whiff" test.

   2. Presence of inflammatory cells in Pap smear.

   3. Direct fluorescent antibody (DFA).

   4. Culture with special media and collection technique.

10. The nurse practitioner is discussing mammography with a group of women. It is important for the nurse practitioner to advise the women:

    1. A mammogram should be done annually for all women of child-bearing age.
    2. All women over 40 years old should have a mammogram on an annual basis.
    3. A mammogram should be done annually after pregnancy, if the woman does not breast-feed.
    4. A mammogram should be done if there is any breast pain or nipple retraction.

11. Which is the most accurate statement regarding a reactive serologic test for syphilis?

    1. All reactive serologic tests require confirmation with a treponemal test.
    2. Reactive serologic tests are highly suspicious for active syphilis.
    3. A false-positive serologic test, though rare, can be unnecessarily traumatizing to a client.
    4. A reactive serologic test most likely implies the need for retreatment.

12. While working-up a client with secondary amenorrhea, the prolactin serum assay results show a level of 24 ng/ml. Appropriate management includes:

    1. Administering medroxyprogesterone acetate 10 mg bid × 5 days.
    2. Referring to an endocrinologist.
    3. Recording the results as within normal limits.
    4. Assessing for nipple discharge.

13. When evaluating an older adult with amenorrhea and normal secondary sex characteristics, the purpose of the progesterone challenge is to determine the presence of:

    1. Endogenous estrogen.
    2. Thyroxine.
    3. Prolactin.
    4. Adequate body fat.

14. Which is **not** a risk factor for heart disease in the postmenopausal female?

    1. Hyperlipidemia.
    2. Cigarette smoking.
    3. Hormone replacement therapy (HRT).
    4. Diabetes mellitus.

15. Which is **not** a risk factor for osteoporosis?

    1. Cigarette smoking.
    2. Caucasian.
    3. Alcohol consumption.
    4. Obesity.

16. A middle-aged female presents with dysfunctional uterine bleeding. A hormonal profile reveals increased follicle-stimulating hormone (FSH) and luteinizing hormone (LH) levels. The most likely cause for these findings is?

    1. Hypothalamic disorder.
    2. Onset of climacteric.
    3. Premature ovarian failure.
    4. Anterior pituitary disorder.

Gynecologic Disorders

17. During a yearly physical examination, a nurse practitioner asks a woman if she has any problems or questions about sexual function or activity. Initially, the client hesitates, but with further questioning and discussion, she states that she is unsure if she has ever experienced an orgasm before. The nurse practitioner suspects:

    1. Vaginismus.
    2. Primary orgasmic dysfunction.
    3. Secondary orgasmic dysfunction.
    4. Dyspareunia.

18. The definition of bacterial vaginosis is:

    1. A syndrome resulting from homeostatic disruption in the vagina.

    2. Vaginitis caused by flagellated protozoan.

    3. A bacterial sexually transmitted disease that can be symptomatic or asymptomatic.

    4. A virus characterized by recurrent outbreaks and remissions.

19. Which is **not** a criterion for the diagnosis of bacterial vaginosis?

    1. Positive amine test (whiff test).

    2. Presence of clue cells.

    3. Vaginal pH >4.5.

    4. Presence of pseudohyphae.

20. The most common cause of dysfunctional uterine bleeding is:

    1. Thyroid disorder.

    2. Blood dyscrasia.

    3. Anovulation.

    4. Uterine tumor.

21. What is a cause of secondary amenorrhea?

    1. Testicular feminization.

    2. Hypogonadotropic hypogonadism.

    3. Congenital absence of uterus.

    4. Extreme exercise.

22. Which is **not** a risk factor for the development of cervical cancer?

    1. Human papillomavirus (HPV).

    2. Virginal status.

    3. Multiple sexual partners.

    4. Previous high-grade squamous intraepithelial lesion (HSIL).

23. A woman is complaining of tenderness and burning of her vulva. On examination the vulva is edematous and excoriated. The nurse practitioner performs a wet mount prep of the vaginal secretions. It reveals pseudohyphae and spores. The diagnosis for this client is:

    1. Vulvovaginal candidiasis.

    2. Chlamydia trachomatis.

    3. Bacterial vaginitis.

    4. Gonorrhea.

24. The leading cause of death in female genital cancers, excluding breast is:

    1. Ovarian cancer.

    2. Endometrial cancer.

    3. Cervical cancer.

    4. Vulvar and/or vaginal cancer.

25. Which is **not** a risk factor for endometrial cancer?

    1. Obesity.

    2. Birth control pill use.

    3. Unopposed estrogen use.

    4. Advancing age, >50 years.

26. What is the most common female genital malignancy, excluding the breast?

    1. Ovary.

    2. Endometrium.

    3. Cervix.

    4. Vulva/vagina.

27. Which is **not** considered to be a risk factor in the development of breast cancer?

    1. Early menopause.

    2. High-fat diet.

    3. Advancing age.

    4. Early menarche.

28. The initial work-up for dysfunctional uterine bleeding (DUB) should include:

    1. Referral for diagnostic dilatation and curettage (D&C).

    2. Referral for endometrial biopsy to rule out cancer.

3. Complete blood count (CBC), pregnancy test (if pre-menopausal), endocrine studies.

4. Coagulation studies, sexually transmitted disease (STD) cultures.

29. Which is **not** a risk factor for breast cancer?

    1. History of maternal breast cancer—premenopausal onset.

    2. First pregnancy after age 35.

    3. Late menopause after age 54.

    4. Fibrocystic breast disease.

30. What is the leading cause of death for females in the United States.

    1. Breast cancer.

    2. Colon cancer.

    3. Heart disease.

    4. Stroke.

31. Reactive cellular changes noted on a Pap smear are most often associated with:

    1. Inflammation.

    2. Use of estrogen vaginal cream.

    3. Drying artifact.

    4. Use of oral contraceptives.

32. Risk factors for cervical disease include:

    1. Pregnancy after 35 years of age.

    2. Viral exposure.

    3. Low parity.

    4. Prolonged contraceptive use.

33. What is the most common cancer in females in the United States?

    1. Breast cancer.

    2. Colon cancer.

    3. Malignant melanoma.

    4. Lung cancer.

34. A 48-year-old female client presents to the clinic with the following list of complaints: hot flashes, no menses for 14 months, insomnia, crying spells, irritability, decreased libido, and fatigue. At the end of her history and physical exam, she begins to cry and tells the nurse practitioner that she thinks she is going crazy; she then begs the nurse practitioner to tell her what is wrong. Which is **inappropriate** for the nurse practitioner to advise the client at this point?

    1. Obtain lab tests including FSH and LH.

    2. Discuss hormone replacement, including risks and benefits, and short- and long-term treatment strategies.

    3. Discuss antidepressant therapy and a referral for counseling sessions for depression.

    4. Provide the client with written information regarding menopause and the options for treatment of symptoms.

35. Follow-up care for a client with chancroid should include:

    1. Screening for human immunodeficiency virus (HIV) as well as syphilis.

    2. Mandatory notification and treatment of all sexual partners.

    3. Screening for lymphogranuloma venereum.

    4. Culture for gonorrhea.

36. During her annual exam, a 45-year-old female complains of recent breast changes. She states that her breasts are painful and frequently feel "lumpy." Because of this, she has stopped doing monthly breast self-examination (BSE) feeling that it is a waste of time. What would be the most appropriate advice to offer her?

    1. Stress the importance of continuing monthly BSE to detect unusual lumps because she knows the feel of her breasts.

    2. Suggest she at least do BSE every 2 months.

    3. Suggest she start getting mammograms to establish some baseline data about her breasts.

    4. Suggest she determine when her breasts are nontender and least "lumpy" and change her schedule for BSE.

37. Which is **not** a risk factor for ovarian cancer?

    1. Family history of ovarian cancer.

    2. Advancing age, >50 years.

    3. Birth control pill use.

    4. Positive BRCA 2 gene.

38. A woman with bilateral breast implants asks if it is really necessary to do monthly BSE because she does not know what to feel for. The most appropriate response would be:

    1. Suggest she involve her sexual partner in assessing her breasts on a regular basis.

    2. Review the steps in BSE until she feels comfortable with the process.

    3. Acknowledge the difficulty of doing BSE after implant surgery.

    4. Explain the usefulness of regular mammograms for implant clients.

39. An adult client comes to the clinic complaining of abnormal vaginal discharge (dark, watery brown) along with postcoital bleeding. The nurse practitioner suspects the possibility of cancer of the cervix. During the vaginal exam, suspicious physical results would be:

    1. Soft, sill-shaped cervix.

    2. Very firm cervix with an ulcer.

    3. Vague lower abdominal discomfort.

    4. Tender, enlarged lymph nodes.

40. A postmenopausal female is worried about pain in the upper outer quadrant of her left breast. The nurse practitioner should:

    1. Do a breast exam and order a mammogram.

    2. Explain that pain is related to hormone fluctuations and order laboratory studies.

    3. Reassure the client that pain is not a presenting symptom of breast cancer and check for proper fit of the brassiere.

    4. Teach the client breast self-examination.

41. An adult female client presents with a history of vaginal itching and heavy white discharge. The client gives a history of no sexual activity. On exam, the nurse practitioner finds a red, edematous vulva and white patches on the vaginal walls. There is no odor to the discharge. The nurse practitioner expects what factors in the client's history?

    1. A vegetarian diet.

    2. Recent diarrhea.

    3. Early menopause.

    4. Recent antibiotic use.

42. The nurse practitioner knows that the majority of breast cancers occur in which area of the breast?

    1. Upper inner quadrant.

    2. Upper outer quadrant.

    3. Beneath the nipple and areola.

    4. Lower outer quadrant.

43. The client presents with dysfunctional uterine bleeding and has been found to have endometrial cancer. She returned to the nurse practitioner, because she does not understand how this is possible when the Pap smear 6 months ago was negative. The best response is:

    1. Uterine cancer develops quickly.

    2. Pap smears are difficult to read and mistakes can happen.

    3. Pap smears are not useful in detecting uterine cancers in most cases.

    4. The previous Pap smear did not have an adequate sample of tissue.

Pharmacology

44. A 42-year-old female client presents to the office with complaints of dysuria, urinary frequency, and urgency. These symptoms began early this morning. She leaves a clean-catch midstream urine which shows the following: white blood cells (WBCs) too numerous to count (TNTC)/high-power field (HPF), 4–5 red blood cells (RBCs)/HPF, positive nitrites. A urine culture is set up and will be ready in 3 days. Which is **not** a correct treatment for an uncomplicated lower urinary tract infection?

    1. Phenazopyridine (Pyridium) 200 mg 1 tab PO tid × 2 days.

    2. Trimethoprim-sulfamethoxazole (Bactrim DS) 1 tab PO bid × 5 days.

    3. Ceftriaxone (Rocephin) 1 gm IM.

    4. Nitrofurantoin (Macrobid) 1 tab PO bid × 5 days.

45. A 46-year-old female client is being seen in the clinic by the nurse practitioner. She was last seen 2 weeks ago for an upper respiratory tract infection and was treated with amoxicillin (Amoxil) 250 mg PO tid × 10 days. She completed her medication last week but now is aware of vaginal itching and a cottage cheese–like vaginal discharge. She states that she has never experienced such intense itching before. She is in a mutually monogamous relationship. Her last menstrual period (LMP) was 2 weeks ago. Her partner had a vasectomy 2 years ago. Wet mount with KOH shows negative whiff test, rate clue cells, positive lactobacilli, positive hyphae and spores, few WBCs, and no trichomonads. She is leaving tomorrow for a week-long cruise. She is not on any medications, and has no known drug allergies. Your treatment for this problem is:

    1. Metronidazole (Flagyl) 500 mg PO bid × 7 days.

    2. Clindamycin (Cleocin) vaginal cream 1 applicator full vaginally qhs × 7 days.

    3. Fluconazole (Diflucan) 150 mg 1 tablet PO one time.

    4. Hydrocortisone (Cortaid) 1% cream, apply sparingly bid × 7 days.

46. A 55-year-old female client is being seen in the clinic for her annual exam. She went through a natural menopause 5 years ago and has never been interested in hormonal therapy. She smokes 1 pack per day, does no formal exercise, works as a secretary, and volunteers her time in community work 4 nights a week. She is a G2 T2 P0 A0 L2. Her family history is positive for osteoporosis in her monther and myocardial infarction in her father and she is negative for any cancers. She had a normal physical exam today and had a negative mammogram yesterday. She is interested now in hormonal therapy but wants to know what her alternatives are. Which choice **has not** been clinically proven for prevention of osteoporosis or cardiovascular disease?

    1. Conjugated equine estrogen (Premarin) 0.625 mg 1 tablet PO qd and medroxyprogesterone acetate (Provera) 2.5 mg 1 tablet PO qd.

    2. Weight-bearing exercise three times weekly, and calcium 1500 mg PO qd.

    3. Discontinue cigarette smoking.

    4. Wild Mexican yam cream; apply to skin tid.

47. An older female client is seen by the nurse practitioner for her annual exam. She has been on HRT for 6 months, having started herself on the pills left over by her deceased mother. She brings the pills with her, as she wants to remain on these and requests a prescription for Estrace 1 mg daily. She has an intact uterus, is in excellent health, and denies any complaints. She does not have any contraindications to the use of HRT. Her exam is normal. Which represents an **incorrect** and potentially dangerous plan for the nurse practitioner to follow?

    1. Endometrial biopsy.

    2. Prescription for Estrace 1 mg daily; plus medroxyprogesterone acetate (Provera) 2.5 mg daily.

    3. Prescription for Estrace 1 mg daily.

    4. Instruct the client on the risks and benefits of HRT.

48. An older adult female client is seen for follow-up to discuss her HRT with the nurse practitioner. She is seeking a refill on her HRT but is not sure it is working right. She continues to feel hot flashes, moodiness, decreased libido, and has many sleep disturbances. She is on Premarin 0.625 mg daily, and Provera 2.5 mg daily. She denies any vaginal bleeding. Which is **not** an acceptable choice for the client?

    1. Premarin 0.9 mg 1 tab PO qd and Provera 5 mg 1 tab PO qd days 1–12.

    2. Premarin 0.9 mg 1 tab PO qd and Provera 5 mg 1 tab PO qd days 16–25.

    3. Premarin 0.3 mg 1 tab PO qd and Provera 2.5 mg 1 tab PO qd.

    4. Premarin 1.25 mg 1 tab PO qd and Provera 10 mg 1 tab PO qd days 1–12.

49. Which is **not** a contraindication to the use of HRT in the postmenopausal female?

    1. Recent deep vein thrombosis.

    2. Chronic active hepatitis.

    3. Controlled hypertension.

    4. Undiagnosed abnormal genital bleeding.

50. Which dose of conjugated equine estrogen (Premarin) is the minimal effective dose to prevent osteoporosis?

    1. 0.3 mg.

    2. 0.625 mg.

    3. 0.9 mg.

    4. 1.25 mg.

51. An older female client is seen by the nurse practitioner for her annual exam and needs a refill on her hormone replacement therapy. She is feeling well and has not voiced concerns. The client had a total abdominal hysterectomy and bilateral salpingo-oophorectomy 2 years ago for benign fibroids. Her exam is normal. She takes conjugated estrogen (Premarin) 0.625 mg days 1–25 and medroxyprogesterone acetate (Provera) 10 mg from days 16–25. What changes would be appropriate for the nurse practitioner to make in the HRT regimen?

    1. No changes needed; the client is doing well on the present regimen.

    2. Premarin 0.625 mg daily; and discontinue the Provera.

    3. Premarin 0.625 mg daily; and Provera 2.5 mg daily.

    4. Premarin 0.625 mg days 1–25; and Provera 5 mg days 16–25.

52. Before prescribing HRT, which clinical approach should have the highest priority?

    1. The decision about use should rest primarily with the client after providing appropriate education and counseling.

    2. For most women, the benefits of HRT far outweigh any possible side effects, so HRT should be actively encouraged.

    3. Involving the sexual partner in the counseling session is likely to lead to a higher compliance rate for HRT.

    4. Education regarding HRT should include a thorough review of risk factors and possible side effects in order to avoid liability issues.

53. The beneficial effects of estrogen on high-density (HDL) and low density (LDL) lipoprotein fractions include:

    1. An increase in HDL and an increase in LDL.

    2. A decrease in HDL and a decrease in LDL.

    3. An increase in HDL and a decrease in LDL.

    4. A decrease in HDL and an increase in LDL.

54. The nurse practitioner is teaching a client about taking alendronate (Fosamax); her information includes:

    1. Take it midmorning.

    2. Take with food.

    3. Take with a full glass of orange juice.

    4. Remain upright after taking medication.

55. The addition of a progesterone to an estrogen regimen in a postmenopausal woman with a uterus reduces the risk of:

1. Endometrial cancer.

2. Cervical cancer.

3. Gallbladder disease.

4. Breast cancer.

56. The treatment of choice for trichomoniasis is:

   1. Azithromycin (Zithromax) 1 gm PO, single dose.

   2. Ofloxacin (Floxin) 500 mg PO, single dose.

   3. Metronidazole (Flagyl) 2 gm PO, single dose.

   4. Clindamycin (Cleocin) 300 mg PO, single dose.

57. A 50-year-old woman comes into the office with complaints of profuse malodorous discharge. The nurse practitioner's diagnosis is bacterial vaginosis. The nurse practitioner would:

   1. Advise the client to notify her sexual contacts regarding the diagnosis.

   2. Treat the problem with metronidazole (Flagyl) 2 gm for single dose.

   3. Initiate a treatment with doxycycline (Vibramycin) 100 mg PO bid × 7 days.

   4. Determine the presence of pregnancy prior to initiating a course of treatment.

58. When assisting the woman to decide whether to initiate HRT, which statement is true?

   1. Estrogen replacement delays the onset of menopause.

   2. Estrogen and progesterone cause vasomotor symptoms.

   3. Estrogen increases HDL cholesterol levels.

   4. Estrogen replacement with progesterone increase the risk of ovarian cancer.

16   Answers & Rationales

Physical Examination & Diagnostic Tests

1. **(3)** Lubricants, such as Vaseline or K-Y gel, should not be used if a cervical specimen is being obtained for analysis. The cervical brush should not be used on pregnant clients. The bimanual exam is performed after the internal vaginal exam.

2. **(2)** To aid in the examination, an empty bladder will provide for client comfort and will assist the nurse practitioner in making a more accurate assessment during the bimanual portion of the exam. Options #1 and #3 help reduce the client's anxiety, which ultimately may assist in the achievement of comfort.

3. **(1)** A nabothian cyst is a small, white or yellow, raised round area on the cervix. The surface of the cervix should be smooth and may have a symmetrical, reddened circle around the os (squamocolumnar epithelium). The other options are all unexpected, abnormal findings.

4. **(3)** A breast ultrasound is used to determine if a lesion is solid or cystic. Ultrasound misses 50% of lesions <2 cm. The test is not sensitive enough to be used for routine screening and cannot replace mammography. The definitive diagnosis of breast cancer is the breast biopsy.

5. **(1)** KOH lyses epithelial and WBC, making it easier to visualize *Candida* (yeast). *Candida* cells are resistant and remain intact. KOH also assists with diagnosing bacterial vaginosis by alkalinizing vaginal discharge, causing a distinct fishy odor. This is a positive amine or whiff test.

6. **(3)** The Pap smear is a screening test for cervical cancer and precancerous states. The diagnostic test needed to confirm the diagnosis of a high-grade lesion is the colposcopy with guided biopsies. The results to this test are clearly abnormal and must be acted upon. Waiting a year could be deleterious to the client's health. This is not the Pap smear report that one would choose to redo in 4 months; the client needs a diagnostic test, not another screening test. This is not a diagnosis of cervical cancer on this Pap smear; therefore, a referral to a gynecologic oncologist is premature at this juncture.

7. **(4)** The abnormal finding in Option #1 is the enlarged lymph nodes. The abnormal finding in Option #2 is the fixed, stellate mass with nipple discharge. In Option #3, asymmetrical size is normal but the different colors of the areola and unilateral nipple inversion are not. Longstanding nevi and Montgomery's tubercles are normal in Option #4.

8. **(2)** Atrophic changes on the cervix of a postmenopausal female are to be expected, as is the paucity of endocervical cells. Due to her past medical history of breast cancer, she is not a candidate for the use of estrogen vaginal cream, nor is the Pap smear interpretation abnormal. Endocervical curettage is used as a biopsy

technique for sampling tissue from the endocervical canal; however, it is not appropriate to recommend this invasive procedure for someone with scant endocervical cells, but rather for one with abnormal endocervical cells. Since this Pap smear report really is not classified as abnormal, there is no need to recommend a diagnostic procedure for the client.

9. **(4)** Culture and DFA are both used. Culture is the only certain or definitive method of diagnosis. It is a collected cervical specimen, and it takes about 2–6 days to obtain the results. However, the DFA is fast and has good sensitivity and specificity.

10. **(2)** Mammography should be done on a regular basis—baseline screening around age 35, then every 2 years. After age 40, it should be done on an annual basis. It should be done regardless of breast-feeding and the client should not wait until a mass or other symptoms are present.

11. **(1)** Serologic tests are good screening tests, but positive results require following up with a treponemal test to detect specific antibodies.

12. **(2)** Serum prolactin assay levels >20 ng/ml indicate the need for medical referral, usually to an endocrinologist. The most common cause of hyperprolactinemia and galactorrhea (milky breast discharge) is a pituitary tumor or lesion of the hypothalamus. Other causes may be hypothyroidism, medications (narcotics, tranquilizers, antihypertensives), and oral contraceptives.

13. **(1)** The initial work-up for this client includes determining the prolactin level by evaluating serum concentrations and determining the presence of endogenous estrogen. If the woman experiences withdrawal bleeding after the administration of oral or intramuscular progesterone and the prolactin level is normal, this woman is producing estrogen and can be considered anovulatory. Absence of withdrawal bleeding with normal prolactin level requires further work-up.

14. **(3)** HRT reduces the risk of heart disease in the postmenopausal female.

15. **(4)** Obesity is not a risk factor for osteoporosis. Cigarette use, Caucasian race, and alcohol consumption, in addition to others not listed here, are considered to be risk factors for osteoporosis.

16. **(2)** As the function of the ovaries declines, and the amount of circulating estrogen begins to fall, the middle-aged female may begin to experience the symptoms commonly associated with menopause. The body's feedback system will attempt to stimulate the ovaries and increase estrogen level. FSH and LH levels rise in response to these effort.

Gynecologic Disorders

17. **(2)** Primary orgasmic disorder is when an individual has never achieved orgasm, usually a lifelong problem. Dyspareunia is painful intercourse and vaginismus is painful vaginal spasms upon penetration. Secondary orgasmic dysfunction refers to an acquired problem of loss of orgasmic function after an individual has experienced orgasm.

18. **(1)** Bacterial vaginosis results when the normal environment in the vagina is disrupted. The normal vaginal lactobacilli are decreased or absent, and there is an overgrowth of many different types of anaerobic bacteria. Trichomoniasis is caused by a flagellated protozoan and gonorrhea is caused by a bacteria and may be asymptomatic. The virus that causes recurrent outbreaks of genital lesions is herpes genitalis type 2 (HSV-2).

19. **(4)** The criteria for the diagnosis of bacterial vaginosis are characteristic milky homogenous discharge, pH >4.5, amine odor (positive whiff) with addition of KOH, and the presence of epithelial cells studded with coccibacilli that obscure the borders (clue cells). Pseudohyphae are present in candidiasis.

20. **(3)** 90% of dysfunctional uterine bleeding is caused by anovulation. The lack of progesterone allows asynchronous, excessive proliferation of the endometrium. This tissue is fragile and the normal hemostatic mechanism is altered. Thyroid disease, blood dyscrasias, and uterine tumors can mimic dysfunctional uterine bleeding and must be excluded.

21. **(4)** Secondary amenorrhea is defined as no menses for three cycle lengths or 6 months in a woman with previously established menses. Exercise can cause an increase in estrogen and endorphin levels, which influence the release of gonadotropin releasing hormone (GnRH). Without appropriate GnRH release, FSH and LH are not released appropriately, resulting in anovulation, which may lead to amenorrhea. The other conditions listed are causes of primary amenorrhea.

22. **(2)** A person who has never engaged in coital activity is not considered to be at risk for cervical cancer, due to the unlikelihood of exposure to HPV. In addition to others not listed here, the presence of HPV, multiple sexual partners, and/or previous HSIL are considered to be risk factors in the development of cervical cancer.

23. **(1)** The pseudohyphae and spores on the wet mount (KOH) are diagnostic for candida. Chlamydia tachomatis is diagnosed by direct immunofluorescence assay (DFA, or by chlamydia culture). Gonorrhea is diagnosed by a cervical culture, and bacterial vaginitis shows clue cells on the wet mount prep.

24. **(1)** Cancer of the ovary is the leading cause of death due to female genital cancer, excluding the breast, in the United States.

25. **(2)** Birth control pills have been shown to reduce the risk of endometrial cancer. Obesity, unopposed estrogen use, and advanced age, in addition to others not listed here, are considered to be risk factors for developing endometrial cancer.

26. **(2)** Endometrial cancer is the most common female genital cancer.

27. **(1)** Early menopause has not been associated with the development of breast cancer. High-fat diet, advancing age, early menarche, and others not listed here have been identified as risk factors for the development of breast cancer.

28. **(3)** Baseline lab work should be obtained to determine the presence of anemia, possible pregnancy, and/or endocrine dysfunction.

29. **(4)** Fibrocystic breast disease is not a risk factor for breast cancer. In addition to others, those listed above are considered to be risk factors for breast cancer.

30. **(3)** Heart disease remains the leading cause of death for females in the United States.

31. **(1)** Reactive cellular changes are most commonly associated with inflammation including typical repair. Other causes include atrophy with inflammation (atrophic vaginitis, intrauterine device (IUD) use, radiation, and diethylstilbestrol-exposed daughters. Oral contraceptives do not cause reactive changes, and estrogen vaginal cream may be used to improve atrophy.

32. **(2)** The exact cause of cervical disease is unknown. Evidence is increasing that sexually transmitted agents act as carcinogens. Viral exposure to herpes genitalis, HPV, and HIV are, therefore, considered risk factors. Other risk factors are related to sexual activity, such as sex prior to 18 years of age, first pregnancy prior to 18 years of age, multiple sexual partners, high parity, and partners with carcinoma in situ (CIS) of the penis.

33. **(4)** Lung cancer is the most common cancer in females in the United States.

34. **(3)** These symptoms are classic for menopausal syndrome, although it is true that there are some depressive symptoms listed. Antidepressant therapy and counseling for depression at this stage of treatment are not appropriate. Testing, teaching, and treatment in this case should be aimed at the menopause. The depressive symptoms will undoubtedly improve with greater understanding and treatment of the menopausal symptoms.

35. **(1)** Chancroid is well established as a cofactor for HIV transmission.

36. **(4)** Monthly BSEs are the most effective way to pick up early breast changes. Educate her regarding increased tenderness during last half of menstrual cycle. BSE should be done 7 days after cycle ends.

37. **(3)** Birth control pill use has been shown to reduce the risk of ovarian cancer. Family history of ovarian cancer, advancing age, and positive BRCA 2 gene, in addition to others not listed here, are considered to be risk factors for developing ovarian cancer.

38. **(2)** She needs to become more knowledgeable about the normal feel of implants as well as her own breast tissue. Mammography is not a substitute for BSE.

39. **(2)** A very firm cervix along with a cervical lesion/ulcer is suspicious for cancer of the cervix, which can be confirmed with a Pap smear.

40. **(1)** This complaint is an indication for breast exam and mammography. Although pain is not a common presenting symptom, it can be. Teaching BSE is important but not the most important action in this situation; hormone levels can explain breast pain but should not be the first place to look for an explanation.

41. **(4)** Almost half of all vaginal infections are due to candidiasis. The majority of women who develop the disease have recently taken antibiotics. It is not a sexually transmitted disease.

42. **(2)** The most common site for breast cancer is the upper outer quadrant, followed by the area beneath the nipple.

43. **(3)** Pap smears are crucial for the detection of cervical cancer but do not diagnose uterine cancer. In the early stages uterine cancer can be asymptomatic and would not be detectable even on bimanual examination.

Pharmacology

44. **(3)** Rocephin is a very effective drug for complicated urinary tract infection but is unnecessary in the uncomplicated lower urinary tract infection. Bactrim DS and Macrobid are both very effective for urinary tract infection treatment. Pyridium will help to make the client more comfortable until the antibiotic reaches effective levels for treatment.

45. **(3)** Fluconazole is now approved for a single-dose oral treatment of uncomplicated vulvovaginal candidiasis. It is most convenient for this client, who is unlikely to be extremely compliant with vaginal creams, given the upcoming travel. She does not have any contraindications to its use. Metronidazole and clindamycin are treatments for bacterial vaginosis and not for *Candida* infections. Hydrocortisone is a topical steroid use for inflammatory dermatologic conditions, and while it may help the itching, it would not treat the candidiasis.

46. **(4)** While some authors may recommend herbal treatments for menopausal symptoms, there have not been any controlled studies regarding prevention of disease with this substance. Traditional medicine supports the use of HRT for prevention of osteoporosis and cardiovascular disease. The use of weight-bearing exercise and calcium intake has been shown to help maintain bone health. Cigarette smoking increases the risk for both osteoporosis and cardiovascular disease. This client can significantly reduce her risk of these diseases by quitting her tobacco habit.

47. **(3)** The use of unopposed estrogen in the client with an intact uterus could put her at risk for endometrial hyperplasia or cancer. The addition of a progestin protects the endometrium adequately. The client is an excellent candidate for endometrial biopsy, to document the status of the endometrium. This client also needs to be educated on the risks and benefits of HRT.

48. **(3)** The regimen of Premarin 0.3 mg has not been proven to be effective for prevention of osteoporosis or heart disease. In addition, lowering the dosage of the estrogen would not help the client's symptoms. The other dosage regimens listed are all acceptable choices for this client, proving that there are many effective ways for one to utilize HRT, allowing for individualization of the regimen to the client.

49. **(3)** Well-controlled hypertension is not a contraindication to the use of HRT.

50. **(2)** 0.625 mg of conjugated equine estrogen (Premarin) is the minimal effective dose to prevent osteoporosis.

51. **(2)** The client no longer requires the use of Provera to protect the endometrium from the potential effects of estrogen; therefore, the progestin can be discontinued and the client given continuous estrogen therapy without concern. The other dosage regimens listed are appropriate for a client with an intact uterus on HRT.

52. **(1)** Informed consent is essential. The pros and cons of HRT should be explained, but the choice is up to the client.

53. **(3)** Repeated studies have demonstrated an increase in HDL and a decrease in LDL levels associated with postmenopausal administration of oral estrogens. This alteration in lipoprotein fractions has a beneficial effect on coronary artery disease and stroke.

54. **(4)** Clients taking Alendronate (Fosamax) are instructed to take the medication upon arising, 30 minutes prior to eating, with a full glass of water. Clients should be instructed to remain erect after taking the medication to prevent esophageal irritation. Taking medication with food (reduces bioavailability by 40%), coffee, or orange juice (decreases bioavailability by 60%) or after eating significantly reduces absorption.

55. **(1)** Women with a uterus taking unopposed exogenous estrogen have an increased risk of endometrial cancer. The addition of progesterone decreases this risk. The addition of progesterone may prompt bleeding, which many women view unfavorably. Progesterone does not affect cervical cancer, breast cancer, or gallbladder disease.

56. **(3)** Metronidazole (Flagyl) in a single 2-gm dose is the treatment of choice for trichomoniasis. An alternative is dividing the 2 gm into divided doses given the same day. This regimen causes less nausea and may improve compliance.

57. **(4)** Metronidazole (Flagyl) is the treatment of choice for bacterial vaginosis. However, pregnancy should be ruled out prior to beginning treatment because metronidazole should not be used if there is any possibility the woman is pregnant. The sexual partners do not have to be treated, and doxycycline is not the drug of choice.

58. **(3)** The American College of Physicians recommends that HRT be considered for all women, as it is believed that it reduces the levels of LDLs while increasing the levels of HDLs.

Mental Health

Psychosocial Examination & Diagnostic Tests

1. The mental status examination enables the nurse practitioner to identify:

   1. Intelligence quotient and reasoning.

   2. Abstract thinking and memory functioning.

   3. Reasoning and psychomotor skills.

   4. Memory functioning and intelligence quotient.

2. A client with a history of psychiatric problems arrives at the clinic at the clinic shouting that he is a messenger of God and knows the meaning of the prophecies in Revelations. This behavior is assessed as:

   1. A delusion.

   2. A hallucination.

   3. Magical thinking.

   4. An illusion.

3. An assessment of a client experiencing auditory hallucinations would most likely reveal:

   1. Client mumbling to self, tilted head, eyes darting back and forth.

   2. Performance of obsessive-compulsive rituals of turning off and on a radio, talking to self.

   3. Hyperactivity, expansive mood, easy distractibility.

   4. Cool, aloof, unapproachable, avoiding enclosed areas.

4. The MAST and the CAGE are screening instruments for which disease process?

   1. Glaucoma.

   2. Depression.

   3. Alcoholism.

   4. Diabetes.

5. When receiving the records from another agency, the nurse practitioner notes on the summary sheet that the client has a dual diagnosis. This means the client has:

1. Both manic and depressive symptoms of bipolar affective disorder.

2. Two closely related psychiatric disorders (e.g., panic disorder and bulimia nervosa).

3. Coexistence of both a psychiatric disorder (e.g., depression) and a substance abuse disorder (e.g., alcohol dependence).

4. Coexistence of a personality disorder (e.g., borderline personality) and a psychiatric disorder (e.g., panic disorder).

6. While completing the history on an older adult, the nurse practitioner understands that when a client "makes up stories or answers" to the questions, this is known as:

1. Perseveration.

2. Confabulation.

3. Echolalia.

4. Alcoholic encephalopathy.

7. In taking a history from a client with depression, which is the most important questions for the nurse practitioner to ask?

1. Have you ever experienced hallucinations, delusions, or illusions?

2. Have you ever been hospitalized in a psychiatric facility?

3. Do you regularly take antidepressants or other medications?

4. Have you thought about or attempted suicide?

8. Which statement is correct about mental health in the older adult and supports research findings in the literature?

1. Self-esteem does not decline as a person ages.

2. Older adults are consistently concerned about their physical appearance.

3. Older adults have a negative self-image compared with younger adults.

4. Learning ability is not maintained due to loss of short-term memory.

Psychiatric Disorders

9. An elderly client has been experiencing confusion. The nurse practitioner is trying to determine whether the confusion is related to depression or dementia. In evaluating this client, what specific assessment finding would be helpful in making this distinction?

1. Determining whether confusion worsens in the evening.

2. Assessing early morning agitation, hyperactivity, and insomnia.

3. Noting signs of anger, hostility, and loss of control.

4. Assessing reality distortions and preoccupation with family matters.

10. An older client calls the clinic and asks to speak to the nurse practitioner. When she answers the telephone, the client states that he is going to commit suicide. The priority goal is to:

1. Refer the client to an appropriate treatment facility.

2. Encourage ventilation of angry and depressed feelings.

3. Assess the lethality of the suicide plan.

4. Establish rapport with the client.

11. An elderly woman answers the nurse practitioner's questions by mumbling in low tones with answers that seem inappropriate. What would be initial findings associated with a diagnosis of dementia?

1. Sees people floating across the ceiling of her room.

2. Has problems with cognition and confusion.

3. Hears voices at night telling her to change her clothes.

4. Shows fear when the nurse makes any movements toward her.

12. The nurse practitioner understands the following about elder abuse:

   1. It is often reported by the victim.

   2. Abuse tends to de-escalate from the perpetrator.

   3. Midshaft fractures of the humerus or femur rarely indicate abuse.

   4. Bruises and lesions are often found on the inner aspects of extremities.

13. The nurse would expect which symptoms in a client with a diagnosis of schizophrenia?

   1. High energy with varying sleep patterns and nonstop conversation.

   2. Extreme and frequent mood swings with hyperactivity and difficulty concentration.

   3. Paranoia, delusions, hallucinations, and diminished self-care.

   4. Antisocial, manipulative, charismatic, and able to lie convincingly.

14. Dementia can be distinguished from delirium by:

   1. Dementia lasts days to weeks compared to delirium, which lasts months to years.

   2. Dementia is often associated with medications or systemic illness.

   3. Dementia exhibits a disturbance in attention that is not present in delirium.

   4. Dementia does not include altered perception, such as illusions.

15. An elderly client is brought to the nurse practitioner by his family for evaluation of increasing confusion over the past few days. The client has a history of dementia; however, the family states that this is a definite change. What course of action would the nurse practitioner consider?

   1. Help the family look for a nursing home.

2. Order an immediate magnetic resonance image (MRI).

3. A comprehensive medication review.

4. A referral to neurology.

16. An elderly client was taken to the clinic in a confused state that began suddenly 24 hours ago. She fails to be oriented to person, time, or place. She as incontinent of urine due to her confusion. She looks apathetic and is drowsy. The nurse practitioner would suspect:

   1. Delirium.

   2. Dementia.

   3. Depression.

   4. A psychotic disorder.

17. An older client comes to your office with the complaint of confusion. The daughter is concerned that her mother is developing Alzheimer's disease. Which of these assessments would indicate this client is experiencing delirium versus dementia?

   1. The confusion has been slowly developing.

   2. The confusion started after she started taking cimetidine (Tagamet).

   3. The client's attention span has not been affected.

   4. The client's memory has been impaired.

18. Which of the following groups of clients fall under mandatory reporting laws for abuse and neglect in a majority of states in the United States?

   1. Children, adult women, dependent elderly.

   2. Children, disabled individuals, adult women.

   3. Disabled individuals, adult women, dependent elderly.

   4. Children, disabled individuals, dependent elderly.

19. All of the following behaviors meet the criteria outlined in the *Diagnostic and Statistical Manual of Mental Disorders, Fourth Edition* (DSM-IV) for substance abuse **except**:

    1. Repeated arrests for drunk driving.

    2. Multiple absences from work due to substance use.

    3. Chronic anxiety attacks.

    4. Recurrent arguments with spouse about his/her drinking behavior.

Pharmacology

20. A client has been receiving fluphenazien (Prolixin) for the past 3 weeks. The nurse practitioner's assessment notes the following: temperature elevated (41°C), marked muscle rigidity, agitation, and confusion. The nurse practitioner understands these findings are often associated with the diagnosis of:

    1. Acute dystonia.

    2. Tardive dyskinesia.

    3. Neuroleptic malignant syndrome.

    4. Extrapyramidal disorder.

21. The preferred antidepressant for an elderly client is:

    1. Amitriptyline (Elavil).

    2. Sertraline (Zoloft).

    3. Trazodone (Desyrel).

    4. Haloperidol (Haldol).

22. A client has been referred to the nurse practitioner. The client's medical history reveals a long-term usage of antianxiety agents that the client considers harmless. The nurse practitioner understands that antianxiety agents can:

    1. Cause drug dependency.

    2. Produce hepatotoxicity and nephrotoxicity.

    3. Lead to functional damage of the cardiopulmonary system.

    4. Cause profound dissociative personality problems.

23. An older female has a diagnosis of dementia and is taking haloperidol (Haldol) 2 mg HS. The nurse practitioner observes her engaging in a restless, repetitive movement with her legs. She states that not only does she have ongoing movement but she also feels jittery. The nurse practitioner would interpret this activity to be:

    1. Ataxia.

    2. Akathisia.

    3. Agitation.

    4. Dyskinesia.

24. What is the best initial treatment plan for a sleep disorder in the elderly client?

    1. Medicate with amitriptyline (Elavil).

    2. Medicate with trazodone (Desyrel).

    3. Discuss the importance of naps daily.

    4. Decrease noise and light in the environment.

25. An elderly client presents with a new symptom of acute confusion over the last 24 hours. Which assessment would be the priority for the nurse practitioner to evaluate during the examination?

    1. Drug history.

    2. Electrocardiogram (ECG).

    3. Mini mental state examination.

    4. Thyroid profile.

26. The nurse practitioner is aware that the following class of drugs is most likely to precipitate a hypertensive crisis in the elderly:

    1. Narcotic analgesics.

    2. Monoamine oxidase (MAO) inhibitors.

    3. Barbiturates.

    4. Phenothiazines.

27. The nurse practitioner knows that the following class of drugs would have the

greatest effect on memory in the elderly client:

1. Phenothiazines.

2. Tricyclic antidepressants.

3. Benzodiazepines.

4. MAO inhibitors.

28. Of the following antidepressants, which one has the most sedating side effects making it a good sleeping agent?

1. Fluoxetine (Prozac).

2. Doxepin (Sinequan).

3. Trazadone (Desyrel).

4. Paroxetine (Paxil).

29. In the management of acute alcohol withdrawal delirium, a nurse practitioner may want to use all of the following drugs **except**:

1. Chlordiazepoxide (Librium).

2. Lorazepam (Ativan).

3. Thiamine.

4. Chlorpromazine (Thorazine).

30. Which laboratory results would be **least** important to assess before placing a client on lithium?

1. Thyroid-stimulating hormone, triiodothyronine, thyroxine.

2. Blood urea nitrogen creatinine.

3. Urinalysis, electrolytes.

4. Alanine aminotransferase, aspartate aminotransferase, lactate dehydrogenase.

31. Benzodiazepines are useful in the treatment of all the disorders below **except**:

1. Alcohol withdrawal.

2. Anxiety.

3. Obsessive-compulsive disorder.

4. Seizures.

32. When starting a psychotropic medication in the elderly, a good rule of thumb is:

1. Start low, go slow.

2. Higher doses are almost always needed.

3. Side effects of psychotropic medications will usually not impact other medications.

4. The same adult dosages can be used initially without any problems.

33. A client is a 20-year, two-pack-a-day smoker with a history of chronic bronchitis. What is the prescription to give to this client who wishes to stop smoking?

1. Nicotine polacrilex (Nicorette) gum 2-mg piece, chew for 30 minutes, q1–2h × 6 weeks, then q2–4h × 3 weeks, then q4–8h × 3 weeks, then discontinue.

2. Nicotine patch (Nicoderm) 21 mg/24 hr qd × 6 weeks, then 14 mg/24 hr qd × 2 weeks, then 7 mg/24 hr × 2 weeks, then discontinue.

3. Bupropion HCI (Zyban) 150 mg qd × 3 days, then 150 mg bid for 7–12 weeks and to stop smoking when medication is started.

4. Nicotine patch (Nicoderm) 14 mg/24 hr qd × 6 weeks, then 7 mg/24 hr qd × 6 weeks, then discontinue.

34. The nurse practitioner understands the following about the use of benzodiazepines in the older adult?

1. Withdrawal symptoms may occur with 24 hours of abruptly stopping the medication.

2. Adverse side effects are minimal and tend to minimize the incidence of falls and other injuries.

3. Long-acting medications (i.e., chlordiazepoxide [Librium]) are preferred over the shorter acting medications (i.e., lorazepam [Ativan]).

4. Larger doses are needed to maintain therapeutic levels for the anxious or agitated client.

17   Answers & Rationales

Psychosocial Examination & Diagnostic Tests

1. **(2)** The mental status examination provides a basic assessment of the client's intellectual functioning (reasoning, abstract thinking, memory). The intelligence quotient (IQ) is determined by psychological testing. Psychomotor skills assessment is part of a neurologic examination.

2. **(1)** Delusions are false, fixed beliefs that can be of a persecutory or grandiose nature. In this instance, the client is experiencing a delusion of grandeur. A hallucination is a false sensory experience. An illusion is a misinterpretation of reality. Magical thinking is when the client feels that his thoughts or wishes can control other people.

3. **(1)** The client experiencing the auditory hallucination will often look out into space and act as if he is listening to someone talking. This is associated with behaviors such as tilting the head, mumbling, and eye movement.

4. **(3)** The Michigan Alcoholism Screening Test (MAST) and the CAGE (Cut down, Annoyed, Guilty, Eye opener) are used to alert providers to the possibility of alcoholism.

5. **(3)** Dual diagnosis involves both a psychiatric diagnosis and a substance abuse diagnosis.

6. **(2)** The fabrication of events or situations to fill in gaps in the memory, usually in a plausible way, is a classic definition of a client who is experiencing dementia due to chronic alcoholism. Clients with alcohol amnesic disorder or Korsakoff's syndrome may experience confabulation. Echolalia is the parroting or automatic, meaningless, repeating of another's words. Perseveration is the involuntary persistent repetition of an idea or response (i.e., the client keeps repeating the same phrase over and over).

7. **(4)** Although the other questions are important to obtain during the initial history, it is most important to ascertain whether or not the client has contemplated suicide. In addition, determination of a specific plan and the means to do it are also involved in the questioning about suicidal ideation.

8. **(1)** According to research, self-esteem along with attitude and morals are maintained as a client ages and older adults tend to have a positive self-image when compared to younger adults. Learning ability is maintained, although more time is often needed for the early phases of the learning process. Retrieval of information in long-term memory is slower and short-term memory is diminished.

Psychiatric Disorders

9. **(1)** Confusion can occur in both dementia and depression. However, with dementia, symptoms worsen at night.

10. **(4)** The nurse practitioner must first establish trust and rapport with the caller before an assessment can be made. If rapport is not established, the client will hang up the phone. The nurse practitioner understands that by keeping the client talking, he is prevented from acting out the suicidal threat.

11. **(2)** Confusion and cognitive function problems (i.e, short-term memory loss) are initial signs of dementia. The severity of the symptoms is dependent upon what stage of cognitive degeneration the client is manifesting. The other options are characteristic of hallucinatory experiences and usually occur later.

12. **(4)** Bruising on the extensor surfaces of the arms is common and usually not considered abuse, while bruising on the inner surfaces of extremities and areas with different stages of resolution are often found in the elderly abused client.

13. **(3)** The characteristics of schizophrenia are delusions, tangential thought, suspiciousness, disorganized behavior, and hallucinations.

14. **(4)** Adults with dementia do not usually have altered perceptions that include illusions. They may experience hallucinations and delusions. Dementia does last months to years. Delirium is often associated with medications or systemic illness and a disturbance in the ability to pay attention.

15. **(3)** Drug effects are one of the most common causes of a sudden increase in dementia in the elderly. Dementia has a gradual increase, and a sudden increase is a cause for concern. The nurse practitioner should question the family about new addition to the client's medications and who helps the client take his medication. It should also include a "brown bag review" of the client's medications, both prescription and over-the-counter.

16. **(1)** Due to the acute confusion state and the incontinence, she is experiencing delirium. This is most likely secondary to a urinary tract infection. Dementia is more insidious versus acute. Depression and psychosis are not consistent with the assessments. The major symptoms in depression would include loss of interest, sleep, decreased appetite, concentration, activity, guilt, energy, or potential suicidal thoughts. Psychotic disorders include thoughts and behavior where the client is not in touch with reality.

17. **(2)** A history of a new medication with an abrupt onset of confusion must be reviewed closely. An adverse reaction of cimetidine (Tagamet) in the elderly is confusion. Dementia results in confusion that slowly develops. The attention span and memory may be affected in each diagnosis.

18. **(4)** The laws in most states require the reporting of suspected or actual abuse and neglect of any person considered to be dependent or with a reduced ability to make life choices. Children, disabled individuals, and dependent elderly fall into these categories. Very few states require reporting for adult women unless a weapon is involved; this is a different situation requiring a report.

19. **(3)** Chronic anxiety attacks are not part of the DSM-IV criteria.

Pharmacology

20. **(3)** The client is experiencing a rare problem called neuroleptic malignant syndrome. This client would require immediate referral and hospitalization. Acute dystonia, parkinsonism, and akathisia are associated with extrapyramidal disorder or acute movement disorder. Tardive dyskinesia occurs late in therapy and is often irreversible. Slow, worm-like movements of the tongue are the earliest symptom, followed by grimacing, lip smacking, and involuntary limb movements.

21. **(2)** Zoloft's favorable side-effect profile makes it a useful alternative to the traditional tricyclic antidepressants. It has the shortest half-life of the currently marketed serotonin reuptake inhibitors. Elavil has the most anticholinergic and sedating side effects of the antidepressants. There may be pronounced effects on the cardiovascular system (hypotension). Geropsychiatrists agree it is best to avoid in the elderly. Desyrel is very sedating for the elderly client. Haldol is an antipsychotic medication.

22. **(1)** Physical dependence can occur, even with low doses of the medication. This is a particular problem in the elderly, who are sensitive to low dose ranges.

23. **(2)** Akathisia is a feeling of restlessness. Clients may complain of a feeling of muscular quivering. Ataxia is a disorder where muscular incoordination occurs with voluntary muscular movements. Agitation is a general assessment that may be part of the psychotic behavior. Dyskinesia is a defect in the voluntary movement.

24. **(4)** Correction of environmental factors and treatment of underlying iatrogenic and medical problems should be addressed initially. Elavil can cause excessive somnolence. Desyrel may be of particular use when sleep disturbance is prominent; however, it does not address the best initial plan. The goal is to begin with good sleep hygiene prior to pharmacologic therapy. Eliminating naps during the day may be useful in facilitating sleep.

25. **(1)** Drug–drug interactions are a common cause of acute confusion in the elderly client. This assessment can minimize the need to do further costly interventions if the client only needs medication adjustment. The other options would be included in the plan after the drug history had been completed and had been ruled out as a potential problem.

26. **(2)** In combination with tyramine-rich foods that have undergone an aging process such as cheese, wine, beer, salami, and yogurt, catecholamines are released from the nerve endings, causing a hypertensive crisis. The other drugs listed cause hypotension.

27. **(3)** The benzodiazepines cause sedation and decreased attention, which in turn affect the memory. Although phenothiazines and antidepressants may also cause sedation, they do not affect memory.

28. **(3)** Trazadone (Desyrel) has sedation as a side effect, which has made it less popular as an antidepressant; however, it is commonly prescribed for insomnia.

29. **(4)** All of the drugs listed above may be used in acute alcohol withdrawal delirium, except chlorpromazine, which is an antipsychotic that has not use in the management.

30. **(4)** It is **not** important to evaluate liver function before initiating treatment with lithium. The adverse side effects of lithium affect renal, cardiac, and thyroid function. Baseline electrolytes are also important to obtain.

31. **(3)** Seizures, alcohol withdrawal, and anxiety are commonly treated with benzodiazepines. They are **not** the first drug of choice for obsessive-compulsive disorder; selective serotonin reuptake inhibitors are usually used.

32. **(1)** Dosages should be reduced by 30–50% to start therapy and gradually increase as necessary. Adverse effects are likely to occur because of slowed drug metabolism, which occurs with aging. These include hypotension, arrhythmias, and sedative and anticholinergic effects.

33. **(2)** A highly nicotine-dependent client benefits from intense counseling and prescription of alternative nicotine delivery during the smoking cessation process. Usually the nicotine patch is the preferred form of replacement, as the gum is noncontinuous and withdrawal symptoms may occur during nonchewing times. The nicotine patch delivers a fixed dose of nicotine on a continual basis, is applied once daily, and eliminates the gastrointestinal upset that often occurs with the gum. If this client insisted on using the gum, the dose should be 4 mg, not 2 mg. Option #4 is too low of a dose to start on this client and is not the correct dosing schedule. Zyban (bupropion HCI) would be used in conjunction with the nicotine patch,

and clients are to quit smoking 1–2 weeks after starting the Zyban, not immediately.

34. **(1)** Benzodiazepines should be tapered slowly in the older adult. Withdrawal symptoms occur within 24 hours in clients taking the shorter acting medications and may not occur for several days in clients taking long-acting medications. The adverse effects of oversedation, dizziness, confusion, and sometimes hypotension contribute to falls and other injuries in the elderly. In Option #3, short-acting medications are preferred. Typically, larger doses are not needed, but rather small initial doses with gradual increments.

18

Emergencies

1. While visiting a rural public school, an older adult was bitten on the hand by a raccoon. At the rural clinic, the nurse practitioner cleansed the wound. The next action would have been:

   1. Administer tetanus antitoxin.

   2. Contact local animal control authorities.

   3. Administer rabies immune globulin (RIG) and human diploid cell vaccine (HDCV).

   4. Teach the family how to do hourly soaks to the hand using normal saline and peroxide.

2. An older adult is brought to the clinic with a history of an insect bite last evening. What presenting symptom would be associated with the bite of a brown recluse spider?

   1. Paresthesias in all extremities.

   2. Edematous, erythematous area with coalescing macules.

   3. Tissue sloughing in the bite area within 8–10 hours.

   4. Development of a central black eschar or "sinking infarct" in 6–12 hours.

3. The nurse practitioner understands that cat bites become infected more often than dog bites because:

   1. Dogs have a "cleaner mouth" than cats.

   2. Cat bites are often deep puncture wounds.

   3. Dog bites are usually on the face, which makes them more susceptible to infection.

   4. Cat bites are usually associated with clawing and spreading of microorganisms.

4. When do bites due to insects, spiders, snakes, and bees most commonly occur?

   1. Fall.

   2. Spring to fall.

   3. Winter.

   4. Any time of the year.

5. An older adult was bitten by a neighbor's dog 3 days ago. He has developed an infection in a large wound on his lower leg. What would be appropriate management of this client?

   1. Prescribe amoxicillin/clavulanate potassium (Augmentin) 250 mg PO tid × 14 days.

   2. Approximate the edges of the wound together with suture.

   3. Prescribe cephalexin (Keflex) 500 PO tid × 7 days.

   4. Have the client return to the clinic for follow-up in 2 weeks.

6. Medical management for a brown recluse spider bite includes:

   1. Warm, moist soaks to the area.

   2. Ice pack and elevate area.

   3. Active and passive range of motion to area.

   4. Avoid use of antihistamines.

7. An elderly client has been bitten by a black widow spider while doing yard work. He is having a severe reaction. The nurse practitioner expects:

   1. Hypotension and shock.

   2. Localized pain, erythema, and edema in the area.

   3. Black eschar of sloughing tissue within 4 hours of the bite.

   4. Abdominal rigidity, nausea, and headache.

18   Answers & Rationales

1. **(3)** Any type of animal bite that might be associated with an animal that may potentially harbor rabies (skunks, bats, raccoons, foxes, coyotes, rats) should be treated with both active and passive rabies immunization. Tetanus antitoxin would be indicated if the adult was not current on the immunization. Animal authorities would be called after the initial treatment to locate the animal and sacrifice it, so that the brain could be examined for rabies.

2. **(4)** Brown recluse spiders produce sharp pain at the instant of the bite with subsequent minor swelling and erythema. Tissue necrosis may occur within 4 hours. A blue-gray to black macular halo may surround the bite with eventual widening and sinking of the center of the lesion leading to a "sinking infarct" that leaves a deep ulcer, which takes weeks or months to heal.

3. **(2)** Deep puncture wounds are more likely to get infected with anaerobic organisms. Bites on the hand have the highest infection rate, whereas bites on the face have the lowest infection rate.

4. **(2)** Insects are more active, reproduce, and are in greater numbers in the warm months (i.e., spring to early fall).

5. **(1)** Prior to developing an infection, prophylactic medication treatment would be penicillin V potassium (Pen-Vee K) 50 mg/kg/day PO qid × 3 days. Keflex is not indicated due to resistant strains of *Pasteurella multocida*, an organism present in 25% of dog bites and 50% of cat bites. An infected bite should be followed up on a daily basis, until the infection clears. Open-wounded management is indicated, not suturing.

6. **(2)** Heat application is contraindicated; ice packs and elevation are preferred to decrease the edema. The area should be immobilized. Tetanus toxoid may be given along with antihistamines to reduce swelling and relieve itching.

7. **(4)** In addition to these symptoms, bronchospasm, hypertension, seizures, and altered mental status may occur. Black eschar is associated with a brown recluse spider bite.

19

Research & Theory

Research

1. When designing a research project that will involve clients, from the options presented below, the most important point to be included in the written consent to participate is:

   1. The directions regarding the use of a black pen.

   2. The anticipated date for publication of the completed research report.

   3. The assurance of privacy and confidentiality.

   4. The number of previously published research studies about this topic.

2. When determining whether to incorporate into your clinical practice a new procedure based on the findings of a recent study, which of the following should you consider?

   1. The statistical significance of the findings.

   2. The statistical relevance of the findings.

   3. The statistical software program used.

   4. The statistical background of the researcher.

3. The research process is similar to the processes nurse practitioners use to provide client care in that both are decision-making processes that include the steps (in the order presented here) of:

   1. Assessing, teaching, evaluating, and discussing.

   2. Defining, planning, implementing, and charting.

   3. Questioning, evaluating, diagnosing, and teaching.

   4. Assessing, planning, implementing, and evaluating.

4. Both descriptive and inferential statistics are used in research. However, their purposes are different in that:

   1. Inferential statistics are used for assigning participant code numbers.

   2. Descriptive statistics are used for assigning participant code numbers.

   3. Inferential statistics are used for hypothesis testing.

   4. Descriptive statistics are used for hypothesis testing.

5. In an ambulatory care setting, the nurse practitioner might find it difficult to utilize nursing research because:

1. The demands of providing primary care leave little time for research utilization.

2. Procedures for research utilization have not been well defined in the literature.

3. Research published in professional journals is too difficult to access by clinicians.

4. Ambulatory care settings have little in common with the settings used for most research.

6. While nursing theories vary greatly in their perspective of nursing care, all nursing theorists explicitly incorporate three key concepts. These three concepts, which are basic to nursing care, are:

1. Individuals, families, and communities.

2. Primary, secondary, and tertiary prevention.

3. Past, present, and future well-being.

4. Person, health, and environment.

7. The scientific method for conducting research uses the null hypothesis, which is statistically based. The correct format for the null hypothesis is:

1. There are no significant differences between two groups.

2. Group "A" is greater than group "B."

3. Group "A" is less than group "B."

4. There is a 95% probability that group "A" is different from group "B."

8. When evaluating claims made on advertisements, such as "Drug X has been used for 5 years with over 1 million doses administered in the United States, Canada, and Great Britain. Drug X stops heartburn, aids in digestion, and prevents esophageal reflux and is the 'treatment of choice' to relieve GERD," the nurse practitioner realizes that the claim is:

1. Invalid, as there is no control or comparison group or statistics stated.

2. Valid, as there are sufficient numbers of users who have had success.

3. Invalid, because the level of significance is not mentioned to be at the 0.05 level.

4. Valid, as the cohort and Hawthorne effect are operating.

9. The utilization of research in nursing practice can be equated with:

1. The nursing process.

2. The change process.

3. Discharge planning.

4. Family planning.

10. You are compiling monthly statistics for your practice, and one of the elements of your analysis is the cultural background of your clients. What level of data is "cultural background"?

1. Nominal level data.

2. Ordinal level data.

3. Interval level data.

4. Ratio level data.

11. A nurse practitioner practicing with a physician in general practice is compiling the practice statistics at the end of the month. The clients who received care range from infants to the elderly. Of the following data from the monthly report, which is most likely to be normally distributed?

1. The lab tests scheduled for the clients.

2. The gender of the clients.

3. The primary diagnosis of the clients.

4. The age of the clients.

12. A nurse practitioner practicing with a physician in general practice is compiling the practice statistics at the end of the month. The clients who received care range from infants to the elderly. The nurse practitioner and the physician want to know the average monthly income of their clients. Which would be the most appropriate statistical measure of the "average income" assuming income was exact in dollars and cents?

1. The mean.

2. The median.

3. The mode.

4. The range.

13. A nurse practitioner is evaluating research articles for a utilization project. The majority of the articles report that either random selection or random assignment was used to select the sample for that study. Because certain procedures in research are used across disciplines, what can be assumed for studies where randomization has been used?

    1. The ages of the research subjects in these studies will be negatively skewed.

    2. The research subjects in these studies will automatically be half male and half female.

    3. The ages of the research subjects in these studies will be positively skewed.

    4. The researchers were attempting to obtain the most representative sample.

14. The ability to predict outcomes of care is desirable both in research and in practice. If a nurse practitioner wanted to create a theoretical model for a specific aspect of his/her practice to predict the client outcomes, which statistical analysis method would be used to analyze the clinical data?

    1. Descriptive statistics.

    2. Repeated measures t-test.

    3. Multiple regression.

    4. Chi-squared for independent samples.

15. Research articles are being evaluated for a utilization project. What can the nurse practitioner do if he/she does not understand the statistical procedures that were used for the analysis of data in an article?

    1. Assume that the correct procedure was used, and read about the method or consult a statistician for an explanation of the statistics.

    2. Assume that the article is beyond his/her ability to understand, so set that one aside and go on to the next article.

3. Assume that the correct procedure was used and instead of reading the results section, read the discussion of the findings section.

4. Assume that the article is beyond his/her ability to understand and use someone else's critique of the reported study.

16. The nurse practitioner has determined that the office procedures for diagnosing and stabilizing new diabetics need to be evaluated and possibly changed. Which would be the best choice for the first phase of the evaluation?

    1. Design and conduct a double-blind clinical trial.

    2. Design and conduct a research utilization project.

    3. Design and conduct a research project comparing men and women.

    4. Design and conduct a study to test Callista Roy's theoretical model.

17. The nurse practitioner was reading a nursing research article in which there were no statistically significant findings. The most appropriate response would be:

    1. "Reading this article was a waste of my time."

    2. "Because of reading this article, there is no reason to conduct similar studies."

    3. "Reading this article raises new questions for my practice."

    4. "Because of reading this article, I will immediately change my practice."

18. The verification of the more abstract nursing theories (e.g., Martha Rogers) is often hampered by:

    1. The lack of adequate measures for the theoretical concepts.

    2. Prior studies that did not support the theory.

    3. The lack of adequate laboratory settings for conducting experiments.

    4. Prior studies that were conducted in other countries.

19. In a recently published study, the researcher reported "the statistical analysis used to identify the differences between the two variables was Pearson's correlation." Which most specifically tells what is wrong with this statement?

    1. Pearson's correlation can be used only with three or more variables.

    2. Pearson's correlation actually identifies the common factors between variables.

    3. Pearson's correlation can be used only when there is a single variable.

    4. Pearson's correlation actually identifies the relationship between variables.

20. Qualitative research studies are conducted by nurse researchers because:

    1. Qualitative studies help to identify and define nursing concepts.

    2. With qualitative methods, there are no concerns about the rights of research subjects.

    3. Qualitative approaches provide precise measures for statistical analysis.

    4. Nurse researchers find qualitative research designs easier to use.

21. The normal ranges of blood chemistry values are most like which statistical concept?

    1. The standard error.

    2. The mean.

    3. The standard deviation.

    4. The median.

22. The five major sequential steps of research utilization are:

    1. Establish a client relationship, complete a health assessment, diagnoses, devise a plan of care, evaluate the treatment.

    2. Identify the problem, assess published research, design the innovation, evaluate, decide whether to adopt the innovation.

    3. Review the popular literature, review the practice's clients, summarize the findings, evaluate, teach the client.

    4. Review the client's lab reports, complete a thorough health assessment, diagnose, implement the treatment, evaluate.

23. Both *qualitative* and *quantitative* research methods are used in nursing research because:

    1. Master's-prepared nurses conduct quantitative studies, while doctorally prepared nurses conduct quantitative studies.

    2. Master's-prepared nurses conduct qualitative studies, while doctorally prepared nurses conduct quantitative studies.

    3. They complement each other because they produce different types of findings about the same concepts.

    4. They complement each other because they produce the same types of findings about different concepts.

24. Nursing research subscribes to the scientific method for the design of research studies. The advantage of this is that:

    1. Nursing research is based on logically constructed arguments.

    2. Nursing research is designed to answer any research questions.

    3. Nursing research findings are precise and need not be duplicated.

    4. Nursing research findings are generalizable to all client populations.

25. With the restructuring of health care delivery and a shift in the provision of nonacute care from the hospital to the ambulatory care settings and the home, previous nursing research that was conducted in hospitals:

    1. Now becomes applicable to all in-hospital providers of care.

    2. Remains relevant in the new settings; client care is unchanged.

    3. Should be applied directly to client care provided in the new settings.

    4. May no longer be applicable to the delivery of client care.

26. Nurse researchers strive to substantiate causality so that client outcomes can be consistently predicted. For the nurse practitioner, the ability to predict the outcomes for every client could mean that:

    1. The appropriate treatment would be prescribed for clients.

    2. No further studies would need to be conducted about treatments.

    3. The client's individual qualities would not need to be considered.

    4. Treatments would not need to be individualized for each client.

27. The reason that quantitative research articles always have a section containing descriptive findings is that descriptive data analysis:

    1. Provides the basis for making inferences about the findings.

    2. May yield statistically significant findings that were unexpected.

    3. Is conducted for predicting client outcomes in nursing settings.

    4. Organizes the data for clearer understanding of subjects and variables.

28. The difference between univariate and multivariate studies is:

    1. The number of subjects in the sample.

    2. The number of variables being studied.

    3. The number of sites for collecting data.

    4. The number of statistical hypotheses.

29. The theoretical basis for nursing practice is:

    1. A relatively new approach to nursing care.

    2. Borrowed from other professions such as medicine.

    3. As old as formal nursing and began with Florence Nightingale.

    4. Unrelated to the conduct of nursing research studies.

30. The independent variable and the dependent variable of a research study might be thought of as:

    1. The cause (the independent variable) and the effect (the dependent variable).

    2. The median (the independent variable) and the mode (the dependent variable).

    3. The outcome (the independent variable) and the treatment (the dependent variable).

    4. The sample (the independent variable) and the population (the dependent variable).

31. *Variance* is a key statistical concept. How would current nursing research methods change if there were no variance?

    1. We would need to increase the sample size in all of our research studies to 100 research subjects or greater.

    2. Since our current research methods do not depend on the presence of variance, we would not need to change our current methods.

    3. We would need to decrease the sample size of all our research studies to 15 research subjects.

    4. Since our current research methods are based on the presence of variance, we would not be able to use our current methods.

Theory

32. Nursing practice based on nursing theory contributes to the professionalization of nursing practice by:

    1. Adapting the medical model to nursing care.

    2. Limiting the choice of treatments for clients.

    3. Determining what type of clients will be seen by the nurse.

    4. Providing a consistent perspective for providing care to clients.

33. A nurse practitioner has decided to incorporate a nursing theoretical model into his/her practice. Which nursing model is most applicable to an ambulatory care setting?

    1. Orem's Model of Self-Care.

    2. Roy's Adaptation Model.

    3. Roger's Unitary Person Model.

    4. King's System Model.

34. Which nurse theorist is considered to have general system theory as philosophical orientation to her model?

    1. Sister Callista Roy.

    2. Martha Rogers.

    3. Rosemarie Parse.

    4. Betty Neuman.

35. Which nurse theorist addresses nursing outcomes in terms of primary, secondary, and tertiary prevention?

    1. Sister Callista Roy.

    2. Betty Neuman.

    3. Imogene King.

    4. Jean Watson.

36. Which nursing theorist's model primarily addresses health promotion?

    1. Jean Watson.

    2. Betty Neuman.

    3. N. J. Pender.

    4. Sister Callista Roy.

Answers & Rationales

Research

1. **(3)** By federal law, clients must be assured of their privacy and confidentiality. The other information is interesting and may be included, but is not required by federal law.

2. **(1)** In published research reports, of the choices listed, only the first choice is consistently reported by researchers. The clinical relevance is considered, not the statistical relevance. The specific program used does not make a difference, since all are based on the same statistical formulas. Researchers frequently work with statistical consultants so that a researcher's background is not a limitation to a published study.

3. **(4)** Only the last choice contains those elements common to both processes, which are assessing, planning, implementing, and evaluating.

4. **(3)** Only Option #3 is true. Neither descriptive nor inferential statistics are used to assign participant code numbers. Descriptive statistics are used to describe the sample.

5. **(1)** Inadequate time can be a barrier to research utilization in any setting. The process of research utilization is well delineated by researchers. With the ever-increasing availability of professional journals via the Internet, access is rarely a problem. There is a considerable body of research that has been conducted in ambulatory care settings.

6. **(4)** All current theories incorporate person, health, and environment. Other concepts may or may not be explicitly included in nursing theories.

7. **(1)** The correct format for the null hypothesis is, "There are no significant differences between two groups." The alternate or research hypothesis may take the other forms.

8. **(1)** Even though the claims detail extensive use of "Drug X," there must be statistical evidence as demonstrated through the use of control or comparison groups that will render a level of significance.

9. **(2)** Incorporating research findings into practice often results in a change in practice. The nursing process is most like conducting research.

10. **(1)** The variable of "cultural background" is categorical data or nominal level data.

11. **4)** The gender and primary diagnosis are nominal level data, and the lab tests would be skewed, while the age would approximate the normal curve.

12. **(2)** The median income would be most representative of the average because the income of 50% of the clients is above and 50% is below the median. The mean could be influenced by one client with very high or very low income, and the mode only identifies the income that is reported most often. The range only identifies the lowest and the highest income and does not present an average.

13. **(4)** Randomization is a research technique used to increase the amount of control in any research design. The other three options are false; they do not occur because of randomization.

14. **(3)** Of the choices, only multiple regression examines the relationship between two or more variables in a way that permits prediction.

15. **(1)** In reviewing research, it is necessary to understand the statistical methods that the researcher used in order to determine the value of the study findings for the practice setting. The researcher's discussion may not provide the full extent of the findings, while someone else's critique may reflect a specific point of view that does not apply in every situation.

16. **(2)** As a first step, a research utilization project would provide a thorough review of the published literature on which to base a change. A full study may not be needed, and testing a theoretical model is not appropriate for this situation.

17. **(3)** The lack of significant findings is an important piece of information about the topic of the research, and definitely is not a waste of time. Particularly when findings are nonsignificant, more studies need to be conducted about this topic. Ideally, changes in practice are based on the findings of more than one study.

18. **(1)** The lack of adequate measures for theoretical concepts is a major roadblock in many areas of research, and particularly so with the more abstract theories. Prior studies always provide information about the theory, even when conducted in other countries. More abstract concepts tend not to be studied in lab settings.

19. **(4)** Correlations identify the relationships between variables. Two or more variables may be used. Factor analysis is used to identify common factors.

20. **(1)** The purpose of qualitative designs is to identify and define nursing concepts. Qualitative designs do not yield precise measures, are usually not analyzed statistically, are more difficult to use, and

carry the same concerns about the rights of subjects as all other research designs.

21. **(3)** The normal ranges of blood chemistry values are based on studies that identified the standard deviation for each blood chemical. The mean and the median are averages, and the standard error is not applicable to this situation.

22. **(2)** This option contains the published steps. All other options are nursing actions taken on behalf of the client (in no particular order).

23. **(3)** The two methods do complement each other because they produce different types of findings about the same concepts. The educational preparation of the researcher does not dictate the research method used.

24. **(1)** The scientific method is highly organized, and is based on logical reasoning. Findings are rarely precise and studies do need to be duplicated. Some questions are not answerable by our current research methods. Because of small samples and other limitations, many findings from nursing research are **not** generalizable.

25. **(4)** Such a drastic change in health care delivery may make previous studies no longer applicable to nursing care. Health care restructuring has changed the way client care is provided.

26. **(1)** The ability to always predict client outcomes would mean that every client would receive the exact treatment for that individual. Treatments would still have to be individualized, and individual qualities would need to be considered. Because new treatments are always being devised, there would be a need for ongoing research.

27. **(4)** Descriptive data analysis does organize the data, and it facilitates understanding. Descriptive statistics cannot be used for significance testing or for making inferences, for which inferential statistics are used. Predictions are made from studies that use inferential statistics.

28. **(2)** "Variate" refers to the number of variables in the study.

29. **(3)** The theoretical basis for nursing practice began with Florence Nightingale and has been used for practice and for research for over a century. Nursing theories are specifically developed for nursing.

30. **(1)** The independent variable may be considered the cause or the treatment, and the dependent variable may be considered the effect or the outcome. The median, mode, sample, and population are not designations for the independent or the dependent variables.

31. **(4)** All our current research and statistical analysis methods rely on the presence of variance or variation; so that if variance is no longer present, our current methods could no longer be used. If there is no variance, a sample of one would be adequate.

Theory

32. **(4)** Theory-based practice contributes the consistent perspective that permits the comparison of care across settings. Theory-based practice does not necessarily limit treatments or determine client types.

Theory-based practice specifically eliminates reliance on the medical model.

33. **(1)** Orem's theory focuses on the client participating and being in control of his/her own health care. Roy's model is most appropriate for acute care settings, Roger's for a holistic health setting, and King's for a mental health setting.

34. **(4)** Betty Neuman's Health Care Systems Model, Imogene King's Systems Interaction Model, and Dorothy Johnson's Behavioral Systems are based on general systems theory. Roy's Adaptation Model is based on stress and adaptation as the framework. Martha Rogers's Science of Unitary Human Beings and Rosemarie Parse's Human Becoming Model are based on a humanistic developmental framework.

35. **(2)** Betty Neuman identified the need to implement nursing interventions through use of one or more of three prevention modalities (primary, secondary, and tertiary prevention).

36. **(3)** Pender's Health Promotion Model is an excellent nursing model that readily fits into a nurse practitioner's scope of practice. The other theorist's models are Betty Neuman's Health Care Systems Model, Jean Watson's Human Science and Human Model of Caring, and Roy's Adaptation Model.

Issues & Trends

1. Considering the four advanced practice roles, clinical nurse specialist, nurse practitioner, certified nurse midwife, and nurse anesthetist, which role became accepted by and included into the practice arena without significant controversy?

   1. Clinical nurse specialist.

   2. Nurse practitioner.

   3. Certified nurse midwife.

   4. Nurse anesthetist.

2. Historically, who was one of the most outspoken opponents of the nurse practitioner role.

   1. Loretta Ford.

   2. Hildegard Peplau.

   3. Martha Rogers.

   4. Dorothea Orem.

3. Who started the first nurse practitioner program?

   1. Hildegard Peplau.

   2. Mary Breckenridge.

   3. Agnes McGee.

   4. Loretta Ford.

4. Which is the most important action in developing health policy skills in the nurse practitioner?

   1. Develop political allies in Congress.

   2. Work on a campaign.

   3. Support causes such as teen pregnancy prevention or AIDS research/prevention.

   4. Write letters and editorials.

5. Which is the least important barrier to collaborative advanced nursing practice?

   1. Prescriptive authority.

   2. Reimbursement privileges.

   3. Legal scope of practice.

   4. Political activism.

6. For the nurse practitioner to obtain reimbursement, an understanding of which is important?

   1. Minimum Nursing Data Set (MNDS).

   2. ICD-9-CM, CPT, and HCPC codes.

   3. HCPC codes and NANDA diagnosis.

   4. Medicare and Medicaid number.

7. Steps of the change process according to Kurt Lewin are:

   1. Unsolving, mobilizing, recruiting, finalizing.

   2. Building relationships, acquiring resources, choosing solution, stabilizing.

   3. Unfreezing, moving, refreezing.

   4. Forming, storming, norming.

8. What was the major impetus for nurse practitioner development?

   1. Need for an expert nurse clinician.

   2. Shortage of primary care physicians.

   3. Trend for specialized nurses to diagnose and manage unstable acute and chronic clients.

   4. Movement of graduate nursing education to diagnosis and treatment of major illness.

9. The nurse practitioner understands that Medicare B provides:

   1. Hospitalization costs for the insured.

   2. Health insurance benefits for low-income families.

   3. Benefits that cover physicians, nurse practitioners, medical equipment, and outpatient services.

   4. Outpatient laboratory, radiography services, and skilled nursing care in appropriate facilities.

10. What is the impact of the Balanced Budget Act of 1997 on nurse practitioner practice?

    1. Authorizes all states to provide nurse practitioners prescriptive authority.

    2. Provides for only well visits and primary care services.

    3. Prevents a physician from billing 100% for a nurse practitioner's services.

    4. Allows direct Medicare payments to nurse practitioners in both rural and urban settings.

11. In the clinic, you have observed the following: one medical assistant is usually pleasant and helpful; the other is often abrasive and angry. The most important basic guideline to be observed by the nurse practitioner nurse who must resolve a conflict between two medical assistants is:

    1. Require the medical assistants to reach a compromise.

    2. Weigh the consequences of each possible solution.

    3. Encourage ventilation of anger and use humor to minimize the conflict.

    4. Deal with issues, not personalities.

12. A male nurse practitioner approaches another nurse practitioner who is his friend and tells him that one of the female physicians at the clinic often follows him into the supplies room and tells him how good looking he is. Yesterday, she patted his hand and said, "I wish we would get to know each other better. I would make it worth your while—better benefits at the clinic, more money." The male staff nurse asks his friend, "What do I do? I don't want to date her, but I don't want to lose my job. I just want her to leave me alone!" The best reply for the friend would be:

    1. "Tell her that her behavior makes you feel uncomfortable and that you want her to stop."

    2. "Go for it!! Date her and see if you get what she promises."

    3. "Go as soon as possible to the human relations office at the agency and relate to them the entire situation."

    4. "Contact your lawyer and get advice as soon as possible, in case she decides to turn the tables and accuse you of advances."

Answers & Rationales

1. **(1)** According to the National commission on Nursing (1983) and the Task Force on Nursing Practice in Hospitals (1983), the clinical nurse specialist (CNS) role was accepted quite rapidly. The psychiatric clinical nurse specialist role is considered the oldest and most highly developed of the CNS specialities and helped initiate the growth of other CNS specialities.

2. **(3)** Martha Rogers argued that the development of the nurse practitioner role was a ploy to lure nurses out of nursing and into medicine, hence weakening and undermining nursing's unique role in health care. This led to a major division within nursing, which led to barriers in the establishment of nurse practitioner education programs within the mainstream of graduate nursing education.

3. **(4)** Loretta Ford, R.N., Ph.D. and Henry Silver, M.D. established the first pediatric nurse practitioner program at the University of Colorado. Mary Breckenridge established the Frontier Nursing Service in the depressed rural mountain area of Kentucky which led to training nurse midwives. Agnes McGee is credited with offering the first postgraduate program for the nurse anesthetist role at St. Vincent's Hospital in Portland, Oregon. Hildegard Peplau started the first psychiatric clinical nurse specialist program at Rutger's University.

4. **(1)** Although all of these answers are important for the nurse practitioner to develop policy skills, the most important is developing political allies. Having political allies in decision-making places (legislature) will enable the nurse practitioner to be active and informed regarding issues surrounding regulation, limitations on admitting privileges and prescriptive authority, and managed care.

5. **(4)** There are three major issues that are central to the expansion of the nurse practitioner role—prescriptive authority, reimbursement privileges, and legal scope of practice. Although political activism is important, it is not specific to collaborative practice.

6. **(2)** The *International Classification of Diseases, 9th Edition* (ICD-9-CM codes identify the condition, illness, or injury to be treated and are used for billing insurance carriers. Physician's Current Procedural Terminology (CPT) codes specify the procedure or medical service given (over 7000 terms). Medicare and state Medicaid carriers are required by law to use CPT codes. The HCFA Common Procedure Coding System (HCPC) is used for reporting supplies and medical equipment.

7. **(3)** Lewin described three processes of change: unfreezing—involves breaking the habit, disturbing the equilibrium; moving—development of new responses based on new information with a change in attitudes, feelings, behaviors, or values; and refreezing—reaching a new status quo, stabilizing and integrating new behaviors with appropriate support that is available to maintain the change. Forming, storming, and norming refer to the stages of group process development. Option #2 is Havelock's change theory steps.

8. **(2)** According to most sources, the nurse practitioner role developed due to a shortage of primary care physicians in the 1960s and 1970s, as medical specialization was the trend.

9. **(3)** Medicare is regulated by the federal government and includes the services described, plus outpatient laboratory and radiography services. Hospitalization costs are covered under Medicare A.

10. **(4)** The Balanced Budget Act is crucial and significant pieces of legislation that allows direct payments to nurse practitioners at "80% of the lesser of either the actual charge or 85% of the fee schedule amount of the same service if provided by a physician." This does not change the "incident to" rule, which allows a physician to bill for 100% for a nurse practitioner's services (i.e., provided the physician is in the suite at the time of the service and readily available to provide assistance).

11. **(4)** Conflict must be addressed directly by the nurse practitioner. The personal characteristics of each of the medical assistants must not enter into the conflict resolution process. Determine what is the issue of conflict and then work on possible solutions to resolve the issue. Compromise is just one method of conflict resolution where both parties must be willing to give up something.

12. **(1)** There are two ways to deal with sexual harassment at work: informally and formally through a grievance procedure. Always start with the direct approach; ask the person to STOP! Tell the harasser in clear terms that the behavior makes you uncomfortable and that you want it to stop immediately.

21

Legal & Ethical Issues

1. An occurrence-form professional liability insurance policy is preferred because:

   1. The amount of insurance money available to pay a claim increases with each renewal of the policy.

   2. The policy proceeds are available to pay claims regardless of when the claim is reported to the carrier.

   3. The carrier will be notified of a potential claim during the policy period.

   4. The coverage is broader than that provided by a claims-made policy form.

2. Early reporting of a potential professional liability claim is advantageous because:

   1. Insurance carriers have a 10-day reporting window after which the coverage is canceled.

   2. Documents and witnesses needed to defend the claim are more likely to be available at the time of the event.

   3. Your insurance premiums will be reduced upon a good-faith showing of cooperation with the carrier.

   4. Risk Management personnel require such reporting in order to comply with Joint Commission on the Accreditation of

Healthcare Organizations (JCAHO) mandates.

3. Your nursing license may be in jeopardy if:

   1. You appropriately delegate medication administration to a trusted RN employee who administers a fatal dose.

   2. You delegate client assessment tasks to an LPN who has been floated to your outpatient clinic for the day.

   3. You provide nursing care services consistent with established standards of practice in your jurisdiction.

   4. The medical assistant in your supervising physician's office exceeds the scope of his/her authority, but you take prompt action to correct the problem.

4. Your client is a 46-year-old mentally retarded man who has been diagnosed with colon cancer. Consent for his corrective surgery should be obtained from:

   1. The client himself.

   2. The client's 84-year-old mother who is his closest relative.

   3. The client's court-appointed guardian.

   4. The administrator of the group home where the client lives.

5. Your client is a 75-year-old woman with metastatic cancer. Her affairs are in order; she has arranged all her finances and her own funeral rites. She has systematically secured enough barbiturates to successfully end her life; she asks you to mix the drugs for her in some pudding to make them palatable for ingestion. Your best course of action would be:

   1. Mix the medications as requested and stay with her while she consumes the preparation.

   2. Consult with family and attending physician to warn them about the client's proposed course of action.

   3. Seek an immediate order for an antidepressant.

   4. Sit down with the client and conduct a physical and psychological needs assessment.

6. The Patient Self-Determination Act, passed by Congress in 1990, resulted in which of the following policy changes:

   1. Hospitals are mandated to assist every client to create a "living will."

   2. Federally funded managed care organizations (MCOs) are required to inform subscribers about their rights under state law to create advance directives.

   3. Home health agencies are required to have "do-not-resuscitate" orders on file for all terminally ill clients.

   4. Hospitalized clients are obligated to select a surrogate decision maker to make health care decisions for them if they become incapacitated.

7. Both the Food and Drug Administration (FDA) and the Department of Health and Human Services (DHHS) have regulations governing research activities on human subjects. The principal investigator is responsible for:

   1. Securing a signed special research consent form.

   2. Reporting back to the Institutional Review Board if a subject is injured during the course of the study.

   3. Appearing before the Institutional Review Board to present the study and secure approval to proceed with subject recruitment at the facility.

   4. All of the above.

8. If you are served with a summons and complaint (i.e., lawsuit documents), the first step you should take is:

   1. Call the client to determine the basis for the action and what you allegedly did wrong.

   2. Call the client's lawyer (listed on the first page of the lawsuit) to get more information about the case.

   3. Call your insurance company for instructions on how to proceed.

   4. Confer with your colleagues and review the chart to see if you need to clarify your notes.

9. As a nurse practitioner in an impoverished rural area, you frequently encounter female clients in situations of domestic violence with few community options for referral. Participating in community education forums and fundraising for a safe house is an example of applying the ethical principle of:

   1. Autonomy.

   2. Nonmaleficence.

   3. Justice.

   4. Veracity.

10. Nurses practicing in expanded roles should carry professional liability insurance for which of the following reasons:

    1. Premiums are often modest and are a tax-deductible business expense.

    2. Even if the employer insures the nurse practitioner, there may be situations of conflict between employer and nurse necessitating separate legal counsel, a covered benefit under the policy.

    3. As roles expand, so does the liability potential.

    4. All of the above.

11. The confidentiality of medical records is always a valid concern, especially in this age of computerization, "smart cards," and fax machines. Release of medical information to third parties is:

    1. Addressed mainly in state laws or statutes.

    2. Prohibited without the informed consent of the client.

    3. Automatic when the requesting party is a third-party payor or insurer.

    4. Disallowed if the records contain proof of a diagnosis of acquired immunodeficiency syndrome (AIDS).

12. Which are **not** included in the definition of disability under the Americans with Disabilities Act?

    1. Profoundly deaf employees.

    2. Persons who are wheelchair bound.

    3. Current users of illegal drugs.

    4. Persons who are mentally retarded.

13. If your client is having a problem with a managed care plan, you can offer to assist in the following way:

    1. Suggest that the client contact the customer service department (may be called "member services") at the plan to resolve the issue; a formal grievance filing may be necessary.

    2. Remind the client who is a member of the "senior" plan for Medicare recipients, that he/she may complain to the federal Office of Personnel Management (OPM).

    3. Remind the client that the state's insurance department also investigates complaints against health plans.

    4. All of the above.

14. Health policy theorist Daniel Callahan believes that our health care system could be improved by:

    1. Making the care of the chronically ill our first priority, so that these individuals are not abandoned by the health care system.

    2. Making preventive care the first priority.

    3. Maintaining the current allocation of dollars to high-tech care.

    4. Leaving the system "as is" and let market forces determine the allocation of health care dollars.

15. If a piece of equipment malfunctions while being used on a hospitalized client, the risk manager would probably recommend the following course of action:

    1. Return the item to the manufacturer with a description of the problem and a request for analysis.

    2. Tag and sequester the item at the facility and defer analysis pending risk management review of the litigation potential.

    3. Send the item to the biomedical engineering department with a request for immediate equipment breakdown and troubleshooting.

    4. Repair the item, either in-house or by an outside contracted firm, and return it to service as soon as possible.

16. Nurse expert witnesses are essential in the adjudication of most professional negligence claims against nurses. The following criteria for nurse experts are sought by attorneys:

    1. Appropriate professional education, preferably at the technical level.

    2. Relevant and recent professional work experience.

    3. Ability to understand and articulate the legal issues involved in the claim.

    4. Published authorship of medical texts in the clinical subject areas.

17. Which federal law mandates the tracking of implantable medical devices?

    1. The Administrative Procedures Act (APA).

    2. The Patient Self-Determination Act (PSDA).

    3. The Safe Medical Devices Act (SMDA).

    4. The Omnibus Budget Reconciliation Act (OBRA) of 1987.

18. Which of the following are elements of a broad-based risk management program?

    1. A hazardous materials compliance program as part of a comprehensive safety and security system.

    2. An early-warning/incident reporting program to identify elements of risk.

    3. A system of contract review to avoid assuming liabilities that should be borne by others.

    4. All of the above.

19. The type of insurance coverage that is purchased (or self-insured) by an organization to handle employee job-related injuries is:

    1. Profession liability insurance.

    2. Business interruption insurance.

    3. Directors and officers (D&O) insurance.

    4. Worker's compensation insurance.

20. While driving your personal vehicle on a job-related errand, you are struck by a semitrailer on the interstate. The car is totaled and you are severely injured. Which insurance policies will respond to these losses?

    1. Your personal auto policy and your employer's worker's compensation policy.

    2. The employer's business auto policy and worker's compensation policy.

    3. Your homeowner's policy.

    4. The semitrailer driver's personal auto policy.

21. Nurse practitioners with hospital privileges may be impacted by the part of the Health Care Quality Improvement Act known as the National Practitioner Data Bank. Which of the following statements about the Data Bank is **not** true?

    1. Professional liability insurance claims payments made on behalf of nurse practitioners must be reported to the Data Bank.

    2. The facility granting medical staff privileges must query the Data Bank

before approving a nurse practitioner's privileges.

    3. The purpose of the Data Bank is to have a national source of information about malpractice claims, licensure actions, and restrictions on privileges so that nurse practitioners may not easily move from one jurisdiction to another to escape quality review.

    4. Insurance companies report all malpractice payments made on behalf of affected nurse practitioners, regardless of the amount of the payment.

22. In 1985 Congress took action against a phenomenon known as "patient dumping" by enacting what was known at the time as the COBRA law, now referred to as the Emergency Medical Treatment and Active Labor Act (EMTALA). Which statement about EMTALA is **not** true?

    1. The original purpose of the statute was to prohibit the transfer of uninsured, untreated clients from the emergency department of one hospital to another (usually the county hospital).

    2. Subsequent rules and case law have expanded the statute so that almost any unauthorized transfer of a client from one facility to another is potentially problematic.

    3. In order to effect a proper transfer, the forwarding facility need not notify or secure the acquiescence of the receiving facility.

    4. The transferring facility must utilize appropriate transport methods and send copies of clients' medical records.

23. You are a nurse practitioner wishing to effect change in the state's laws regarding the dispensing of prescription medications by nurse practitioners. You would take your case to:

    1. The state legislature.

    2. The state board of nursing.

    3. The state board of pharmacy.

    4. The nursing specialty organization.

24. The common meaning of "gag clauses" or "gag orders" in the managed care arena is:

    1. The MCO declines to publish, in its subscriber contracts, the treatments that are excluded from coverage under the plan.

    2. The MCO refuses to allow its member services personnel to answer certain subscriber questions about covered benefits.

    3. MCO contracts with providers disallow the offering of treatment alternatives that the providers know are not covered by clients' plans.

    4. Providers are prohibited from offering experimental treatment to clients.

25. Under the Safe Medical Devices Act of 1990, the following health care providers or organizations are required to report the death of a client to the FDA if the death is related to the use of a medical device:

    1. Physicians' office staff.

    2. Hospitals, home health agencies, and ambulance companies.

    3. Nurse family members treating clients without compensation.

    4. Physicians making home visits.

26. A client receives a medication that was intended for another person. An appropriate way to document this event in the medical record would be:

    1. "Client was given *x* mg of *y* drug in error."

    2. "*x* mg *y* drug administered to client. No adverse effects noted. Physician notified."

    3. "Client received wrong medication. Incident report filed. Practitioner disciplined."

    4. "Practitioner inadvertently administered *y* drug to wrong client. Supervisor notified. Family threatening litigation."

27. The one reason that clients offer, above all others, for suing practitioners for medical negligence is:

    1. The care they received was substandard.

    2. The provider made an honest mistake.

    3. The client was not "heard" when he/she attempted to communicate with the provider.

    4. The client participated fully in all aspects of medical decision making, but the results were disappointing.

28. Informed consent is based upon the ethical principle of:

    1. Beneficence.

    2. Respect for persons.

    3. Nonmaleficence.

    4. Autonomy.

29. The four elements of a professional negligence claim are:

    1. Duty, fulfillment of duty, professional relationship, and wrongful act.

    2. Professional responsibility, fault, harm to the client, and wrongful act.

    3. Duty, breach of duty, causal connection between the act and the harm, and harm to the client.

    4. Professional relationship, intentional wrongful act, proximate cause, and damage to the client.

30. You are making an initial home health care visit to an elderly lady whose spouse tells you that she is often confused. He answers all your questions and dominates the discussion. You proceed to do your initial assessment; the wife does seem to be oriented to time, place and person. Who is the proper party to sign the written form to request/consent for services?

    1. The husband.

    2. The wife/client.

    3. The attending physician.

    4. The home health aide who will be providing continuing care.

31. An expert witness is usually required in a nursing negligence case because:

    1. Knowledge of medical or nursing facts is not considered intuitive to a lay jury.

    2. Jurors are allowed to use their "sixth sense" regarding the facts presented to them.

    3. Fact witnesses are not able to present an unbiased account of the circumstances in dispute.

    4. Appropriately credentialed experts have more credibility in the eyes of lay jurors.

32. The standard of care for a nurse practitioner, in a trial, will be established by expert witness(es). The expert opinion will be based upon:

    1. National norms for the speciality.

    2. Facility policies and procedures.

    3. Professional literature.

    4. All of the above.

33. Alternative Dispute Resolution (ADR) is a process where the parties to a dispute resolve their differences outside of a court trial. Advantages to this system of problem solving include all **except**:

    1. The parties usually prefer the process because they have opportunity to be heard in a less formal and less intimidating environment.

    2. The process is often less time consuming and less costly than traditional litigation.

    3. Damage awards are less likely to include nonfinancial compensation.

    4. Insurers are amenable to working with mediators with a track record of fairness and successful case resolution.

34. The statute of limitations is:

    1. The state law that prescribes the time frames within which a nursing negligence action may be filed.

    2. The law that states that minors have no legal authority to sue nurses for malpractice.

    3. The law that limits the right of clients to sue nurse practitioners for negligent acts.

    4. The federal law that limits a nurse practitioner's right to countersue a client for malicious prosecution.

35. You are a family nurse practitioner driving along the interstate on your way to a nursing seminar. You observe a head-on collision and decide to stop to render aid. Which statement is **false** with respect to your potential liability for malpractice:

    1. You had no legal obligation to stop to render assistance; if you had driven by the accident, there would be no liability on your part.

    2. If you provide appropriate nursing care, gratuitously, you will be protected from liability under your state's Good Samaritan law.

    3. Even if you act in a grossly negligent manner, the Good Samaritan law will shield you from liability.

    4. The protections afforded by the Good Samaritan law may differ from state to state; you should research your state's law on the subject.

36. If you are subpoenaed to appear for a deposition in a nursing negligence case, appropriate preparation is prudent. One of the following tips would probably not be suggested by your attorney. Which piece of advice is **not** appropriate?

    1. Discretely chew gum to calm your nerves and dress for dinner because depositions usually take all day and you will not have time to change.

    2. Review the client's medical record and any other materials suggested by your attorney prior to your appearance for questioning.

    3. Take as much time as you need to think about your response before answering; do not let an attorney put words in your mouth.

    4. Be straightforward and truthful; remember that "I don't know" and "I don't remember" are acceptable responses.

37. Which of the following documentation tips is **not** a good idea?

    1. Carefully document your criticism of a fellow provider's clinical decision in the client's medical record. This will protect you if your treatment decisions need to be defended later.

    2. Use standard abbreviations in the medical record so that subsequent readers will have no doubt as to your meaning and intent.

    3. Document telephone conversations with the client and/or the family in the medical record. Be particularly vigilant about recording changes in the client's medications.

    4. Document noncompliant client behaviors in the medical record; be thorough, yet factual.

28. In 1987, and again in 1994, Congress acted to update many of the regulations that govern the provision of long-term care services. If you are an employer or nurse manager in this environment, you need to know that:

    1. Nursing assistants working in long-term care facilities must be formally trained and certified.

    2. Clients or residents have specific rights, such as information about their physical condition, medical benefits, and associated costs.

    3. New and swifter sanctions are available to reviewers to impose upon facilities with deficiencies.

    4. All of the above.

39. You are employed as a nurse practitioner in a private medical office. You notice all the activity at the front desk where some clients are checking in for appointments; staff is scheduling tests; and telephone advice triage is in progress. To preserve client confidentiality, you could implement which of the following changes?

    1. Orient the fax machine and computer monitor such that incoming reports or other data cannot be read by nonstaff members.

    2. Do all telephone scheduling from a more secure location, such as a conference room in the back office.

    3. Create a more private space to confer with clients who need follow-up information or explanations of tests or treatments.

    4. All of the above.

40. As a nurse-employer, you would be well advised to have procedures in place to appropriately terminate an employee. To avoid a charge of discrimination, or a claim for wrongful termination, you should be particularly sensitive to the protections afforded to select groups. Which of the following is **not** a protected class under the antidiscrimination statutes?

    1. Pregnant women.

    2. Gay men.

    3. Those age 40 and older.

    4. The handicapped.

41. Which activity could be considered grounds for a sexual harassment claim?

    1. A male employee tells an off-color joke to another man. The joke is overheard by a female co-worker who seems to appreciate the humor in it. The joke-telling is an isolated incident.

    2. A nurse-supervisor conducts an employee performance review. The supervisor does not mention a prior social relationship with the employee; the ratings are appropriate for the level of performance; the employee receives a salary increase.

    3. A co-ed locker room is decorated with multiple centerfold photos from a popular men's magazine. The female employees find this offensive and have filed several complaints.

    4. A nurse is complimented on her appearance and asked on a date by her boss. She informs the boss that she is married and not seeking another relationship. The incident is forgotten.

42. Your client is a comatose lady who needs a feeding tube inserted for long-term nutritional needs. Her husband presents you with a document which he says is his wife's living will. It is signed by him, and sets out, so he says, the wishes of his wife with respect to the feeding tube. The living will is not a legally binding document because:

    1. The wife did not sign the document.

    2. The husband is not authorized to execute a living will on behalf of his wife.

    3. This type of advance directive must be signed by the individual while he/she is legally competent to execute documents.

    4. All of the above.

43. A nurse practitioner is helping out at a clinic for homeless women. A diabetic client, in her third trimester of pregnancy, has been reasonably compliant with respect to insulin therapy. Now, however, she has announced her intent to abandon her insulin regimen because she has heard on the streets that some drugs are harmful to fetuses. Which option is not legally appropriate for the nurse practitioner, as her health care provider, to consider?

    1. Seek the support of the clinic's attorney to file a petition for court-ordered treatment for the client.

    2. Attempt to engage the client in dialogue to provide her with accurate medical information.

    3. Detain the client in the homeless shelter and administer the insulin, with or without her consent.

    4. Confer with social services to find an appropriate interim placement for the client until her medical and legal issues can be sorted out.

44. The purpose of the Americans with Disabilities Act is:

    1. To level the playing field with respect to employment and other opportunities for disabled people.

    2. To create a federal entitlement program for people with AIDS.

    3. To guarantee wheelchair access to every residential and commercial building.

    4. To authorize interpreters for deaf employees at all private businesses.

45. As a result of the U.S. Supreme Court's ruling on assisted suicide, the current state of the law on this topic is:

    1. Assisted suicide is still a criminal offense in most jurisdictions.

    2. A physician may prescribe a fatal dose of medication with the concurrence of the ethics committee.

    3. A nurse practitioner may prescribe a fatal dose of medication with the concurrence of the supervising physician.

    4. A pharmacist may instruct a client how to mix and ingest a fatal dose of prescription medication.

46. A professional negligence or medical malpractice case is a civil action. The difference between a civil lawsuit and a criminal lawsuit is:

    1. The damages sought in a civil suit are monetary; one private party sues another for money.

    2. If you are convicted in a criminal case, you are still covered by your professional liability insurer.

    3. In a criminal case, your state sues you for money; other penalties do not apply.

    4. In a civil suit, if you do not prevail you could be incarcerated.

47. Which of the following is **not** a form of alternative dispute resolution (ADR)?

    1. Mediation.

    2. Binding and nonbinding arbitration.

    3. Settlement conference.

    4. A jury trial.

48. A health care provider has a duty to disclose certain information to the client as part of the informed consent process.

Exceptions to this duty would include all of the following **except**:

1. The client has waived the right to receive the data.

2. It is a bona fide emergency situation.

3. The provider believes that the information would be harmful to the client and invokes the therapeutic privilege.

4. The client is 80 years old and the elderly are unable to comprehend complex medical facts.

49. Before providing a detailed reference on a former employee, the nurse practitioner should consider the following:

1. Check the requirements of the Human Resources Department of your employer.

2. If the comments are perceived as negative, and the former employee becomes aware of them, you could subject yourself to suit for defamation.

3. If the employee exhibits unsafe client care practices, it may be wiser to risk legal action from the employee than to subject future clients to this unsafe practitioner.

4. All of the above.

50. The primary purpose of a pre-employment physical is:

1. To identify existing health problems that might adversely affect the company's insurance rates.

2. To determine the mental status of the applicant.

3. To determine if the applicant is physically capable of doing the job.

4. To document any existing disabilities and recommend accommodations.

51. A nurse practitioner involved in work-related surveillance knows that the records related to this activity must be held for how many years after employment?

1. 5 years.

2. 25 years.

3. 30 years.

4. Can be destroyed only after the employee's death.

52. The nurse practitioner knows that when treating a work-related injury it is required that he/she:

1. Document thoroughly because of the high probability of legal action.

2. Communicate directly with the client's employeer.

3. File a report with the industrial commission documenting the injury and treatment.

4. Notify the Occupations Safety and Health Administration.

53. Which situation would be considered reportable under the Occupational and Safety Health Act?

1. 3-cm abrasion of the forearm.

2. A warehouse worker with back strain reassigned to office work for a week.

3. A twisted ankle that responded to ice and ACE wrap.

4. A minor closed head injury with no loss of consciousness.

54. The purpose of an Occupational and Safety Health Administration 200 log is to record:

1. Occupational injuries and illnesses.

2. Only work-related deaths.

3. Dangerous workplace situations.

4. Lost work days.

55. The American Disabilities Act (ADA) regulates how employers treat the disabled. Under the ADA, disability is defined as a physical or mental impairment that substantially limits one or more major life activities of an individual or a record of a situation in which an individual is regarded as having such an impairment. This would include:

1. A history of addiction.

2. Paralysis.

3. Bipolar disorder.

4. All of the above.

56. Bioethical practice dilemmas are best described as situations in which proposed treatment alternatives are:

    1. Ranked from most to least acceptable.

    2. Not appealing to involved parties.

    3. Lacking acceptance by anyone.

    4. Less than perfect approaches to the situation.

21 Answers & Rationales

1. **(2)** The most important advantage of an occurrence policy is that, assuming the policy is in effect at the time of the occurrence, the coverage is available regardless of how long it takes to become aware of a claim (the long "tail" of a medical malpractice claim). The limits do not automatically increase. The carrier need not be notified during the policy period as is required with claims-made coverage. The coverage under each policy may be as broad as the carrier allows.

2. **(2)** Fact witnesses and necessary paperwork are always easier to discover the closer in time you seek them after a medical misadventure. Memories are fresh and documents are less likely to be misplaced or destroyed. There is no rigid reporting window required by insurance carriers; they do want to be notified in a timely manner. Insurance premiums may be reduced if an insured's track record is clean (i.e., no claims), but not by mere compliance with policy requirements. Risk management employees prefer early notification so that damage control efforts may be implemented promptly, not for regulatory reasons.

3. **(2)** Assessment skills are presumed to be within the purview of the professional nurse, not those with fewer years of nursing education. Also, in this scenario, the LPN is an unknown entity to the delegator. Delegating to the LPN should be done cautiously after determining that person's skill level. Your license is not in jeopardy if you delegated appropriately, as in Option #1, but an error was made, and is attributed to the delegatee. Activities in

Options #3 and #4 are appropriate for the role.

4. **(3)** The client's capacity to consent is questionable; therefore, alternatives must be sought. If the client has a court-appointed guardian, as set out in Option #3, then that person is the decision maker. The court has already made a determination of the client's legal incapacity and appointed the person to whom you will look for consent. If there were no guardian, you would analyze whether the client himself may be able to consent or whether you would look to his mother as the most appropriate surrogate decision maker. The group home employee has no automatic legal authority to consent to treatment for any resident.

5. **(4)** Assisted suicide is still a criminal activity in most states (and in legal limbo in the others). Circumventing the client may seem to be an appealing option, but it substitutes paternalism for the autonomy we all claim as our due. A diagnosis of depression can hardly be made with inadequate data; the necessary information can only be determined by conferring with the client herself.

6. **(2)** MCOs are one group of health care organizations impacted by this law. All subscribers must be provided with the stated information at the time of enrollment. Advance directive documents, though extremely helpful in the health care setting, are never mandatory.

7. **(4)** These are the basic requirements for conducting research at health care facilities.

8. **(3)** Your insurance carrier is thoroughly familiar with the processes of handling a claim. They will assist you with every step of this fearsome activity; the first significant obligation they will meet is to put you in touch with your lawyer. Conferring with the client or the client's lawyer is never a wise move. Your colleagues can only offer moral support at this state; your lawyer is the professional of choice at this time. Never, never even think about altering a record; it can turn a defensible case into a nondefensible one.

9. **(3)** Lobbying for underserved clients is an example of justice, which is the duty to treat all clients fairly, without regard to age, socioeconomic status, or other variables. Autonomy is the client's right to self-determination without outside control. Nonmaleficence is the duty to prevent or avoid doing harm whether intentional or unintentional. Veracity is the duty to tell the truth.

10. **(4)** These are all valid reasons to protect your assets in the event of litigation. There is an opposing view regarding the need for professional liability insurance. Some professionals feel that if there are few assets to protect, insurance is an unnecessary expense. Nurses with professional liability coverage ("deep pockets") could be retained as defendants in a case for a longer period of time.

11. **(1)** Look to state law to define the circumstances under which confidential medical information may be disclosed. There may be additional requirements imposed by federal regulations (e.g., the handling of certain psychiatric records), but the bulk of the rule making on this issue is accomplished at the state level. There are exceptions to the requirement of client consent, such as communicable disease reporting to public health authorities, and court-ordered record production. Third-party payors, although powerful with their fiscal controls, must produce some proof of client consent to acquire records. An AIDS diagnosis does not shield a record from production, although many states have enacted extra levels of protection for this information. Again, knowledge of state laws is helpful.

12. **(3)** The ADA does not protect this group of people. In fact, employers may test for illegal drug use; this is not considered a medical examination, which ordinarily is subject to specific requirements under the law.

13. **(4)** These are all ways to get satisfaction from a health plan. You could also offer to help explain clinical issues to plan personnel who may not be clinically oriented.

14. **(1)** Callahan believes that health care priorities need to be re-evaluated. He advocates spending first on chronic care (those who cannot be cured), then preventive care, and lastly on the high-cost, high-tech modalities that benefit few but consume enormous resources.

15. **(2)** The best immediate solution is to identify the item and remove it from service to avoid further client injury. Then, the risk manager, in consultation with the facility's attorneys and/or insurers, will determine how to proceed with equipment analysis. Returning the item to the manufacturer removes it from your control and diminishes your opportunity to defend against a charge of user error. Immediate repair may fail to uncover the real cause of the client injury and impair a successful defense of a claim. If the litigation potential is high, the parties may wish to pool their efforts (and costs) to conduct a third-party review of the equipment. If litigation is likely, then it is also likely that the manufacturer and others in the distribution chain will be co-defendants with the facility and its staff.

16. **(2)** The level of education preferred is that of an advanced degree. The legal issues are the province of the attorneys and the judge; the nurse is expected to be the expert in the clinical issues. Published authors, on nursing issues, can add credibility, but specific work experience coupled with the education credentials are minimally required.

17. **(3)** The APA describes the workings of federal agencies. The PSDA deals with advance directives; and the OBRA of 1987 changed the rules dealing with long-term care.

18. **(4)** These and other elements combine to produce a program of systematic risk identification, analysis, treatment, and evaluation, with the overall goal of loss prevention.

19. **(4)** Liability insurance is acquired to protect the organization from suits by clients arising from negligent acts of employees. Business interruption coverage is usually purchased in tandem with fire insurance. It reimburses an organization for losses sustained while the business is partially or completely shut down after a catastrophic event. The organization's management team (CEO and senior staff) is insured against losses based upon business judgment errors through D&O coverage. Worker's compensation is the line of coverage that protects employees after on-the-job injuries. It is a no-fault system (negligence is not a factor) that covers employee medical bills and pays a percentage of wages while an employee is unable to work.

20. **(1)** You were driving your personal vehicle, so your own auto insurer is "primary"; that is, it responds first to a loss. Since you were on company business, your injuries were sustained "within the course and scope of your employment," so there is coverage under the employer's worker's compensation policy for your medical bills and wage replacement. Depending on the circumstances, and policy definitions, there could be some "excess" or additional coverage available under the employer's auto policy, but, in no event would that carrier be primarily responsible for your losses. This is not the type of incident that homeowner's insurance is intended to cover. The semitrailer presumably in use as a business vehicle, would not be insured under a driver's personal auto policy.

21. **(1)** At this point, the mandatory reporting affects only dentists and doctors. Other licensed practitioners are subject to permissive reporting.

22. **(3)** The forwarding facility needs to know whether the receiving facility has space for the new arrival and, more importantly, the ability to treat the particular illness for which the client needs therapy. A familiar example of a client transfer is that of the burn victim for whom specialty care is mandatory; the locations of that specialty care are usually limited.

23. **(1)** Health care policy within the states is codified or enacted into law by the respective state legislatures. The boards have significant input (hopefully) in the process, providing the research data and expert "testimony" that the legislatures need in order to make informed decisions. Nursing organizations should also be willing to provide background information and nurse experts to educate the lawmakers.

24. **(3)** The MCO's cost-containment strategy is enhanced if providers practice within the treatment guidelines suggested by the plans. Providers who inform clients that a certain treatment regimen is the preferred alternative create difficulties if that alternative is excluded from coverage. MCOs usually clearly set out the exclusions in the plan documents, and member services personnel are expected to be able to explain the coverage to subscribers. Experimental treatment, if excluded, would be listed as such in the plan documents.

25. **(2)** These are three of the agencies required to report. Events occurring in the other settings are exempt from reporting requirements under this federal law.

26. **(2)** This is the most factual note; the writer does not apportion blame or assume liability. The other notes would be "red flags" for a chart reviewer. The mention of an incident report makes it virtually impossible to protect these documents from disclosure, especially in those jurisdictions that still afford some protection to these internal early warning documents that seek to alert risk management personnel to a potential claim.

27. **(3)** Clients are often unable to evaluate the quality of the care they receive, but they do react to the way in which the care is delivered. Perceptions by clients of rudeness or "uncaring" on the part of the provider often spur clients to pursue legal action. Clients tend to be more forgiving of less-than-optimal outcomes if they have been involved in the process and are treated with respect.

28. **(4)** Making one's own decisions is the basis for informed consent and the ethical underpinning of the Patient Self-Determination Act. "Doing good" (Option #1) and its corollary "avoiding harm" (Option #3) are ethics principles usually cited as the bases for other health care activities such as maintaining profession competency. Respect for persons is a more global ethical principle supporting much of a nurse's personal philosophy of caring.

29. **(3)** Usually phrased as duty, breach, proximate cause, and damages, these are the four elements of proof required to prevail in a medical negligence action. Intentional acts are not synonymous with negligent acts. Duty presumes a professional relationship and obligation to provide services. The breach is the error or mistake ascribed to the provider that results in the harm to the client.

30. **(2)** A competent adult client is the person to whom you look for consent to treat. It is only when the client is unable to consent that surrogate decision makers are sought. Individual states' laws need to be checked for the selection and priority of surrogate decision makers.

31. **(1)** Lay jurors are not expected to know the clinical facts and circumstances involved in a professional negligence claim. The expert witness is necessary to educate the jurors about those medical facts and to testify to the standard of care to be applied. Witnesses with direct involvement in the case are no less credible because of their involvement; their testimony, and personal bias, if any, will be evaluated by the jurors in the context of their roles.

32. **(4)** With respect to nursing specialties, the standard of care is usually a national one. Facility policies, books, and journals are important to review, and physician input may be sought. In some cases, physicians may even be allowed to testify about the standard of care.

33. **(3)** One particular advantage of ADR is the flexibility of the system. In mediation, for example, the mediator can assist with crafting a solution package that meets all the needs of a party, including such things as an apology from the health care provider. Money is not always the only answer. Insurers' goals, however, usually do focus on cash: avoiding huge damage awards to plaintiffs. If a mediator is successful in facilitating case settlements, the costs are usually significantly lower than the costs of a court trial. Insurers with an eye on the bottom line are not averse to these advantages.

34. **(1)** Statutes of limitations set out each state's rules for the timing of the filing of lawsuits, including malpractice actions. These statutes are procedural laws, in that they describe the "how-to" parameters within which legal rights may be exercised. Minority is considered a legal disability; other state laws usually define it and describe its effects. Rights to sue are not governed by statutes of limitations.

35. **(3)** Statutes may indeed differ from state to state with respect to the breadth of the protection, but most will protect a nurse who renders aid, without expectation of compensation, in a competent manner. Gross negligence will usually void the statutory protections.

36. **(1)** A professional appearance boosts your credibility as a witness. inappropriate attire and gum-chewing detract from the professional demeanor that you will want to project. Preparation is critical before your words are recorded and transcribed as part of the official litigation transcript. Review documents as noted, but refrain from bringing any materials with you to the deposition without your attorney's approval. Always ask for clarification of ambiguous questions. Speculation is not appropriate. Your professional work history is always asked; so, a copy of your curricula vitae (CV) is a useful tool to bring along to a deposition.

37. **(1)** Jousting in the client's medical record is never a good idea. It provides fodder for plaintiffs' lawyers but does not contribute to quality nursing care. If you have a conflict with another provider, deal with the provider directly, preferably in person. Another arena for resolving such disputes is the quality review process.

38. **(4)** Long-term care is a specialized area with layers of regulatory requirements, most stemming from the federal government. Nurses who work in this environment need to be vigilant about learning the rules and maintaining compliance. Ongoing, effective communication with regulators is essential.

39. **(4)** We have a tendency to get very careless with our information management and the way we interact with clients and their very personal data. The often wide-open and very frantic front-desk atmosphere of an office does little to calm client fears that their information will be too-easily accessible to those without a need to know.

40. **(2)** Sexual preference is not a protected classification. The other options refer to different federal laws that provide varying degrees of protection to those groups. It is prudent to check with your business attorney to determine if the policies you have drafted for your office are in compliance with federal guidelines. The Equal Employment Opportunity Commission (EEOC), which enforces the laws, publishes guidelines about the various statutes. These publications are available, either free or at minimal cost, from the agency. Some may be available on the Internet.

41. **(3)** This seems to fit the criteria for a hostile environment, a form of sexual harassment. The harassment seems to be pervasive and longstanding; the women have complained and apparently no action has been taken. The isolated incident and single date request do not rise to the level of harassment. The participants did not find the actions objectionable; and job performance was not affected. In Option #2, although the potential was there for the nurse to use the prior relationship as a club to either downgrade the employee or deny a benefit, this result did not occur.

42. **(4)** Advance directives are documents crafted by individuals who personally decide how they wish their future health care decisions to be handled. The documents must be prepared while the signer is fully capable of understanding their content and importance. Since the wife in this scenario is already comatose, she has missed her opportunity to prepare advance directives. This does not mean that the spouse is unable to decide on her medical treatment, it just means that a different consent process needs to be employed.

43. **(3)** This option would create liability potential for the nurse practitioner under at least two legal theories (e.g., battery and false imprisonment). Obviously, Option #2 would be the first prong of a planned approach to convince this client that she needs the prescribed medical therapy. Option #4 would be the next choice. Court-ordered treatment is a consideration with a viable fetus.

44. **(1)** This is the overall goal of the ADA. It is not another entitlement program, and it cannot impose wheelchair ramp requirements on every building owner in America. Access ramps and interpreters may be required as a "reasonable accommodation" to qualified people in certain defined circumstances. There is no across-the-board mandate for these types of aid to the handicapped.

45. **(1)** The Supreme Court essentially deferred to the states to legislate on this topic. In most states, the activity is not permitted. In one of the states involved in the high court's case, a statute permitting assisted suicide is being challenged. Nurse practitioners need to look at their states' laws on this topic for guidance. The other providers referenced in Options #2, #3, and #4 would act at their peril if their states' laws followed the current majority view.

46. **(1)** The purpose of a medical malpractice action is to make the claimant whole by the awarding of money damages. The award compensates the claimant or plaintiff for the wrong (or tort) he has suffered at the hands of the defendant. On the criminal side, the state sues on behalf of society for violations of society's criminal laws. The punishment is fines, imprisonment, or both. Professional liability insurance usually excludes criminal and intentional acts, so coverage for these types of activities is unlikely.

47. **(4)** The full-blown jury trial is what ADR seeks to avoid. Mediation and arbitration are the most well-known forms of ADR. Some jurisdictions use the settlement conference as a technique to attempt settlement after a lawsuit has been filed but before a trial begins. Another type of ADR is called a summary jury trial, which is a private, shortened version where the parties share some evidence and get a sense of the strengths and weaknesses of each side's position. There are also hybrids such as "med-arb" where a proceeding starts out as a mediation; but if the case does not settle, it is referred to an arbitrator for resolution.

48. **(4)** All clients are entitled to medical information in order to make an informed decision about treatment. Age, in and of itself, is not an exclusionary criterion. Providers may treat in the other circumstances.

49. **(4)** If the Human Resources Department has established guidelines for the handling of references, it would be wise to follow them. It is also an effective mechanism to deflect potentially problematic queries by passing requests to the department most equipped to handle them. Most employers will be very circumspect about the information released, often limiting the data to dates of employment only. Absent some protective state legislation, employers should be prudent about sharing comments on former employees' work histories.

50. **(3)** The purpose is to determine the appropriateness of the applicant for the job.

Identifying health problems to prevent hiring an individual is discriminatory. The mental status and disabilities may also be a part of the pre-employment physical but are not the primary purpose.

51. **(3)** The Occupational Safety and Health Administration requires that these records be held for 30 years after termination of employment.

52. **(3)** It is required by law that a report of any work-related injury be filed with the industrial commission of the state in which the injury occurred.

53. **(2)** The Occupational Health and Safety Administration requires the report of any injury or illness that requires more than first aid treatment, involves loss of work time, causes limited work status, or causes loss of consciousness or death.

54. **(1)** The purpose is to record occupational injuries and illnesses and would also include death reports and lost work days, which would also reveal dangerous working conditions.

55. **(4)** All of the conditions listed would qualify under the ADA and may require accommodation in the workplace.

56. **(4)** The crux of a bioethical dilemma is that the proposed solution(s) is not perfect, and therefore creates some aspect of moral conflict.